# ANTISOCIAL BEHAVIOUR AND CONDUCT DISORDERS IN CHILDREN AND YOUNG PEOPLE

## RECOGNITION, INTERVENTION AND MANAGEMENT

National Clinical Guideline Number 158

**National Collaborating Centre for Mental Health and Social Care Institute for Excellence**

*commissioned by the*

**National Institute for Health and Care Excellence**
*published by*

**The British Psychological Society and The Royal College of Psychiatrists**

**British Library Cataloguing-in-Publication Data**

A catalogue record for this book is available from the British Library.

**ISBN-: 978-1-908020-61-1**

Printed in Great Britain by Stanley L. Hunt (Printers) Ltd.

Additional material: data CD-Rom created by Pix18 (www.pix18.co.uk)


*developed by* National Collaborating Centre for Mental Health
The Royal College of Psychiatrists
4th Floor, Standon House
21 Mansell Street
London
E1 8AA
www.nccmh.org.uk

*commissioned by* National Institute for Health and Care Excellence
1st Floor
10 Spring Gardens
London
SWIX 8PG
www.nice.org.uk

*published by* The British Psychological Society
St Andrews House
48 Princess Road East
Leicester
LE1 7DR
www.bps.org.uk

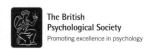

The British
Psychological Society
Promoting excellence in psychology

*and*

The Royal College of Psychiatrists
17 Belgrave Square
London
SW1X 8PG
www.rcpsych.ac.uk

RC
PSYCH
ROYAL COLLEGE OF
PSYCHIATRISTS

# CONTENTS

*Contents*

# GUIDELINE DEVELOPMENT GROUP MEMBERS

**Professor Stephen Scott (Chair)**
Professor of Child Health and Behaviour, Institute of Psychiatry, King's College London;
Consultant Child and Adolescent Psychiatrist & Head, National Conduct Problems Clinic and National Adoption and Fostering Clinic, Maudsley Hospital, London;
Director, Multidimensional Treatment Foster Care Project in England;
Director, National Academy for Parenting Research

**Professor Stephen Pilling (Facilitator)**
Director, National Collaborating Centre for Mental Health;
Director, Centre for Outcomes Research and Effectiveness, University College London

**Professor Nick Gould (Deputy Guideline Chair, representing the Social Care Institute for Excellence)**
Consultant, Social Care Institute for Excellence;
Emeritus Professor of Social Work, University of Bath;
Professor of Social Work, Griffith University, Queensland, Australia

**Ms Beth Anderson**
Senior Research Analyst, Social Care Institute for Excellence, London

**Dr Benedict Anigbogu**
Health Economist, National Collaborating Centre for Mental Health

**Ms Sara Barratt**
Consultant Systemic Psychotherapist; Team Leader, Fostering, Adoption and Kinship Care Team, Tavistock Centre, London

**Ms Ruth Braidwood**
Research Assistant (from May 2012), National Collaborating Centre for Mental Health

**Mrs Maria Brewster**
Service user and carer representative

**Dr Barbara Compitus**
General Practitioner, Bristol

*Guideline development group members*

**Dr Moira Doolan**
Consultant Systemic Psychotherapist;
Lead for interventions: Helping Children Achieve and Safe Studies, National Academy for Parenting Research, Institute of Psychiatry, King's College London

**Professor Peter Fonagy**
Chief Executive, Anna Freud Centre, London;
Freud Memorial Professor of Psychoanalysis, University College London

**Ms Laura Gibbon**
Project Manager (until December 2011), National Collaborating Centre for Mental Health

**Ms Naomi Glover**
Research Assistant (until July 2011), National Collaborating Centre for Mental Health

**Ms Bronwyn Harrison**
Research Assistant (until March 2012), National Collaborating Centre for Mental Health

**Ms Flora Kaminski**
Research Assistant (until July 2011), National Collaborating Centre for Mental Health

**Dr Daphne Keen**
Consultant Developmental Paediatrician, St George's Hospital, London;
Honorary Senior Lecturer, St George's, University of London

**Dr Paul McArdle**
Consultant and Senior Lecturer Child and Adolescent Psychiatry, Newcastle

**Dr Paul Mitchell**
Clinical Lead, Hindley Young Offenders Institution Mental Health Team, Manchester

**Ms Maryla Moulin**
Project Manager (from January 2012), National Collaborating Centre for Mental Health

**Dr Rosa Nieto-Hernandez**
Systematic Reviewer (until September 2011), National Collaborating Centre for Mental Health

**Ms Melinda Smith**
Research Assistant (until April 2012), National Collaborating Centre for Mental Health

**Ms Sarah Stockton**
Senior Information Scientist, National Collaborating Centre for Mental Health

**Dr Clare Taylor**
Senior Editor, National Collaborating Centre for Mental Health

**Dr Jenny Taylor**
Consultant Clinical Psychologist;
Supervisor of the Hackney site of the Department of Health's Multi-Systemic Therapy National Research Trial, London

**Dr Amina Yesufu-Udechuku**
Systematic Reviewer (until June 2011), National Collaborating Centre for Mental Health

**Dr Craig Whittington**
Associate Director (Clinical Effectiveness) and Senior Systematic Reviewer (from October 2011), National Collaborating Centre for Mental Health

**Mrs Philippa Williams**
Service user and carer representative

**Mr Tony Wootton**
Retired Head Teacher, Millthorpe School, York

## EDITORIAL ASSISTANCE

**Ms Liz Allison**
Deputy Director, Psychoanalysis Unit, Research Department of Clinical, Educational and Health Psychology, University College London

**Ms Lucy Burt**
Research Assistant, National Collaborating Centre for Mental Health

**Dr Ifigeneia Mavranezouli**
Senior Health Economist, National Collaborating Centre for Mental Health

## COPY EDITING

**Ms Nuala Ernest**
Assistant Editor, National Collaborating Centre for Mental Health

# 1    PREFACE

This guideline, which is a collaboration between NICE and the Social Care Institute for Excellence (SCIE), has been developed to advise on the recognition, identification and management of conduct disorders (including oppositional defiant disorder) and associated antisocial behaviour in children and young people. The guideline updates and replaces *Parent-Training/Education Programmes in the Management of Children with Conduct Disorders*, NICE technology appraisal guidance 102 (NICE, 2006). The guideline recommendations have been developed by a multidisciplinary team of healthcare professionals, people with conduct disorders and their carers, and guideline methodologists after careful consideration of the best available evidence. It is intended that the guideline will be useful to clinicians and service commissioners in providing and planning high-quality care for people with conduct disorders and antisocial behaviour while also emphasising the importance of the experience of care for people with conduct disorders and their carers (see Appendix 1 for more details on the scope of the guideline).

Although the evidence base is rapidly expanding there are a number of major gaps, and future revisions of this guideline will incorporate new scientific evidence as it develops. The guideline makes a number of research recommendations specifically to address gaps in the evidence base. In the meantime, it is hoped that the guideline will assist clinicians, and people with conduct disorders and their carers by identifying the merits of particular treatment approaches where the evidence from research and clinical experience exists.

## 1.1    NATIONAL CLINICAL GUIDELINES

### 1.1.1    What are clinical guidelines?

Clinical guidelines are 'systematically developed statements that assist clinicians and service users in making decisions about appropriate treatment for specific conditions' (Mann, 1996). They are derived from the best available research evidence, using pre-determined and systematic methods to identify and evaluate the evidence relating to the specific condition in question. Where evidence is lacking, the guidelines incorporate statements and recommendations based upon the consensus statements developed by the Guideline Development Group (GDG).

Clinical guidelines are intended to improve the process and outcomes of healthcare in a number of different ways. They can:

- provide up-to-date evidence-based recommendations for the management of conditions and disorders by healthcare professionals
- be used as the basis to set standards to assess the practice of healthcare professionals
- form the basis for education and training of healthcare professionals
- assist service users and their carers in making informed decisions about their treatment and care

- improve communication between healthcare professionals, service users and their carers
- help identify priority areas for further research.

### 1.1.2    Uses and limitations of clinical guidelines

Guidelines are not a substitute for professional knowledge and clinical judgement. They can be limited in their usefulness and applicability by a number of different factors: the availability of high-quality research evidence, the quality of the methodology used in the development of the guideline, the generalisability of research findings and the uniqueness of individuals.

Although the quality of research in this field is variable, the methodology used here reflects current international understanding of the appropriate practice for guideline development (Appraisal of Guidelines for Research and Evaluation Instrument [AGREE]; www.agreetrust.org) (AGREE Collaboration, 2003), ensuring the collection and selection of the best research evidence available and the systematic generation of treatment recommendations applicable to the majority of people with conduct disorders. However, there will always be some people for whom and situations for which clinical guideline recommendations are not readily applicable. This guideline does not, therefore, override the individual responsibility of healthcare professionals to make appropriate decisions in the circumstances of the individual, in consultation with the person with conduct disorders or their carer.

In addition to the clinical evidence, cost-effectiveness information, where available, is taken into account in the generation of statements and recommendations of the clinical guidelines. While national guidelines are concerned with clinical and cost effectiveness, issues of affordability and implementation costs are to be determined by the National Health Service (NHS).

In using guidelines, it is important to remember that the absence of empirical evidence for the effectiveness of a particular intervention is not the same as evidence for ineffectiveness. In addition, and of particular relevance in mental health, evidence-based treatments are often delivered within the context of an overall treatment programme including a range of activities, the purpose of which may be to help engage the person and those who care for them so as to provide an appropriate context for the delivery of specific interventions. It is important to maintain and enhance the service and relational contexts in which these interventions are delivered, otherwise the specific benefits of effective interventions may be lost. Indeed, the importance of organising care in order to support and encourage a good therapeutic relationship and to promote the young person's close personal relationships is at times as important as the specific treatments offered.

### 1.1.3    Why develop national guidelines?

The National Institute for Health and Care Excellence (NICE; previously National Institute for Health and Clinical Excellence) was established as a Special Health

Authority for England and Wales in 1999, with a remit to provide a single source of authoritative and reliable guidance for service users, professionals and the public. NICE guidance aims to improve standards of care, diminish unacceptable variations in the provision and quality of care across the NHS, and ensure that the health service is person-centred. All guidance is developed in a transparent and collaborative manner, using the best available evidence and involving all relevant stakeholders.

NICE generates guidance in a number of different ways three of which are relevant here. First, national guidance is produced by the Technology Appraisal Committee to give robust advice about a particular treatment, intervention, procedure or other health technology. Second, NICE commissions public health intervention guidance focused on types of activity (interventions) that help to reduce people's risk of developing a disease or condition, or help to promote or maintain a healthy lifestyle. Third, NICE commissions the production of national clinical guidelines focused upon the overall treatment and management of a specific condition. To enable this latter development, NICE has established four National Collaborating Centres in conjunction with a range of professional organisations involved in healthcare.

SCIE was launched in October 2001 as part of the government's drive to improve social care. It is an independent registered charity, governed by a board of trustees, whose role is to develop and promote knowledge about good practice in social care. SCIE works with people and organisations throughout the social care sector to identify useful information, research and examples of good practice. Using this information, SCIE produces resources that evaluate practice in a particular area of social care, draws out key messages for good practice and identifies areas where more research is needed to inform good practice.

### 1.1.4    From national clinical guidelines to local protocols

Once a national guideline has been published and disseminated, local healthcare groups will be expected to produce a plan and identify resources for implementation, along with appropriate timetables. Subsequently, a multidisciplinary group involving commissioners of healthcare, primary care and specialist mental health professionals, service users and carers should undertake the translation of the implementation plan into local protocols, taking into account both the recommendations set out in this guideline and the priorities set out in the National Service Framework for Mental Health (Department of Health, 1999) and related documentation. The nature and pace of the local plan will reflect local healthcare needs and the nature of existing services; full implementation may take a considerable time, especially where substantial training needs are identified.

### 1.1.5    Auditing the implementation of clinical guidelines

This guideline identifies key areas of clinical practice and service delivery for local and national audit. Although the generation of audit standards is an important and necessary step in the implementation of this guidance, a more broadly-based imple-mentation strategy will be developed. Nevertheless, it should be noted that the Care Quality Commission will monitor the extent to which commissioners and providers of health and social care have implemented these guidelines.

## 1.2    THE NATIONAL CONDUCT DISORDERS IN CHILDREN AND YOUNG PEOPLE GUIDANCE

### 1.2.1    Who has developed this guideline?

This guideline has been commissioned by NICE and developed within the National Collaborating Centre for Mental Health (NCCMH). The NCCMH is a collaboration of the professional organisations involved in the field of mental health, national ser-vice-user and carer organisations, a number of academic institutions and NICE. The NCCMH is funded by NICE and is led by a partnership between the Royal College of Psychiatrists and the British Psychological Society's Centre for Outcomes Research and Effectiveness, based at University College London.

The GDG was convened by the NCCMH and supported by funding from NICE. The GDG included carers of children and young people with conduct disorders, and professionals from psychiatry, clinical psychology, psychotherapy, paediatrics, gen-eral practice, nursing, education, social work, and the private and voluntary sectors.

Staff from the NCCMH provided leadership and support throughout the process of guideline development, undertaking systematic searches, information retrieval, appraisal and systematic review of the evidence. Members of the GDG received train-ing in the process of guideline development from NCCMH staff, and the service users and carers received training and support from the NICE Patient and Public Involvement Programme. The NICE Guidelines Technical Adviser provided advice and assistance regarding aspects of the guideline development process.

All GDG members made formal declarations of interest at the outset, which were updated at every GDG meeting. The GDG met a total of 12 times throughout the process of guideline development. It met as a whole, but key topics were led by a national expert in the relevant topic. The GDG was supported by the NCCMH technical team, with additional expert advice from special advisers where needed. The group oversaw the production and synthesis of research evidence before presentation. All statements and recommendations in this guideline have been generated and agreed by the whole GDG.

### 1.2.2    For whom is this guideline intended?

This guideline will be relevant for children and young people with conduct disorders and antisocial behaviour (with an intelligence quotient [IQ] of 60 and above). It covers the care provided by primary, community, secondary, tertiary and other healthcare professionals who have direct contact with, and make decisions concerning the care of, children and young people with conduct disorders and antisocial behaviour.

The guideline will also be relevant to the work, but will not cover the practice, of those in:
● occupational health services
● social services
● the independent sector.


### 1.2.3 Specific aims of this guideline

The guideline makes recommendations for recognition, intervention and management of conduct disorders. It aims to:
● improve access and engagement with treatment and services for children and young people with conduct disorders and antisocial behaviour (including oppositional defiance disorder)
● evaluate the role of specific psychological, psychosocial, educational and pharmacological interventions in the treatment of conduct disorders
● evaluate the role of psychological, psychosocial and physical (such as diet) interventions in combination with pharmacological interventions in the treatment of conduct disorders
● integrate the above to provide best-practice advice on the care of individuals throughout the course of their conduct disorder
● promote the implementation of best clinical practice through the development of recommendations tailored to the requirements of the NHS in England and Wales.


### 1.2.4 The structure of this guideline

The guideline is divided into chapters, each covering a set of related topics. The first three chapters provide a summary of the clinical practice and research recommendations, and a general introduction to guidelines and to the methods used to develop them. Chapter 4 to Chapter 8 provide the evidence that underpins the recommendations about the treatment and management of conduct disorders.

Each evidence chapter begins with a general introduction to the topic that sets the recommendations in context. Depending on the nature of the evidence, narrative reviews or meta-analyses were conducted, and the structure of the chapters varies accordingly. Where appropriate, details about current practice, the evidence base and any research limitations are provided. Where meta-analyses were conducted, information is given about the interventions included and the studies considered for review. Further sub-sections are used to present Grading of Recommendations Assessment, Development, and Evaluation (GRADE) summaries of findings tables, clinical summaries and health economic evidence. A sub-section called 'From evidence to recommendations' is used to explain how the GDG moved from the evidence to the recommendations. Finally, recommendations (clinical and research) related to each topic are presented at the end of each chapter. On the CD-ROM, full details about the included studies can be found in Appendix 16; where meta-analyses were conducted, the data are presented using forest plots in Appendix 17; full GRADE evidence profiles are presented in Appendix 18; evidence tables for economic studies are presented in Appendix 20; evidence tables for the review of access and experience of care are presented in Appendix 21 (see Text Box 1 for details).

**Text Box 1:  Appendices on CD-ROM**

| | |
|---|---|
| Search strategies for the identification of clinical studies | Appendix 7 |
| Search strategies for the identification of health economic evidence | Appendix 10 |
| Review protocols | Appendix 15 |
| Clinical evidence study characteristics tables:<br>• Prevention and treatment<br>• Case identification<br>• Pharmacological interventions | Appendix 16a<br>Appendix 16b<br>Appendix 16c |
| Clinical evidence forest plots | Appendix 17 |
| GRADE evidence profiles | Appendix 18 |
| Methodology checklists for economic studies | Appendix 19 |
| Evidence tables for economic studies on interventions | Appendix 20 |
| Evidence tables for the access to and experience of care | Appendix 21 |

In the event that amendments or minor updates need to be made to the guideline, please check the NCCMH website (nccmh.org.uk) where these will be listed and a corrected PDF file available to download.

# 2 ANTISOCIAL BEHAVIOUR AND CONDUCT DISORDERS IN CHILDREN AND YOUNG PEOPLE

## 2.1 INTRODUCTION

This guideline is concerned with the management of conduct disorder and oppositional defiant disorder, as defined in the *International Classification of Diseases, 10th Revision* (ICD-10) (World Health Organization, 1992) and the *Diagnostic and Statistical Manual of Mental Disorders, 4th Edition Text Revision* (DSM-IV-TR) (American Psychiatric Association, 2000), and associated antisocial behaviour in primary, community and secondary care. Conduct disorder is an overarching term used in psychiatric classification that refers to a persistent pattern of antisocial behaviour in which the individual repeatedly breaks social rules and carries out aggressive acts that upset other people. Oppositional defiant disorder is a milder variant mostly seen in younger children. The term 'conduct disorders' (or 'a conduct disorder') is used in this guideline to encompass both disorders. Because the term is not well known among the public, or even among healthcare professionals, the guideline title includes the term 'antisocial behaviour' to make it clear to as wide a range of people as possible what the guideline addresses.

Globally, conduct disorders are the most common mental health disorders of childhood and adolescence, and they are the most common reason for referral to child and adolescent mental health services (CAMHS) in Western countries. A high proportion of children and young people with conduct disorders grow up to be antisocial adults with impoverished and destructive lifestyles; a significant minority will develop antisocial personality disorder, among whom the more severe will meet criteria for psychopathy. Conduct disorders in childhood and adolescence are becoming more frequent in Western countries and place a large personal and economic burden on individuals and society, involving not just healthcare services and social care agencies but all sectors of society including the family, schools, police and criminal justice agencies. It is therefore appropriate that this guideline has been developed by NICE jointly with SCIE.

### 2.1.1 Medicalising a social problem?

Infringement of the rights of other people is a requirement for the diagnosis of a conduct disorder. Because manifestations of conduct disorders and antisocial behaviour include a failure to obey social rules despite relatively intact mental and social capacities, many have seen the disorders as principally socially determined. It could therefore be argued that the responsibility for their cause and elimination lies solely with people who can influence the socialisation process, such as parents, schoolteachers, social service departments and politicians, rather than by healthcare professionals. Additionally, because the disorders are so prevalent, it would be logistically impossible for CAMHS to see all children and young people – adding a further reason not to medicalise the problem. Certainly, all of the above mentioned agencies have major roles to play in the recognition, assessment and management of conduct disorders/antisocial behaviour.

However, there are several reasons why CAMHS services also have a role to play. First, advances in the last three decades have shown that in addition to social causes there are substantial genetic and biological contributions to conduct disorders/antisocial behaviour; therefore, the contribution of these factors needs to be assessed and factored into intervention plans. Second, many children and young people exhibiting conduct disorders/antisocial behaviour have coexistent mental health and learning problems, or disorders that require recognition and assessment, including for example attention and concentration problems (attention deficit hyperactivity disorder [ADHD]), attachment problems, traumatic memories (post-traumatic stress disorder [PTSD]), autistic traits and dyslexia. Third, the quality of the parent–child relationship needs to be assessed systematically using well-validated constructs; this will include assessment of mental health problems in the parents such as depression and alcohol and drug problems. Fourth, all of these factors need to be weighted and judged for their relative contribution in the individual concerned, and an appropriate intervention plan drawn up taking these into account, including personal meanings and cultural sensitivities. Finally, it is mainly work from the fields of child and adolescent psychology and mental health that has clarified many of the mechanisms contributing to the development and persistence of antisocial behaviour, and has led this discipline to develop notably effective treatments, mostly psychosocial in nature, which are often not available from other agencies. This knowledge needs to be disseminated more widely so that more children can benefit; at present fewer than a quarter of affected children and young people receive any specific help (Vostanis et al., 2003), and much of this is likely to be ineffective (Scott, 2007). There is therefore a need for mental health professionals to work closely alongside other professionals and agencies and contribute to the planning and delivery of humane and effective services. Failure to achieve this will mean that great numbers of children and young people will have their lives avoidably blighted.

## 2.2    THE DISORDER

This guideline is concerned with the management of conduct disorder in the community and in prison as defined in ICD-10 (World Health Organization, 1992) and DSM-IV-TR (American Psychiatric Association, 2000) (see Section 2.3 for details about the classification of both conduct disorder and oppositional defiant disorder).

Aggressive and defiant behaviour is an important part of normal child and adolescent development, which ensures physical and social survival. Indeed, some parents may express concern if a child is too acquiescent and unassertive. The level of aggressive and defiant behaviour varies considerably among children, and it is probably most usefully seen as a continuously distributed trait. Empirical studies do not suggest a level at which symptoms become qualitatively different, nor is there a single cut-off point at which they become impairing for the child or a clear problem for others. There is no 'hump' towards the end of the distribution curve of severity to suggest a categorically distinct group who might on these grounds warrant a diagnosis of conduct disorder.

Picking a particular level of antisocial behaviour to call conduct disorder or oppositional defiant disorder is therefore necessarily arbitrary (Moffitt et al., 2008). For all children, the expression of any particular behaviour also varies with age; physical hitting, for example, is at its peak at around 2 years of age and declines to a low level over the ensuing years. Therefore any judgement about the significance of the level of antisocial behaviour has to be made in the context of the child's age. Before deciding that the behaviour is atypical or a significant problem, a number of other clinical features have to be considered:

- *level*: severity and frequency of antisocial acts, compared with children of the same age and gender (see Sections 2.2.1 and 2.2.2)
- *pattern*: the variety of antisocial acts, and the setting in which they are carried out (see Section 2.2.3)
- *persistence*: duration over time (see Section 2.2.3)
- *impact*: distress and social impairment of the child; disruption and damage to others (see Section 2.2.4).

It should be noted that the making of a diagnosis of a conduct disorder only means that at the time, the individual concerned has been behaving in a way that meets the specified criteria. It is purely a phenomenological description and carries no implications about the cause in any particular case. The child may spontaneously change over time and so no longer meet criteria for a diagnosis. In some, the origins might be entirely outside the child, with the child reacting as any child might to a coercive, traumatic or abusive upbringing. In others, it might be that the child had had a completely benign upbringing but was born with callous-unemotional traits that were displayed in all social encounters. Thus the use of a diagnosis is fully consistent with a biopsychosocial approach to the understanding and treatment of the presenting phenomena.

## 2.2.1    Changes in clinical features with age

*Younger children* aged 3 to 7 years usually present with general defiance of adults' wishes, disobedience of instructions, angry outbursts with temper tantrums, physical aggression to other people (especially siblings and peers), destruction of property, arguing, blaming others for things that have gone wrong, and a tendency to annoy and provoke others.

In *middle childhood*, from 8 to 11 years, the above features are often present, but as the child grows older and stronger, and spends more time outside the home, other behaviours are seen. They include: swearing, lying about what they have been doing, stealing others' belongings outside the home, persistent breaking of rules, physical fights, bullying other children, being cruel to animals and setting fires.

In *adolescence*, from 12 to 17 years, more antisocial behaviours are often added: being cruel to and hurting other people, assault, robbery using force, vandalism, breaking and entering houses, stealing from cars, driving and taking away cars without permission, running away from home, truanting from school, and misusing alcohol and drugs.

Not all children who start with the type of behaviours listed in early childhood progress on to the later, more severe forms. Only about half continue from those in early childhood to those in middle childhood; likewise, only about a further half of those with the behaviours in middle childhood progress to show the behaviours listed for adolescence (Rowe et al., 2002). However, the early onset group are important as they are far more likely to display the most severe symptoms in adolescence, and to persist in their antisocial tendencies into adulthood. The most antisocial 5% of children aged 7 years are 500 to 1000% more likely to display indices of serious life failure at 25 years, for example drug dependency, criminality, unwanted teenage pregnancy, leaving school with no qualifications, unemployment and so on (Fergusson et al., 2005). Follow-back studies show that most children and young people with conduct disorders had prior oppositional defiant disorder and most (if not all) adults with antisocial personality disorder had prior conduct disorders. Likewise about 90% of severe, recurrent adolescent offenders showed marked antisocial behaviour in early childhood (Piquero et al., 2010). In contrast, there is a large group who only start to be antisocial in adolescence, but whose behaviours are less extreme and who tend to become less severe by the time they are adults (Moffitt, 2006).

## 2.2.2    Gender

Severe antisocial behaviour is less common in girls than in boys; they are less likely to be physically aggressive and engage in criminal behaviour, but more likely to show spitefulness and emotional bullying (such as excluding children from groups and spreading rumours so others are rejected by their peers), and engage in frequent unprotected sex (which can lead to sexually transmitted disease and pregnancy), drug abuse and running away from home. Whether there should be specific criteria for diagnosing conduct disorder in girls is debated (Moffitt et al., 2008).

## 2.2.3    Pattern of behaviour and setting

The severity of conduct disorder is not determined by the presence of any one symptom or any particular constellation, but is due to the overall volume of symptoms, determined by the frequency and intensity of antisocial behaviours, the variety of types, the number of settings in which they occur (for example home, school, in public) and their persistence. For general populations of children, the correlation between parent and teacher ratings of conduct problems on the same measures is low (only 0.2 to 0.3), which means that there are many children who are perceived to be mildly or moderately antisocial at home but well behaved at school, and vice versa. However, for more severe antisocial behaviour there are usually manifestations both at home and at school.

### 2.2.4     Impact

At home, the child or young person with a conduct disorder is often exposed to high levels of criticism and hostility, and sometimes made a scapegoat for a catalogue of family misfortunes. Frequent punishments and physical abuse are not uncommon. The whole family atmosphere is often soured and siblings also affected. Maternal depression is often present, and families who are unable to cope may, as a last resort, give up the child to be cared for by the local authority. At school, teachers may take a range of measures to attempt to control the child or young person, bring order to the classroom and protect the other pupils, including sending the child or young person out of the class, which sometimes culminates in permanent exclusion from the school. This may lead to reduced opportunity to learn subjects on the curriculum and poor examination results. The child or young person typically has few, if any, friends, and any friends become annoyed by their aggressive behaviour. This often leads to exclusion from many group activities, games and trips, thus restricting the child or young person's quality of life and experiences. On leaving school, the lack of social skills, low level of qualifications and, possibly, a police record make it harder to gain employment.

### 2.3      CLASSIFICATION

### 2.3.1     Diagnosis

The ICD-10 classification has a category for conduct disorders (F91). The ICD-10 'Clinical Descriptions and Diagnostic Guidelines' (World Health Organization, 1992) states:

> *Examples of the behaviours on which the diagnosis is based include the follow-ing: excessive levels of fighting or bullying; cruelty to animals or other people; severe destructiveness to property; fire-setting; stealing; repeated lying; truancy from school and running away from home; unusually frequent and severe tem-per tantrums; defiant provocative behaviour; and persistent severe disobedi-ence. Any one of these categories, if marked, is sufficient for the diagnosis, but isolated dissocial acts are not. (F91)*

An enduring pattern of behaviour should be present, but no time frame is given and there is no impairment or impact criterion stated.

The ICD-10 'Diagnostic Criteria for Research' (World Health Organization, 1992) differ, requiring symptoms to have been present for at least 6 months, and the intro-ductory rubric indicates that impact upon others (in terms of violation of their basic rights), but not impairment of the child, can contribute to the diagnosis. The research criteria take a menu-driven approach whereby a certain number of symptoms have to be present. Fifteen behaviours are listed to be considered for a diagnosis of conduct disorder, which usually but by no means exclusively apply to older children and young people. The behaviours can be grouped into four classes:

### a) Aggression to people and animals:
1. often lies or breaks promises to obtain goods or favours or to avoid obligations
2. frequently initiates physical fights (this does not include fights with siblings)
3. has used a weapon that can cause serious physical harm to others (for example bat, brick, broken bottle, knife, gun)
4. often stays out after dark despite parental prohibition (beginning before 13 years of age)
5. exhibits physical cruelty to other people (for example ties up, cuts or burns a victim)
6. exhibits physical cruelty to animals.

### b) Destruction of property:
7. deliberately destroys the property of others (other than by fire-setting)
8. deliberately sets fires with a risk or intention of causing serious damage).

### c) Deceitfulness or theft:
9. steals objects of non-trivial value without confronting the victim, either within the home or outside (for example shoplifting, burglary, forgery).

### d) Serious violations of rules:
10. is frequently truant from school, beginning before 13 years of age
11. has run away from parental or parental surrogate home at least twice or has run away once for more than a single night (this does not include leaving to avoid physical or sexual abuse)
12. commits a crime involving confrontation with the victim (including purse-snatching, extortion, mugging)
13. forces another person into sexual activity
14. frequently bullies others (for example deliberate infliction of pain or hurt, including persistent intimidation, tormenting, or molestation)
15. breaks into someone else's house, building or car.

To make a diagnosis, at least three behaviours from the 15 listed above have to be present, one for at least 6 months. There is no impairment criterion. There are three subtypes: 'conduct disorder confined to the family context' (F91.0), 'unsocialised conduct disorder' (F91.1, where the young person has no friends and is rejected by peers) and 'socialised conduct disorder' (F91.2, where peer relationships are normal). It is recommended that age of onset be specified, with childhood-onset type manifesting before 10 years and adolescent-onset type after 10 years. Severity should be categorised as mild, moderate or severe according to the number of symptoms or impact on others, for example causing severe physical injury, vandalism or theft.

For younger children, usually up to 9 or 10 years old (although it can in theory be used up to 18 years), there is a list of eight symptoms for the subtype known as 'oppositional defiant disorder' (F91.3):

1. has unusually frequent or severe temper tantrums for his or her developmental level
2. often argues with adults
3. often actively refuses adults' requests or defies rules
4. often, apparently deliberately, does things that annoy other people
5. often blames others for his or her own mistakes or misbehaviour
6. is often 'touchy' or easily annoyed by others
7. is often angry or resentful
8. is often spiteful or resentful.

To make a diagnosis of the oppositional defiant type of conduct disorder, four symptoms from either this list or the conduct disorder 15-item list must be present, but no more than two from the latter. Unlike for the conduct disorder variant, there is an impairment criterion for the oppositional defiant type: the symptoms must be maladaptive and inconsistent with the child or young person's developmental level.

Where there are sufficient symptoms of a comorbid disorder to meet diagnostic criteria, ICD-10 discourages the application of a second diagnosis, and instead offers a single, combined category for the most common combinations. There are two major kinds: mixed disorders of conduct and emotions, of which depressive conduct disorder (F92.0) is the best researched; and hyperkinetic conduct disorder (F90.1). There is modest evidence to suggest these combined conditions may differ somewhat from their constituent elements.

DSM-IV-TR follows the ICD-10 research criteria very closely and does not have separate clinical guidelines. The same 15 behaviours are given for the diagnosis of conduct disorder (312.8, American Psychiatric Association, 2000), with almost identical wording. As in ICD-10, three symptoms need to be present for diagnosis. Severity and childhood or adolescent onset are also specified in the same way. However, unlike ICD-10, there is no division into socialised/unsocialised or family context, only into types, and there is a requirement for the behaviour to cause 'clinically significant impairment in social, academic, or social functioning'. Comorbidity in DSM-IV-TR is handled by giving as many separate diagnoses as necessary, rather than by having single, combined categories.

In DSM-IV-TR, oppositional defiant disorder is classified as a separate disorder, not as a subtype of conduct disorder. Diagnosis requires four from a list of eight behaviours, which are the same as ICD-10; but, unlike ICD-10, all four have to be from the oppositional list and none may come from the conduct disorder list. In older children it is debated whether oppositional defiant disorder is fundamentally different from conduct disorder in its essential phenomena or any associated characteristics, and the value of designating it as a separate disorder is arguable. In this guideline, the term 'conduct disorders' will henceforth be used as it is in ICD-10, to refer to all variants including oppositional defiant disorder. The term 'conduct problems' will be used for less severe antisocial behaviour.

'Juvenile delinquency' is a legal term referring to an act by a young person who has been convicted of an offence that would be deemed a crime if committed by an adult. Most but not all recurrent juvenile offenders have conduct disorder.

### 2.3.2 Differential diagnosis

Making a diagnosis of conduct disorder is usually straightforward, but comorbid conditions are often missed. Differential diagnosis may include:

1. *Hyperkinetic syndrome and attention deficit hyperactivity disorder.* These are the names given by ICD-10 and DSM-IV-TR, respectively, for similar conditions, except that the former is more severe. For convenience, the term 'hyperactivity' will be used here. It is characterised by impulsivity, inattention and motor overactivity. Any of these three sets of symptoms can be misconstrued as antisocial, particularly impulsivity, which is also present in conduct disorders. However, none of the symptoms of conduct disorders are a part of hyperactivity so excluding conduct disorders should not be difficult. A frequently made error, however, is to miss comorbid hyperactivity when conduct disorder is definitely present. Standardised questionnaires are very helpful here, such as the Strengths and Difficulties Questionnaire (SDQ), which is brief and just as effective at detecting hyperactivity as much longer alternatives (Goodman & Scott, 1999).
2. *Adjustment reaction to an external stressor.* This can be diagnosed when onset occurs soon after exposure to an identifiable psychosocial stressor such as divorce, bereavement, trauma, abuse or adoption. The onset should be within 1 month for ICD-10 and 3 months for DSM-IV-TR, and symptoms should not persist for more than 6 months after the cessation of the stress or its sequelae.
3. *Mood disorders.* Depression can present with irritability and oppositional symptoms, but, unlike typical conduct disorder, mood is usually clearly low and there are vegetative features (difficulties with basic bodily processes, such as eating, sleeping and feeling pleasure); also, more severe conduct problems are absent. Early bipolar disorder can be harder to distinguish because there is often considerable defiance and irritability combined with disregard for rules, and behaviour that violates the rights of others. Low self-esteem is the norm in conduct disorders, as is a lack of friends or constructive pastimes. Therefore it is easy to overlook more pronounced depressive symptoms. Systematic surveys reveal that around a third of children with a conduct disorder have depressive or other emotional symptoms severe enough to warrant a diagnosis.
4. *Autistic spectrum disorders.* These are often accompanied by marked tantrums or destructiveness, which may be the reason for seeking a referral. Enquiring about other symptoms of autistic spectrum disorders should reveal their presence.
5. *Dissocial and antisocial personality disorder.* In ICD-10 it is suggested that a person should be 17 years or older before dissocial personality disorder can be considered. Because from the age of 18 years most diagnoses specific to childhood and adolescence no longer apply, in practice there is seldom a difficulty in terms of formal diagnosis. In DSM-IV-TR, conduct disorder can be diagnosed in people over 18 years, so there is potential overlap. A difference in emphasis is the severity and pervasiveness of the symptoms of those with personality disorder, whereby all the individual's

relationships are affected by the behaviour pattern, and the individual's beliefs about his antisocial behaviour are characterised by callousness and lack of remorse.

In contrast to a formal diagnosis of dissocial or antisocial personality disorder, however, there has been an explosion of interest in the last decade in what have been termed psychopathic traits in childhood. The characteristics of the adult psychopath include grandiosity, callousness, deceitfulness, shallow affect and lack of remorse. Can the 'fledgling psychopath' be identified in childhood? Certainly there are now instruments that reliably identify callous-unemotional traits such as lack of guilt, absence of empathy and shallow, constricted emotions in children (Farrington, 2005). Further research has shown that callous-unemotional traits in childhood are associated with a failure to inhibit aggression in response to signs of distress in others, arising from a deficit in processing victims' distress cues, and reduced ability to recognise fear and sadness (Blair et al., 2005). In longitudinal studies such children go on to be more aggressive and antisocial than others without such traits (Moran et al., 2009), and they are harder to treat, responding less well to interventions (Haas et al., 2011; Hawes & Dadds, 2005).

6. *Subcultural deviance.* Some young people are antisocial and commit crimes but are not particularly aggressive or defiant. They are well-adjusted within a deviant peer culture that approves of recreational drug use, shoplifting and so on. In some areas, one third or more of young males fit this description and would meet ICD-10 diagnostic guidelines for socialised conduct disorder. Some clinicians are unhappy to label such a large proportion of the population with a psychiatric disorder. Using DSM-IV-TR criteria would preclude the diagnosis for most young people like this due to the requirement for significant impairment.

### 2.3.3 Multiaxial assessment

ICD-10 recommends that multiaxial assessment be carried out for children and young people, while DSM-IV-TR suggests it for all ages. In both systems Axis 1 is used for psychiatric disorders that have been discussed above. The last three axes in both systems cover general medical conditions, psychosocial problems and level of social functioning; these topics will be discussed in Section 2.5. In the middle are two axes in ICD-10, which cover specific (Axis 2) and general (Axis 3) learning disabilities; and one in DSM-IV-TR (Axis 2), which covers personality disorders and general learning disabilities.

Both specific and general learning disabilities are essential to assess in children and young people with a conduct disorder. A third of children with a conduct disorder have a reading level two standard deviations (SDs) below that predicted by the person's IQ (Trzesniewski et al., 2006). While this may in part be due to lack of adequate schooling, there is good evidence that the cognitive deficits often precede the behavioural problems. General learning disability is often missed in children and young people with a conduct disorder unless IQ testing is carried out. The rate of conduct disorder increases several-fold in those with an IQ below 70.

This chapter describes the general pattern of behaviour that comprises conduct disorder and alternative diagnoses. When considering an individual child or young person, the assessment, formulation and management plan will, of course, not only consider the presence or absence of behaviours but will also cover many other issues, including the particular circumstances and influences that led to the presentation, the family's strengths and resources, and the meanings ascribed to the situation.

## 2.4    EPIDEMIOLOGY

In the large 1999 and 2004 British surveys carried out by the Office of National Statistics, 5% of children and young people aged 5 to 15 years met the ICD-10 criteria for conduct disorders with a strict impairment requirement (Green et al., 2005). A modest rise in diagnosable conduct disorder over the second half of the twentieth century has also been observed when comparing assessments of three successive birth cohorts in Britain (Collishaw et al., 2004). In terms of class, there is a marked social class gradient with conduct disorders more prevalent in social classes D and E compared with social class A (Green et al., 2005). With regard to ethnicity, young people's self-reports of antisocial behaviours as well as crime victim survey reports of perpetrators' ethnicity show an excess of offenders of black African ancestry, whereas children and young people of British Asian ancestry show lower rates compared with their white counterparts (Goodman et al., 2010).

### 2.4.1    Gender differences in prevalence

The gender ratio is approximately 2.5 males for each female, with males further exceeding females in the frequency and severity of behaviours. On balance, research suggests that the causes of conduct problems are the same for both genders, but males have more conduct disorders because they experience more of its individual-level risk factors (for example hyperactivity and neurodevelopmental delays). However, in recent years there has been increasing concern among clinicians about treating antisocial behaviour among girls (Pullatz & Bierman, 2004).

### 2.4.2    Lifecourse differences

There has been much evidence to support a distinction between antisocial behaviour first seen in early childhood versus that seen first in adolescence, and these two subtypes are included in the DSM-IV-TR. Early onset clearly predicts continuation through childhood. Those with early onset have a lower IQ, more ADHD symptoms, lower scores on neuropsychological tests, greater peer difficulties and are more likely to come from dysfunctional family backgrounds (Moffitt, 2006). Those with later onset become antisocial mainly as a result of social influences, including association with a deviant peer group, and typically have no neuropsychological abnormalities. Findings from the follow-ups of large cohorts show poorer adult outcomes for the early-onset group in domains of violence, mental health, substance misuse, work and family life (Moffitt, 2006). However, the adolescent-onset group, who were originally named 'adolescence limited', were not without adult difficulties, hence the name change. As adults they still engaged in self-reported offending, and they also had problems with alcohol and drugs. Thus the age-of-onset subtype distinction has strong predictive validity, but adolescent-onset antisocial behaviours may have more long-lasting consequences than previously supposed.

## 2.5    AETIOLOGY

### 2.5.1    Individual-level characteristics

*Genes*

Fewer than 10% of the families in any community account for more than 50% of that community's criminal offences, which reflects the coincidence of genetic and environmental risks. There is now solid evidence from twin and adoption studies that conduct problems assessed both dimensionally and categorically are substantially heritable (Moffitt, 2005). However, knowing that conduct problems are under some genetic influence is less useful clinically than knowing that this genetic influence appears to be reduced, or enhanced, depending on interaction with circumstances in the child or young person's environment. Several genetically sensitive studies have allowed interactions between family genetic liability and rearing environment to be examined. Both twin and adoption studies have reported an interaction between antisocial behaviour in the biological parent and adverse conditions in the adoptive home that predicted the adopted child's antisocial outcome, so that the genetic risk was modified by the rearing environment. For example, one twin study (Jaffee et al., 2003) found the experience of maltreatment was associated with an increase of 24% in the probability of diagnosable conduct disorder among children at high genetic risk, but an increase of only 2% among children at low genetic risk. Such gene–environment interactions are being increasingly discovered (Dodge et al., 2011). It is important to emphasise that because conduct disorders are partially genetically caused does not mean that environmental or psychosocial interventions will not work. The opposite is true: awareness of a familial liability toward psychopathology increases the urgency to intervene to improve a child or young person's social environment (Odgers et al., 2007).

The search for specific genetic polymorphisms is a fairly new scientific initiative. The candidate gene that is most studied in relation to conduct problems is the monoamine oxidase type A (MAOA) promoter polymorphism. The gene encodes the MAOA enzyme, which metabolises neurotransmitters linked to aggressive behaviour. Positive and negative replication studies have appeared, and a meta-analysis of these studies showed the association between MAOA genotype and conduct problems is modest but statistically significant (Kim-Cohen et al., 2006). Little replication has yet been accomplished using genome-wide association studies (Dick et al., 2011).

*Perinatal complications and temperament*

Recent large-scale general population studies have found associations between life-course persistent-type conduct problems and perinatal complications, minor physical anomalies and low birth weight (Brennan et al., 2003). Most studies support a bio-social model in which obstetric complications might confer vulnerability to other co-occurring risks such as hostile or inconsistent parenting. Smoking in pregnancy is a statistical risk predictor of offspring conduct problems (Brennan et al., 2003), but a causal link between smoking and conduct problems has not been established. Several prospective studies have shown associations between irritable temperament and conduct problems (Keenan & Shaw, 2003).

*Neurotransmitters*
In general, the findings with children have not been consistent. For example, in the Pittsburgh Youth cohort, boys with long-standing conduct problems showed downward changes in urinary adrenaline level following a stressful challenge task, whereas prosocial boys showed upward responses (McBurnett et al., 2005). However other studies have failed to find an association between conduct disorder and measures of noradrenaline in children (Hill, 2002). It should be borne in mind that neurotransmitters in the brain are only indirectly measured, that most measures of neurotransmitter levels are crude indicators of activity and that little is known about neurotransmitters in the juvenile brain.

*Cognitive deficits*
Children with conduct problems have been shown consistently to have increased rates of deficits in language-based verbal skills (Lynam & Henry, 2001). The association holds after controlling for potential confounds such as race, socioeconomic status, academic attainment and test motivation. Children who cannot reason or assert themselves verbally may attempt to gain control of social exchanges using aggression (Dodge, 2006); there are also likely to be indirect effects in which low verbal IQ contributes to academic difficulties, which in turn means that the child or young person's experience of school becomes unrewarding rather than a source of self-esteem and support.

Children and young people with conduct problems have been shown consistently to have poor tested executive functions (Ishikawa & Raine, 2003); (Hobson et al., 2011). Executive functions are the abilities implicated in successfully achieving goals through appropriate and effective actions. Specific skills include learning and applying contingency rules, abstract reasoning, problem solving, self-monitoring, sustained attention and concentration, relating previous actions to future goals, and inhibiting inappropriate responses. These mental functions are largely, although not exclusively, associated with the frontal lobes.

*Autonomic nervous system*
A low resting pulse rate or slow heart rate is associated with antisocial behaviour, (Ortiz & Raine, 2004). Also, a slow skin-conductance response to aversive stimuli is found (Fung et al., 2005).

*Social perception*
Dodge (Dodge, 2006) proposed a model for the development of antisocial behaviours in social interactions. Children liable to behave aggressively focus on threatening

aspects of others' actions, see them as hostile when they are neutral, and are more likely to choose an aggressive solution to social challenges. Several studies have supported these processes (Dodge, 2006).

### 2.5.2    Risks within the family

*Family disadvantage*
There is an association between severe disadvantage and antisocial behaviour in children. The association between disadvantage and childhood antisocial behaviour is indirect, mediated via family relationships such as interparental discord and parenting quality, which is discussed below.

*Parenting style*
Parenting styles related to antisocial behaviour were described by Patterson in his major work *Coercive Family Process* (Patterson, 1982). Parents of children with conduct problems were less consistent in their use of rules, gave more vague commands, were more likely to react to their children based on how they felt (for example more bad mood) rather than based on what the child was actually doing, were less likely to check their children's whereabouts and were unresponsive to their children's sociable behaviour. Patterson proposed a specific mechanism for the promotion of oppositional and aggressive behaviours in children whereby a parent responds to mild irritating child behaviour with a prohibition to which the child responds by escalating their behaviour, and each then raises their anger until the parent backs down, thus negatively reinforcing the child's behaviour. Conduct problems are associated with hostile, critical, punitive and coercive parenting.

Of course, other explanations need to be considered: first, that the associations reflect familial genetic liability toward children's psychopathology and parents' coercive discipline; second, that they represent the effects of children's behaviours on parents; and third, that harsh parenting may be a correlate of other features of the parent–child relationship or family functioning that influence children's behaviours. There is considerable evidence that children's difficult behaviours do indeed evoke parental negativity. The fact that children's behaviours can evoke negative parenting does not however mean that negative parenting has no impact on children's behaviour. The E-Risk longitudinal twin study of British families (Trzesniewski et al., 2006) examined the effects of fathers' parenting on young children's aggression. As expected, a prosocial father's *absence* predicted more aggression by his children. But in contrast, an antisocial father's *presence* predicted more aggression by his children, and his harmful effect was exacerbated the more time each week he spent taking care of the children.

The strong contribution of harsh, inconsistent parenting with lack of warmth to the causation of conduct problems provides an opportunity for intervention. As evidence presented in this guideline will show, parenting programmes that reverse less optimal patterns of parenting and promote positive encouragement of children with the setting of clear boundaries that are calmly enforced lead to improvement of conduct problems.

*Child attachment*

The quality of the parent–child relationship is crucial to later social behaviour, and if the child does not have the opportunity to make attachments, for example due to being taken into institutional care, this typically leads to subsequent problems in relating: antisocial behaviour can arise from infant attachment difficulties. One study found that ambivalent and controlling attachment predicted externalising behaviours after controlling for baseline externalising problems; disorganised child attachment patterns seem to be especially associated with conduct problems. Although it seems obvious that poor parent–child relations in general predict conduct problems, it has yet to be established whether attachment difficulties as measured by observational paradigms have an independent causal role in the development of behaviour problems; attachment classifications could be markers for other relevant family risks. However, in adolescence there is evidence that attachment representations independently predict conduct symptoms over and above parenting quality (Scott et al., 2011).

*Witnessing interparental or partner violence*

Several researchers have found that children exposed to domestic violence between adults are subsequently more likely to themselves become antisocial. In one study, the authors (Cummings & Davies, 2002) proposed that marital conflict influences children's behaviour because of its effect on emotional regulation. Thus, a child may respond to fear arising from marital conflict by controlling their reactions through denial of the situation. This in turn may lead to inaccurate appraisal of other social situations and ineffective problem solving. Repeated exposure to family fighting or violence increases children's emotional dysregulation, resulting in greater reaction under stress. Children's antisocial behaviour may also be increased by partner discord because children are likely to imitate aggressive behaviour modelled by their parents. Through parental fights, children may learn that aggression is a normal part of family relationships, that it is an effective way of controlling others and that aggression is sanctioned not punished.

*Abuse*

Many parents use physical punishment, and parents of children with antisocial behaviour frequently resort to it out of desperation. Overall, associations between physical abuse and conduct problems are well established. In the Christchurch longitudinal study, child sexual abuse predicted conduct problems after controlling for other childhood adversities (Fergusson et al., 1996). However, sometimes some parents resort to severe and repeated beatings that are clearly abusive. This typically terrifies the child, causes great pain and overwhelms the ability of the child to stay calm. It leads the children to be less able to regulate their anger and teaches them a violent way of responding to stress. Unsurprisingly, elevated rates of conduct disorder result (Jaffee et al., 2003).

### 2.5.3    Risks in the community

*Risks in the local community*

It has been difficult to establish any direct link between neighbourhood characteristics and antisocial child behaviour. Thus, neighbourhood characteristics were seen in overly simple ways, such as percentage of ethnic minority residents or percentage of lone-parent households. Moreover, it could not be disproved that families whose members are antisocial tend selectively to move into 'bad' neighbourhoods. Recent neighbourhood research is attempting to address these issues, and suggests that the neighbourhood factors that are important include social processes such as 'collective efficacy' and 'social control'.

*Friendship groups*
Children and young people with antisocial behaviour have poorer peer relationships and associate with other children with similar antisocial behaviours. They have more aggressive and unhappy interactions with other children and they experience more rejection by children without conduct disorders (Coie, 2004).

### 2.5.4    Moving from association to causation

The evidence above shows many associations between antisocial behaviour and a wide range of risk factors. The exact role in causation of most of these risk factors is unknown: while we know what, statistically, predicts conduct-problem outcomes, we do not entirely know how or why. Establishing a causal role for a risk factor is by no means straightforward, particularly as it is unethical to experimentally expose healthy children to risk factors to observe whether those factors can generate new conduct problems. The use of genetically sensitive designs and the study of within-individual change in natural experiments and treatment studies have considerable methodological advantages for suggesting causal influences on conduct problems.

## 2.6    COURSE AND PROGNOSIS

### 2.6.1    Factors predicting poor outcome

Of those with early onset conduct disorder (before the age of 8 years), about half have serious problems that persist into adulthood. Of those with adolescent onset, the great majority (over 85%) desist in their antisocial behaviour by their early twenties. Many of the factors that predict poor outcome are associated with early onset (see Table 1).

To detect protective factors, children who do well despite adverse risk factors have been studied. These so-called 'resilient' children, however, have been shown to have lower levels of risk factors, for example a boy with antisocial behaviour and low IQ living in a rough neighbourhood but living with supportive, concerned parents. Protective factors are mostly the opposite end of the spectrum of the same risk factor, thus good parenting and high IQ are protective. Nonetheless, there are factors associated with resilience that are independent of known adverse influences. These include a good relationship with at least one adult (who does not necessarily have to be the parent), a sense of pride and self-esteem, and skills or competencies.

**Table 1: Factors predicting poor outcome**

| Factor | Outcome |
|---|---|
| *Onset* | Early onset of severe problems, before 8 years old. |
| *Phenomenology* | Antisocial acts which are severe, frequent and varied. |
| *Comorbidity* | Hyperactivity and attention problems. |
| *Intelligence* | Lower IQ. |
| *Family history* | Parental criminality; parental alcoholism. |
| *Parenting* | Harsh, inconsistent parenting with high criticism, low warmth, low involvement and low supervision. |
| *Wider environment* | Low income family in poor neighbourhood with ineffective schools. |

### 2.6.2    Adult outcome

Studies of groups of children with early-onset conduct disorder indicate a wide range of problems that are not only confined to antisocial acts as shown in Table 2. What is clear is that there are not only substantially increased rates of antisocial acts but also that the general psychosocial functioning of adults who had conduct disorder is strikingly poor. For most of the characteristics shown in Table 2, the increase compared with controls is three- to ten-fold (Fergusson et al., 2005). Thus conduct disorder has widespread ramifications in most of the important domains of life, affecting work and relationships. The strength of the effects emphasises the extensive benefits that can accrue from successful treatment, and the importance of making this available to affected children and young people.

### 2.6.3    Pathways

The path from childhood conduct disorder to poor adult outcome is neither inevitable nor linear.

Different sets of influences impinge as the individual grows up and shape the life course. Many of these can accentuate problems. Thus a toddler with an irritable temperament and short attention span may not learn good social skills if they are raised in a family lacking them, and where the child can only get their way by behaving antisocially and grasping for what they need. At school they may fall in with a deviant crowd of peers, where violence and other antisocial acts are talked up and give them a sense of esteem. The child's generally poor academic ability and difficult behaviour

**Table 2:  Adult outcomes**

| Characteristic | Outcome |
|---|---|
| *Antisocial behaviour* | More violent and non-violent crimes, for example mugging, grievous bodily harm, theft, car crimes, fraud. |
| *Psychiatric problems* | Increased rates of antisocial personality, alcohol and drug abuse, anxiety, depression and somatic complaints, episodes of deliberate self-harm and completed suicide, time in psychiatric hospitals. |
| *Education and training* | Poorer examination results, more truancy and early school leaving, fewer vocational qualifications. |
| *Work* | More unemployment, jobs held for shorter time, jobs with low status and income, increased claiming of benefits and welfare. |
| *Social network* | Few (if any) significant friends; low involvement with relatives, neighbours, clubs and organisations. |
| *Intimate relationships* | Increased rate of short-lived, violent, cohabiting relationships; partners often also antisocial. |
| *Children* | Increased rates of child abuse, conduct problems in offspring, children taken into care. |
| *Health* | More medical problems, earlier death. |

in class may lead them to truant increasingly, which in turn makes them fall farther behind. They may then leave school with no qualifications and fail to find a job, and resort to drugs. To fund their drug habit they may resort to crime and, once convicted, find it even harder to get a job. From this example, it can be seen that adverse experiences do not only arise passively and independently of the young person's behaviour; rather, the behaviour predisposes them to end up in risky and damaging environments. Consequently, the number of adverse life events experienced is greatly increased (Champion et al., 1995). The path from early hyperactivity into later conduct disorder is also not inevitable. In the presence of a warm supportive family atmosphere conduct disorders are far less likely than if the parents are highly critical and hostile.

Other influences can, however, steer the individual away from and antisocial path. For example, the fascinating follow-up of delinquent boys to up to the age of 70 years (Laub & Sampson, 2003) showed that the following led to desistence: being separated from a deviant peer group; marrying to a non-deviant partner; moving away from a poor neighbourhood; military service that imparted skills.

## 2.7     TREATMENT

The evidence for the effectiveness of treatments is the subject of the analyses in ensuing chapters. Singly or in combination, they address parenting skills, family functioning, child interpersonal skills, difficulties at school, peer group influences and medication for coexistent hyperactivity.

### 2.7.1     Parenting skills

Parent training aims to improve parenting skills (Scott, 2008). As the following chapters show, there are scores of randomised controlled trials (RCTs) suggesting that it is effective for children up to about 10 years old. Parenting interventions based on social learning theory address the parenting practices that were identified in research as contributing to conduct problems. Typically, they include five elements:

1)  **Promoting play and a positive relationship**
    To cut into the cycle of defiant behaviour and recriminations, it is important to instil some positive experiences for both child and parent and begin to mend the relationship. Helping parents learn the techniques of how to play in a constructive and non-hostile way with their children helps them recognise their needs and respond sensitively. The children in turn begin to like and respect their parents more, and become more secure in the relationship.
2)  **Praise and rewards for sociable behaviour**
    Parents are helped to reformulate difficult behaviour in terms of the positive behaviour they wish to see, so that they encourage wanted behaviour rather than criticise unwanted behaviour. For example, instead of shouting at the child not to run, they would praise him whenever he walks quietly; then he will do it more often. Through hundreds of such prosaic daily interactions, child behaviour can be substantially modified. When some parents find it hard to praise, and fail to recognise positive behaviour when it happens, the result is that the desired behaviour becomes less frequent.
3)  **Clear rules and clear commands**
    Rules need to be explicit and consistent; commands need to be firm and brief. Thus, shouting at a child to stop being naughty does not tell him what he *should* do, whereas, for example, telling him to play quietly gives a clear instruction which makes compliance easier.
4)  **Consistent and calm consequences for unwanted behaviour**
    Disobedience and aggression need to be responded to firmly and calmly by, for example, putting the child in a room for a few minutes. This method of 'time out from positive reinforcement' sounds simple, but requires considerable skill to administer effectively. More minor annoying behaviours such as whining and shouting often respond to being ignored, but again parents often find this hard to achieve in practice.

**5) Reorganising the child's day to prevent trouble**

There are often trouble spots in the day which will respond to fairly simple measures. For example putting siblings in different rooms to prevent fights on getting home from school, banning television in the morning until the child is dressed and so on.

Treatment can be given individually to the parent and child which enables live feedback in light of the parent's progress and the child's response. Alternatively, group treatments with parents alone have been shown to be equally effective. Trials show that parent management training is effective in reducing child antisocial behaviour in the short term for half to two-thirds of families, with little loss of effect at 1- to 3-year follow-up. However, research is now needed on clinical proposals of what interventions can be used for those who do not respond (Scott & Dadds, 2009).

### 2.7.2 Improving family functioning

Functional family therapy, multisystemic therapy and multidimensional treatment foster care (MTFC) aim to change a range of difficulties which impede effective functioning of young people with conduct disorder. These programmes use a combination of social learning theory, cognitive and systemic family therapy interventions. Functional family therapy addresses family processes, including high levels of negativity and blame, and characteristically seeks to improve communication between parent and young person, reduce interparental inconsistency, tighten up on supervision and monitoring, and negotiate rules and the sanctions to be applied for breaking them. Most other varieties of family therapy have not been subjected to controlled trials for young people with conduct disorder or delinquency so cannot be evaluated for their efficacy. Functional family therapy is an assertive outreach model and sessions typically take place in the family home. There is a manual for the therapeutic approach and adherence is checked weekly by the supervisor.

In multisystemic therapy the young person's and family's needs are assessed in their own context at home and in related systems such as at school and with peers. Following the assessment, proven methods of intervention are used to address difficulties and promote strengths. As for functional family therapy, treatment is delivered in the situation where the young person lives. Second, the therapist has a low caseload (four to six families) and the team is available 24 hours a day. Third, the therapist is responsible for ensuring appointments are kept and for effecting change – families cannot be blamed for failing to attend or 'not being ready' to change. Fourth, regular written feedback on progress towards goals from multiple sources is gathered by the therapist and acted upon. Fifth, there is a manual for the therapeutic approach and adherence is checked weekly by the supervisor.

MTFC is another intervention which has been shown to improve the quality of encouragement and supervision that young people with conduct disorder receive. This is an intensive 'wrap around' intervention. The young person temporarily lives with foster carers who are specially trained and, in addition, receives help from individual therapists at school and in the community. The child's parents are also helped to learn more effective parenting skills.

### 2.7.3      Anger management and child interpersonal skills

Most of the programmes to improve child interpersonal skills derive from cognitive behavioural therapy (CBT). What the programmes have in common is that the young people are trained to:
● slow down impulsive responses to challenging situations by stopping and thinking
● recognise their own level of physiological arousal, and their own emotional state
● recognise and define problems
● develop several alternative responses
● choose the best alternative response based on anticipation of consequences
● carry out the chosen course of action
● shortly afterwards, give themselves credit for staying in control and review how it went.
    Over the longer term, the programmes aim to increase positive social behaviour by teaching the young person to:
● learn skills to make and sustain friendships
● develop social interaction skills such as turn-taking and sharing
● express viewpoints in appropriate ways and listen to others.


### 2.7.4      Overcoming difficulties at school

These can be divided into learning problems and disruptive behaviour. There are proven programmes to deal with specific learning problems, such as specific reading difficulties, including Reading Recovery[1]. However, few of the programmes have been specifically evaluated for their ability to improve outcomes in children with conduct disorder, although at the time of writing trials are in progress.

    There are several schemes for improving classroom behaviour, including those that stress improved communication such as 'circle time' and those which work on behavioural principles or are part of a multimodal package. Some of these schemes specifically target children with conduct problems.


### 2.7.5      Ameliorating peer group influences

A few interventions have aimed to reduce the bad influence of deviant peers. A number attempted this through group work with other conduct disordered youths, but outcome studies showed a worsening of antisocial behaviour. Current treatments therefore either see youths individually and try to steer them away from deviant peers, or work in small groups (of around three to five youths) where the therapist can control the content of sessions. Some interventions place youths with conduct disorder in groups with well-functioning youths.

---

[1]http://readingrecovery.ioe.ac.uk/index.html

### 2.7.6    Medication

Where there is comorbid hyperactivity in addition to conduct disorder, several studies attest to a large reduction in both overt and covert antisocial behaviour with the use of medication, both at home and at school (NCCMH, 2010). Medication for pure conduct disorders is less well-established and is reviewed in this guideline.

## 2.8    GENERAL ISSUES WHEN PLANNING TREATMENT

Engagement of the family is particularly important for this group of children and families because dropout from treatment is high, at around 30 to 40%. Practical measures such as assisting with transport, providing childcare, and holding sessions in the evening or at other times to suit the family will all help. Many of the parents of children with conduct disorder may themselves have difficulty with authority and officialdom, and be very sensitive to criticism. Therefore, the approach is more likely to succeed if it is respectful of their point of view, does not offer overly prescriptive solutions and does not directly criticise parenting style. Practical homework tasks increase changes, as do problem-solving telephone calls from the therapist between sessions.

Parenting interventions may need to go beyond skill development to address more distal factors which prevent change. For example, drug or alcohol abuse in either parent, maternal depression and a violent relationship with the partner are all common. Assistance in claiming welfare and benefits and help with financial planning may reduce stress from debts.

A multimodal approach is likely to see greater changes. Therefore, involving the school or the local education authority in treatment by visiting and offering strategies for managing the child in class is usually helpful, as is advocating for extra tuition where necessary. If the school seems unable to cope despite extra resources, consideration could be given to moving the child to a unit that specialises in the management of behavioural difficulties, where skilled staff may be able to improve child functioning so a later return to mainstream school may be possible. Avoiding antisocial peers and building self-esteem may be helped by the child attending after-school clubs and holiday activities.

Where parents are not coping or a damaging abusive relationship is detected, it may be necessary to liaise with the social services department to arrange respite for the parents or a period of foster care. It is important during this time to work with the family to increase their skills so that the child can return to the family. Where there is permanent breakdown, long-term fostering or adoption may be recommended.

## 2.9    PREVENTION

Conduct disorder should offer good opportunities for prevention because it can be detected early reasonably well, early intervention is more effective than later and there are a number of effective interventions.

In the US a number of comprehensive interventions have been tested. One of the best known is the Fast Track project (Conduct Problems Prevention Research Group, 2011). Here, the most antisocial 10% of 5- to 6-year-olds in schools in disadvantaged areas were selected, as judged by teacher and parent reports. They were then offered intervention which was given for 1 year in the first instance and comprised:

● weekly parent training in groups with videotapes
● an interpersonal skills training programme for the whole class
● academic tutoring twice a week
● home visits from the parent trainer
● a pairing programme with sociable peers from the class.

From across the US, 891 children were randomised to receive this treatment or be assigned to the control group and the project has cost over $100 million, with the treatment continuing to be given over 10 years on a tailored basis. However, outcomes have been modest. By age 18 there was no overall improvement of antisocial behaviour, although in the most severe cases a diagnosis of conduct disorder was reduced by 50% (Conduct Problems Prevention Research Group, 2011). In the UK, there has been a drive to disseminate parenting programmes widely (Scott, 2010).

Although a review of universal prevention interventions (that is, those aimed at the general population) is outside the scope of this guideline, a range of selective preventions (that is, those aimed at individuals who are at high risk for developing the disorder or are showing very early signs or symptoms) are reviewed.


## 2.10     ECONOMIC COST

The economic consequence of conduct disorder is characteristically huge, with considerable resource inputs from several government and private sectors. Though the condition can be considered primarily to be a mental health problem (American Psychiatric Association, 2000), the healthcare service provisions for conduct disorder and the resulting healthcare costs are rather small when compared with costs incurred by other sectors such as the criminal justice system (Scott et al., 2001). This is as a result of associated crime committed by the individuals, with resultant significant social costs and harm to individuals and their victims, families and carers, and to society at large (Welsh et al., 2008). Overall, evidence for the cost estimates incurred due to conduct disorder varies widely and tends to be great when a societal perspective is taken.

The cost of conduct disorder, like other health problems, often includes both direct service costs and indirect costs, such as productivity loss as a result of health problems. The extent of direct costs is closely related to the quantity of services utilised by the individual. In comparison with other common types of psychiatric disorders in children and adolescents, those with conduct disorder are more likely to be heavy users of social services than those with emotional disorders or hyperkinetic disorder, and they are also more likely to utilise primary healthcare and specialist education services than those with emotional disorders (Shivram et al., 2009). Similarly, in an earlier work on service utilisation by this population (Vostanis et al., 2003), children with conduct disorder, with or without comorbidity, were observed to be heavy users of health, education and social services compared with those with other form of psychiatric disorders.

Depending on the setting where service is delivered and the prevailing health condition of the individual (for example a child or young person with conduct disorder, conduct problems, oppositional defiant disorder or if they are a juvenile offender), there is considerable variation in the total cost of the services incurred by people with conduct disorders. In a UK study by Scott and colleagues (2001), the cumulative cost of services to individuals diagnosed with conduct disorder at the age of 10 years, over a period of about 18 years, was £70,000 (1998 prices). Costs accumulated by individuals with conduct disorder are about ten times more than those with no conduct problem and three times that of the costs incurred by individuals with conduct problems. Similarly, in a US study comparing the costs of children with conduct disorder, oppositional defiant disorder, elevated levels of problem behaviour and those without any of these disorders (Foster et al., 2005), the mean annual cost of services for the conduct disorder group was estimated as $12,547 (2000 prices), which was about twice the cost of those with oppositional defiant disorder and three times the cost of those without conduct disorder.

Few of the cost studies included costs from all relevant sectors, such as health, education, social services, criminal justice, family and carer, and voluntary sectors, and some studies reported separate cost estimates for services provided to juvenile offenders who were already in contact with the criminal justice system. On average, the annual cost of services incurred by people with conduct disorders and associated problems is between £6,000 (2002/03 prices) and $180,000 (2008 prices) (Romeo et al., 2006; Welsh et al., 2008). Criminal justice service costs are the most significant cost component in most of the studies, accounting for between 19% and 64% of the total costs (Foster et al., 2005; Scott et al., 2001). Other than criminal justice system costs, costs to family and carers, where reported, are the second most significant costs of conduct disorder. In a UK study, the annual cost per child with antisocial behaviour problems without criminal justice costs was estimated to be about £5,960 (2002/03 prices) with the cost to family accounting for about 79% of the total cost, and health service, education and voluntary services accounting for about 8%, 1% and 3%, respectively. The cost to social services was estimated to be less than 1% of the total cost (Romeo et al., 2006). Similarly, Knapp and colleagues (1999) estimated the annual mean cost of services for ten children aged 4 to 10 years to be £15,270 (1996/97 prices) and described the cost to families as accounting for about 31% of the mean costs, and health service costs as accounting for 16%.

There is little evidence on the annual mean cost of services for individuals who have conduct disorder in addition to other co-existing health problems. Knapp and colleagues reported annual mean service costs per patient with conduct disorder and major depressive disorder to be £1,085, which is about 2.4 times more than those with major depressive disorder only (Knapp et al., 2002). Service domains included in the estimate were health and the criminal justice system, and therefore greatly under-estimate the actual mean service costs for such individuals. Another UK study (Barrett et al., 2006) looked at the cost of services provided to younger offenders (aged 13 to 18 years), either in a community setting or in custody over a 6-month period, and reported an average annual cost of services (excluding costs to families) of

£40,000 (2001/02 prices). Services provided in secured accommodation were found to be around three times higher than those provided in the community.

The cost of crime has huge policy implications in estimating the costs of conduct disorder. Because of the strong link between conduct disorder and probable criminal activities, the high cost of crime is often estimated to quantify the extent of the economic consequences of treating conduct disorder. A report by the Sainsbury Centre for Mental Health (2009) estimated that about 80% of all criminal activity is attributable to people who had conduct problems in childhood and adolescence. Methods of crime cost estimation and cost components differ greatly among studies. However, crime costs are generally estimated to include three basic cost categories: costs in the anticipation of crime (for example government crime prevention costs), costs as a consequence of crime (for example victim support services) and costs in response to crime (for example police and court costs), according to the Centre for Criminal Justice (2008) report. Often estimated are costs as a consequence of crime and costs in response to crime, such as tangible service costs and intangible costs (for example pain, suffering or grief suffered by victims of crime) (Cohen, 1998; McCollister et al., 2010). Given the variation in the methods used in crime cost estimation and the cost components included in the estimate, the reported costs of crime are also associated with wide variations. In the US, the reported lifetime costs of crime attributable to a typical offender are in the range of $2.1 to $3.7 million in 2007 US dollars (Cohen & Piquero, 2009) when discounted back to birth. In England and Wales, the lifetime costs of crime per prolific offender are put at around £1.5 million (Sainsbury Centre for Mental Health, 2009). The total cost of crime against individuals and households in 2003/04 pounds was estimated to be around £36.2 billion (Dubourg et al., 2005), and for youths aged between 10 and 21 years the estimated cost of crime in 2009 for Great Britain was reported to be in excess of £1.2 billion, or about £23 million a week (Prince's Trust, 2010).

Taking into consideration the overall lifetime costs of conduct problems, the Sainsbury Centre for Mental Health (2009) estimated that crime-related costs comprise about 71% of the total lifetime costs of people with conduct disorder and 29% for other non-crime related costs. For people with mild or moderate conduct problems, a significant percentage of their lifetime costs is also related to crime (61%). Notwithstanding the extensive literatures on crime costs, there are difficulties in accurately estimating the overall crime costs attributable to children and young people with conduct disorders or the subsequent adverse outcomes in adulthood. Such difficulties are often related to uncertainties in accurately quantifying the value of intangible costs such as fear of crime, pain, suffering or grief suffered by victims of crime (Loomes, 2007; Semmens, 2007; Shapland & Hall, 2007), and other indirect costs such as productivity loss. Aside from the immediate physical health needs of crime victims, mental health needs of crime victims can impose huge costs on both the criminal justice and the health systems when about 20 to 25% of people visiting mental healthcare professionals do so as a result of being victims of crime, at a cost of between $5.8 and $6.8 billion (Cohen & Miller, 1998). As a result, current estimates of the economic cost of conduct disorder can be assumed to be conservative and the actual cost is more likely to exceed the values reported in the literature when all attributed costs are considered.

# 3     METHODS USED TO DEVELOP THIS GUIDELINE

## 3.1     OVERVIEW

The development of this guideline followed *The Guidelines Manual* (NICE, 2009c). A team of health and social care professionals, lay representatives and technical experts known as the Guideline Development Group (GDG), with support from the NCCMH staff, undertook the development of a person-centred, evidence-based guideline. There are seven basic steps in the process of developing a guideline:

1. Define the scope, which lays out exactly what will be included (and excluded) in the guidance.
2. Define review questions that cover all areas specified in the scope.
3. Develop a review protocol for the systematic review, specifying the search strategy and method of evidence synthesis for each review question.
4. Synthesise data retrieved, guided by the review protocols.
5. Produce evidence profiles and summaries using the GRADE approach.
6. Consider the implications of the research findings for clinical practice and reach consensus decisions on areas where evidence is not found.
7. Answer review questions with evidence-based recommendations for clinical practice.

   The clinical practice recommendations made by the GDG are therefore derived from the most up-to-date and robust evidence for the clinical and cost effectiveness of the treatments and services used in the recognition, intervention and management of conduct disorders and antisocial behaviour. Where evidence was not found or was inconclusive, the GDG discussed and attempted to reach consensus on what should be recommended, factoring in any relevant issues. In addition, to ensure a service user and carer focus, the concerns of service users and carers regarding health and social care have been highlighted and addressed by recommendations agreed by the whole GDG.

## 3.2     THE SCOPE

Guideline topics are referred by the Secretary of State and the letter of referral defines the remit, which defines the main areas to be covered; see *The Guidelines Manual* (NICE, 2009c) for further information. The NCCMH developed a scope for the guideline based on the remit. The purpose of the scope is to:

- provide an overview of what the guideline will include and exclude
- identify the key aspects of care that must be included
- set the boundaries of the development work and provide a clear framework to enable work to stay within the priorities agreed by NICE and the National Collaborating Centre, and the remit from the Department of Health/Welsh Assembly Government

- inform the development of the review questions and search strategy
- inform professionals and the public about expected content of the guideline
- keep the guideline to a reasonable size to ensure that its development can be carried out within the allocated period.

An initial draft of the scope was sent to registered stakeholders who had agreed to attend a scoping workshop. The workshop was used to:

- obtain feedback on the selected key clinical issues
- identify which population subgroups should be specified (if any)
- seek views on the composition of the GDG
- encourage applications for GDG membership.

The draft scope was subject to consultation with registered stakeholders over a 4-week period. During the consultation period, the scope was posted on the NICE website (www.nice.org.uk). Comments were invited from stakeholder organisations. The NCCMH and NICE reviewed the scope in light of comments received, and the revised scope was signed off by NICE.

## 3.3 THE GUIDELINE DEVELOPMENT GROUP

During the consultation phase, members of the GDG were appointed by an open recruitment process. GDG membership consisted of: professionals in psychiatry, clinical psychology, nursing, social care and general practice; academic experts in psychiatry and psychology; and carers of children and young people with a conduct disorder. The guideline development process was supported by staff from the NCCMH, who undertook the clinical and health economics literature searches, reviewed and presented the evidence to the GDG, managed the process and contributed to drafting the guideline.

### 3.3.1 Guideline Development Group meetings

Twelve GDG meetings were held between 13 April 2011 and 31 October 2012. During each day-long GDG meeting, in a plenary session, review questions and clinical and economic evidence were reviewed and assessed, and recommendations formulated. At each meeting, all GDG members declared any potential conflicts of interest, and service user and carer concerns were routinely discussed as a standing agenda item.

### 3.3.2 Topic groups

The GDG divided its workload along clinically relevant lines to simplify the guideline development process, and GDG members formed smaller topic groups to undertake guideline work in that area of clinical practice. Topic Group 1 covered questions relating to prevention, Topic Group 2 covered interventions and Topic Group 3 covered health economics. These groups were designed to efficiently manage the large volume of evidence appraisal prior to presenting it to the GDG as a whole. Each topic group was chaired by a GDG member with expert knowledge of the topic area (one of the healthcare professionals). Topic groups refined the review questions and the clinical definitions of treatment interventions, reviewed and prepared the evidence with the systematic reviewer before presenting it to the GDG as a whole, and helped the GDG to identify further expertise in the topic. Topic group leaders reported the status of the group's work as part of the standing agenda. They also introduced and led the GDG discussion of the evidence review for that topic and assisted the GDG Chair in drafting the section of the guideline relevant to the work of each topic group.

### 3.3.3    Service users and carers

Individuals with direct experience of services gave an integral service-user focus to the GDG and the guideline. The GDG included two carers, who contributed as full GDG members to writing the review questions, helping to ensure that the evidence addressed their views and preferences, highlighting sensitive issues and terminology relevant to the guideline, and bringing service-user research to the attention of the GDG. In drafting the guideline, they contributed to writing the guideline's introduction and identified recommendations from the service user and carer perspective.

### 3.3.4    National and international experts

National and international experts in the area under review were identified through the literature search and through the experience of the GDG members. These experts were contacted to identify unpublished or soon-to-be published studies, to ensure that up-to-date evidence was included in the development of the guideline. They informed the group about completed trials at the pre-publication stage, systematic reviews in the process of being published, studies relating to the cost effectiveness of treatment and trial data if the GDG could be provided with full access to the complete trial report. Appendix 4 lists researchers who were contacted.

### 3.4    REVIEW QUESTIONS

Review (clinical) questions were used to guide the identification and interrogation of the evidence base relevant to the topic of the guideline. Before the first GDG meeting, draft review questions were prepared by NCCMH staff based on the scope and an overview of existing guidelines, and discussed with the GDG Chair. The draft review questions were then discussed by the GDG at the first few meetings and amended as necessary. Where appropriate, the questions were refined once the evidence had been searched and, where necessary, sub-questions were generated. Questions submitted by stakeholders were also discussed by the GDG and the rationale for not including any questions was recorded in the minutes. The final list of review questions can be found in Appendix 5.

For questions about interventions, the PICO (population, intervention, comparison and outcome) framework was used (see Table 3).

Questions relating to case identification do not involve an intervention designed to treat a particular condition; therefore, the PICO framework was not used. Rather, the questions were designed to pick up key issues specifically relevant to clinical utility, for example their accuracy, reliability, safety and acceptability to the service user.

In some situations, the prognosis of a particular condition is of fundamental importance over and above its general significance in relation to specific interventions. Areas where this is particularly likely to occur relate to assessment of risk, for example in terms of behaviour modification or screening and early intervention. In addition, review questions related to issues of service delivery are occasionally specified in the remit from the Department of Health/Welsh Assembly Government. In these cases, appropriate review questions were developed to be clear and concise.

To help facilitate the literature review, a note was made of the best study design type to answer each question. There are four main types of review question of relevance to NICE guidelines. These are listed in Table 4. For each type of question, the best primary study design varies, where 'best' is interpreted as 'least likely to give misleading answers to the question'.

However, in all cases, a well-conducted systematic review (of the appropriate type of study) is likely to always yield a better answer than a single study.

Deciding on the best design type to answer a specific review question does not mean that studies of different design types addressing the same question were discarded.

**Table 3:  Features of a well-formulated question on effectiveness intervention – the PICO guide**

| Population | Which population of service users are we interested in? How can they be best described? Are there subgroups that need to be considered? |
|---|---|
| Intervention | Which intervention, treatment or approach should be used? |
| Comparison | What is/are the main alternative/s to compare with the intervention? |
| Outcome | What is really important for the service user? Which outcomes should be considered: intermediate or short-term measures; mortality; morbidity and treatment complications; rates of relapse; late morbidity and readmission; return to work, physical and social functioning and other measures such as quality of life; general health status? |

**Table 4: Best study design to answer each type of question**

| Type of question | Best primary study design |
| --- | --- |
| Effectiveness or other impact of an intervention | RCT; other studies that may be considered in the absence of RCTs are the following: internally/externally controlled before and after trial, interrupted time series |
| Accuracy of information (for example risk factor, test, prediction rule) | Comparing the information against a valid gold standard in a randomised trial or inception cohort study |
| Rates (of disease, service user experience, rare side effects) | Prospective cohort, registry, cross-sectional study |

## 3.5 SYSTEMATIC CLINICAL LITERATURE REVIEW

The aim of the clinical literature review was to systematically identify and synthesise relevant evidence from the literature in order to answer the specific review questions developed by the GDG. Thus, clinical practice recommendations are evidence based, where possible, and, if evidence is not available, informal consensus methods are used to try and reach general agreement (see Section 3.5.9) and the need for future research is specified.

### 3.5.1 The review process

*Scoping searches*
A broad preliminary search of the literature was undertaken in November 2010 to obtain an overview of the issues likely to be covered by the scope, and to help define key areas. Searches were restricted to clinical guidelines, health technology assessment reports and key systematic reviews, and conducted in the following databases and websites:
● BMJ Clinical Evidence
● Canadian Medical Association Infobase (Canadian guidelines)
● Clinical Policy and Practice Program of the New South Wales Department of Health (Australia)
● Clinical Practice Guidelines (Australian guidelines)
● Cochrane Central Register of Controlled Trials
● Cochrane Database of Abstracts of Reviews of Effects
● Cochrane Database of Systematic Reviews
● Excerpta Medica Database (Embase)
● Guidelines International Network
● Health Evidence Bulletin Wales

- Health Management Information Consortium
- Health Technology Assessment (HTA) database (technology assessments)
- Medical Literature Analysis and Retrieval System Online (MEDLINE/MEDLINE in Process)
- National Health and Medical Research Council
- New Zealand Guidelines Group
- NHS Centre for Reviews and Dissemination
- Organizing Medical Networked Information Medical Search
- Scottish Intercollegiate Guidelines Network
- Turning Research Into Practice
- US Agency for Healthcare Research and Quality
- Websites of NICE (including NHS Evidence) and the National Institute for Health Research HTA Programme for guidelines and HTAs in development.

Further information about this process can be found in The Guidelines Manual (NICE, 2009c).

*Systematic literature searches*

After the scope was finalised, a systematic search strategy was developed to locate as much relevant evidence as possible. The balance between sensitivity (the power to identify all studies on a particular topic) and specificity (the ability to exclude irrelevant studies from the results) was carefully considered, and a decision made to utilise a broad approach to searching to maximise retrieval of evidence to all parts of the guideline. Searches were restricted to systematic reviews, RCTs and observational studies, and conducted in the following databases:

- Australian Education Index
- Applied Social Services Index and Abstracts
- British Education Index
- Campbell Collaboration
- Cumulative Index to Nursing and Allied Health Literature
- Cochrane Database of Systematic Reviews
- Central (centralised database of RCTs and other controlled studies)
- Database of Abstracts and Reviews of Effectiveness
- Embase
- Education Resources in Curriculum
- Health Management Information Consortium
- HTA database (technology assessments)
- International Bibliography of Social Sciences
- MEDLINE/in-process database for MEDLINE (PreMEDLINE)
- National Criminal Justice Reference Service
- PsycBOOKS, the full-text database of books and chapters in the American Psychological Association's electronic databases
- PsycEXTRA, a grey literature database, which is a companion to PsycINFO
- Psychological Information Database (PsycINFO)
- Social Science Abstracts
- Social Science Citation Index

- Sociological Abstracts
- Web-based searches for additional evidence were performed in Social Care Online.
    The search strategies were initially developed for MEDLINE before being trans-lated for use in other databases/interfaces. Strategies were built up through a number of trial searches, and discussion of the results of the searches with the review team and GDG, to ensure that all possible relevant search terms were covered. To assure com-prehensive coverage, search terms for the main population were kept purposely broad to help counter dissimilarities in database indexing practices and imprecise report-ing of study populations by authors in the titles and abstracts of records. For stan-dard mainstream bibliographic databases (Embase, MEDLINE, PreMEDLINE and PsycINFO), search terms for main population were combined with the intervention(s), together with a research-based filter for the study design of interest. For smaller, topic-specific databases (for example education and sociological databases), a search, modified to be more precise, was conducted for the main population and study design of interest only. The search terms for each search are set out in full in Appendix 7.

*Reference Management*
Citations from each search were downloaded into the reference management software (EndNote) and duplicates removed. Records were then screened against the eligibility criteria of the reviews before being appraised for methodological quality (see 'Study selection and quality assessment' section, below). The unfiltered search results were saved and retained for future potential re-analysis, to help keep the process both rep-licable and transparent.

*Search filters*
To aid retrieval of relevant and sound studies, filters were used to limit a number of searches to systematic reviews, RCTs and observational studies. The search filters for systematic reviews and RCTs are adaptations of filters designed by the Centre for Reviews and Dissemination, York, the Health Information Research Unit of McMaster University, Ontario, and the University of Alberta. The observational study filter is an in-house development. Each filter comprises index terms relating to the study type(s) and associated textwords for the methodological description of the design(s).

*Date and language restrictions*
Systematic database searches were initially conducted in June 2011 up to the most recent searchable date. Search updates were generated on a 6-monthly basis, with the final re-runs carried out in July 2012 ahead of the guideline consultation. After this point, studies were only included if they were judged by the GDG to be exceptional (for example if the evidence was likely to change a recommendation).
    Although no language restrictions were applied at the searching stage, foreign language papers were not requested or reviewed unless they were of particular impor-tance to a review question.
    Date restrictions were not applied, except for searches of systematic reviews which were limited to research published from 1995. This restriction was put in place because older reviews were thought to be less useful.

*Other search methods*

Other search methods involved: (a) scanning the reference lists of all eligible publications (systematic reviews, stakeholder evidence and included studies) for more published reports and citations of unpublished research; (b) sending lists of studies meeting the inclusion criteria to subject experts (identified through searches and the GDG) and asking them to check the lists for completeness, and to provide information of any published or unpublished research for consideration (see Appendix 4); (c) checking the tables of contents of key journals for studies that might have been missed by the database and reference list searches; (d) tracking key papers in the Science Citation Index (prospectively) over time for further useful references; (e) conducting searches in ClinicalTrials.gov for unpublished trial reports; (f) contacting included study authors for unpublished or incomplete data sets. Searches conducted for existing NICE guidelines were updated where necessary. Other relevant guidelines were assessed for quality using the AGREE instrument (AGREE Collaboration, 2003). The evidence base underlying high-quality existing guidelines was utilised and updated as appropriate.

Full details of the search strategies and filters used for the systematic review of clinical evidence are provided in Appendix 7.

*Study selection and quality assessment*

All primary-level studies included after the first scan of citations were acquired in full and re-evaluated for eligibility at the time they were being entered into the study information database. More specific eligibility criteria were developed for each review question and are described in the relevant clinical evidence chapters. Eligible systematic reviews and primary-level studies were critically appraised for methodological quality (see Appendix 9 for further information). The eligibility of each study was confirmed by at least one member of the appropriate topic group.

For some review questions, it was necessary to prioritise the evidence with respect to the UK context (that is, external validity). To make this process explicit, the topic groups took into account the following factors when assessing the evidence:

● participant factors (for example gender, age and ethnicity)
● provider factors (for example model fidelity, the conditions under which the intervention was performed and the availability of experienced staff to undertake the procedure)
● cultural factors (for example differences in standard care and differences in the welfare system).

It was the responsibility of each topic group to decide which prioritisation factors were relevant to each review question in light of the UK context and then decide how they should modify their recommendations.

*Unpublished evidence*

The GDG used a number of criteria when deciding whether or not to accept unpublished data. First, the evidence must have been accompanied by a trial report containing sufficient detail to properly assess the quality of the data. Second, the evidence must have been submitted with the understanding that data from the study and a summary of the study's characteristics would be published in the full guideline. Therefore, the GDG did not accept evidence submitted as commercial in confidence. However, the GDG recognised that unpublished evidence submitted by investigators might later be retracted by those investigators if the inclusion of such data would jeopardise publication of their research.

### 3.5.2    Data extraction

Study characteristics and outcome data were extracted from all eligible studies that met the minimum quality criteria, using Review Manager 5.1 (The Cochrane Collaboration, 2011) and an Excel-based form (see Appendix 8).

In most circumstances, for a given outcome (continuous and dichotomous), where more than 50% of the number randomised to any group were missing or incomplete, the study results were excluded from the analysis (except for the outcome 'leaving the study early', in which case the denominator was the number randomised). Where there was limited data for a particular review the 50% rule was not applied. In these circumstances the evidence was downgraded due to the risk of bias.

Where possible, outcome data was used from an intention-to-treat (ITT) analysis (that is, a 'once-randomised-always-analyse' basis). For dichotomous efficacy outcomes the effect size was re-calculated if ITT had not been used. When making the calculations, if there was good evidence that those participants who ceased to engage in the study were likely to have an unfavourable outcome, early withdrawals were included in both the numerator and denominator. Adverse effects were entered into Review Manager as reported by the study authors because it is usually not possible to determine whether early withdrawals had an unfavourable outcome.

Consultation with another reviewer or members of the GDG was used to overcome difficulties with coding. Data from studies included in existing systematic reviews were extracted independently by one reviewer and cross-checked with the existing data set. Double data extraction of new data was only undertaken for studies reporting very large effect sizes. Masked assessment (that is, blind to the journal from which the article comes, the authors, the institution and the magnitude of the effect) was not used since it is unclear that doing so reduces bias (Berlin, 1997; Jadad et al., 1996).

### 3.5.3    Synthesising the evidence for the effectiveness of interventions

*Outcome measures*
Many studies include a wide range of outcome measures from different sources (researchers, parents, teachers, clinicians and self) to explore the clinical and social benefits of interventions for conduct disorders. In addition to being of research interest, this wider approach to outcomes mirrors the breadth of contexts within which conduct disordered behaviour is presented, although this heterogeneity brings challenges in determining the relative reliability of measures made by different categories of informant.

For the purposes of the meta-analyses, the GDG established a list of outcomes that it rated as critical and focused on these when making recommendations. For children and young people this included the following outcome categories: agency contact (for example residential care, criminal justice system); antisocial behaviour (at home, at school, in the community); drug/alcohol use; educational attainment (that is, the highest level of education completed); offending behaviour; and school exclusion due to antisocial behaviour.

For each outcome category, where available, data were extracted for parent-, teacher-, researcher-/clinician- and observer-reported outcomes. Only outcome measures that were judged to be established and valid were used in the analysis; less recognised measures, for instance those developed for a particular study were therefore not used.

*Meta-analysis*

Where possible, meta-analysis was used to synthesise evidence from trials of interventions using Comprehensive Meta-Analysis, version 2.2.048 (Borenstein et al., 2005) and Stata, version 12 (StataCorp, 2012).

Dichotomous outcomes were analysed as relative risks (RR) with the associated 95% confidence interval (CI) (see Figure 1 for an example of a forest plot displaying dichotomous data). A relative risk (also called a risk ratio) is the ratio of the treatment event rate to the control event rate. An RR of 1 indicates no difference between treatment and control. In Figure 1, the overall RR of 0.73 indicates that the event rate (that is, non-remission rate) associated with intervention A is about three-quarters of that of the control intervention or, in other words, the relative risk reduction is 27%.

The CI shows a range of values within which there is 95% confidence that the true effect will lie. If the effect size has a CI that does not cross the 'line of no effect', then the effect is commonly interpreted as being statistically significant.

Continuous outcomes were analysed using the standardised mean difference (SMD) when different measures were used in different studies to estimate the same underlying effect (see Figure 2 for an example of a forest plot displaying continuous data). If reported by study authors, ITT data, using a valid method for imputation of missing data, were preferred over data only from people who completed the study.

Because the outcomes of interest have often been measured using different scales within a single study, and the GDG were interested in the effect of an intervention when rated by different people (for example observer and parent), the following procedures were employed. First, relevant data were categorised by rater (that is, observer, researcher/clinician, teacher, parent, self). Second, within each rater category, data from multiple outcomes were pooled using Comprehensive Meta-Analysis (one effect size per study for post-treatment results, and where available, another effect size for the longest follow-up). These data were transferred to Stata, which was used to synthesise results across studies.

*Heterogeneity*

To check for consistency of effects among studies, both the $I^2$ statistic and the chi-squared test of heterogeneity, as well as a visual inspection of the forest plots, were used. The $I^2$ statistic describes the proportion of total variation in study estimates that is due

## Figure 1: Example of a forest plot displaying dichotomous data

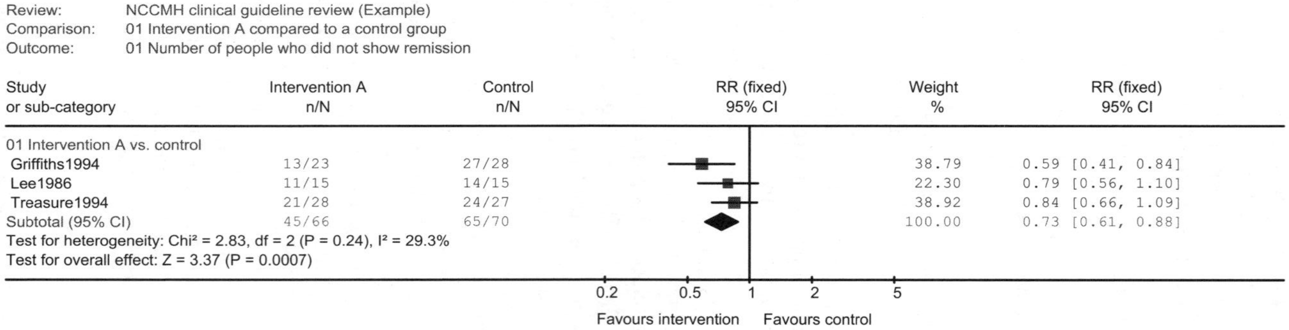

Review: NCCMH clinical guideline review (Example)
Comparison: 01 Intervention A compared to a control group
Outcome: 01 Number of people who did not show remission

| Study or sub-category | Intervention A n/N | Control n/N | RR (fixed) 95% CI | Weight % | RR (fixed) 95% CI |
|---|---|---|---|---|---|
| 01 Intervention A vs. control | | | | | |
| Griffiths1994 | 13/23 | 27/28 | | 38.79 | 0.59 [0.41, 0.84] |
| Lee1986 | 11/15 | 14/15 | | 22.30 | 0.79 [0.56, 1.10] |
| Treasure1994 | 21/28 | 24/27 | | 38.92 | 0.84 [0.66, 1.09] |
| Subtotal (95% CI) | 45/66 | 65/70 | | 100.00 | 0.73 [0.61, 0.88] |

Test for heterogeneity: Chi² = 2.83, df = 2 (P = 0.24), I² = 29.3%
Test for overall effect: Z = 3.37 (P = 0.0007)

0.2  0.5  1  2  5
Favours intervention    Favours control

## Figure 2: Example of a forest plot displaying continuous data

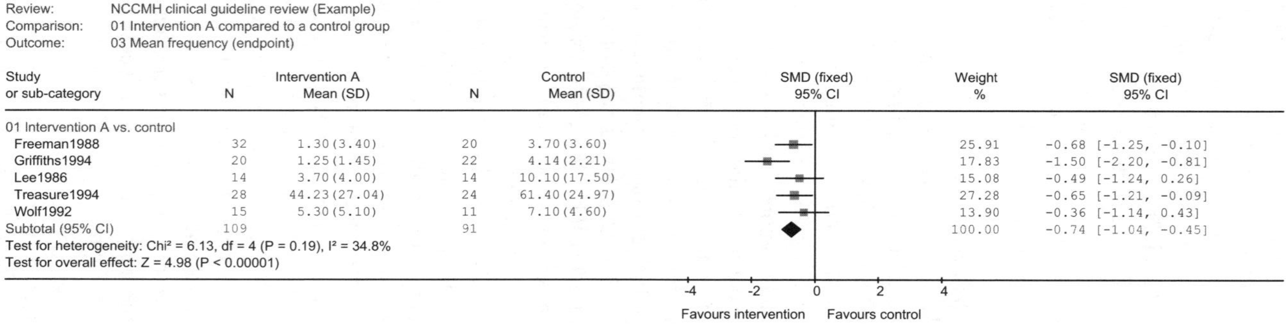

Review: NCCMH clinical guideline review (Example)
Comparison: 01 Intervention A compared to a control group
Outcome: 03 Mean frequency (endpoint)

| Study or sub-category | N | Intervention A Mean (SD) | N | Control Mean (SD) | SMD (fixed) 95% CI | Weight % | SMD (fixed) 95% CI |
|---|---|---|---|---|---|---|---|
| 01 Intervention A vs. control | | | | | | | |
| Freeman1988 | 32 | 1.30 (3.40) | 20 | 3.70 (3.60) | | 25.91 | -0.68 [-1.25, -0.10] |
| Griffiths1994 | 20 | 1.25 (1.45) | 22 | 4.14 (2.21) | | 17.83 | -1.50 [-2.20, -0.81] |
| Lee1986 | 14 | 3.70 (4.00) | 14 | 10.10 (17.50) | | 15.08 | -0.49 [-1.24, 0.26] |
| Treasure1994 | 28 | 44.23 (27.04) | 24 | 61.40 (24.97) | | 27.28 | -0.65 [-1.21, -0.09] |
| Wolf1992 | 15 | 5.30 (5.10) | 11 | 7.10 (4.60) | | 13.90 | -0.36 [-1.14, 0.43] |
| Subtotal (95% CI) | 109 | | 91 | | | 100.00 | -0.74 [-1.04, -0.45] |

Test for heterogeneity: Chi² = 6.13, df = 4 (P = 0.19), I² = 34.8%
Test for overall effect: Z = 4.98 (P < 0.00001)

-4  -2  0  2  4
Favours intervention    Favours control

to heterogeneity (Higgins & Thompson, 2002). The $I^2$ statistic was interpreted in the follow way based on the *Cochrane Handbook for Systematic Reviews of Interventions* (Higgins & Green, 2011):

0 to 40%: might not be important

30 to 60%: may represent moderate heterogeneity

50 to 90%: may represent substantial heterogeneity

75 to 100%: considerable heterogeneity.

The Cochrane Collaboration advice suggests that overlapping categories are less misleading than simple thresholds since the importance of inconsistency depends on (1) the magnitude and direction of effects, and (2) the strength of evidence for heterogeneity (for example, *p* value from the chi-squared test, or a CI for $I^2$).

Where important heterogeneity was detected, random effects univariate meta-regression models were used to examine whether any reported factors explained any of the variance. Then, a multivariate meta-regression model was created including all factors that were shown in the univariate models to explain at least some of the variance.

To examine how much of the heterogeneity was accounted for by the factor(s) included in each model, the adjusted $R^2$ produced by the revised metareg command in Stata was used. Sensitivity analyses were also used to explore the effect of removing studies with high risk of bias, and studies of attenuated interventions (that is, those interventions judged by the GDG to be very brief or because they were self-administered versions of an intervention usually administered by a therapist/researcher).

### Publication bias

The GDG assessed the possibility of publication bias using the Stata metabias command. Where there was evidence of significant asymmetry in the funnel plot (as judged by the Begg and Mazumdar adjusted rank correlation test) (Begg & Mazumdar, 1994), the Stata metatrim command was used to perform the Duval and Tweedie non-parametric 'trim and fill' method (Duval & Tweedie, 2000). This method was used to examine the impact of the missing studies by adjusting the meta-analysis to take into account the theoretically missing studies. Data were only reported where possible publication bias was detected.

### 3.5.4    Synthesising the evidence from test accuracy studies

### Meta-analysis

Review Manager 5 was used to summarise test accuracy data from each study using forest plots and summary receiver operator characteristic (ROC) plots. Where more than two studies reported appropriate data, a bivariate test accuracy meta-analysis was conducted using Meta-DiSc (Zamora et al., 2006) in order to obtain pooled estimates of sensitivity, specificity, and positive and negative likelihood ratios.

### Sensitivity and specificity

The sensitivity of an instrument refers to probability that it will produce a true positive result when given to a population with the target disorder (as compared with a reference or 'gold standard'). An instrument that detects a low percentage of cases will not be very helpful in determining the numbers of service users who should receive further assessment or a known effective treatment because many individuals who should receive the treatment will not do so. This would lead to an underestimation of the prevalence of the disorder, contribute to inadequate care and make for poor planning and costing of the need for treatment. As the sensitivity of an instrument increases, the number of false negatives it detects will decrease.

The specificity of an instrument refers to the probability that a test will produce a true negative result when given to a population without the target disorder (as determined by a reference or 'gold standard'). This is important so that healthy people are not offered further assessment or treatments they do not need. As the specificity of an instrument increases, the number of false positives will decrease.

To illustrate this: from a population in which the point prevalence rate of anxiety is 10% (that is, 10% of the population has anxiety at any one time), 1000 people are given a test which has 90% sensitivity and 85% specificity. It is known that 100 people in this population have anxiety, but the test detects only 90 (true positives), leaving ten undetected (false negatives). It is also known that 900 people do not have anxiety, and the test correctly identifies 765 of these (true negatives), but classifies 135 incorrectly as having anxiety (false positives). The positive predictive value of the test (the number correctly identified as having anxiety as a proportion of positive tests) is 40% (90/90 + 135), and the negative predictive value (the number correctly identified as not having anxiety as a proportion of negative tests) is 98% (765/765 +10). Therefore, in this example, a positive test result is correct in only 40% of cases, while a negative result can be relied upon in 98% of cases.

The example above illustrates some of the main differences between positive predictive values and negative predictive values in comparison with sensitivity and specificity. For both positive and negative predictive values, prevalence explicitly forms part of their calculation (Altman & Bland, 1994b). When the prevalence of a disorder is low in a population this is generally associated with a higher negative predictive value and a lower positive predictive value. Therefore although these statistics are concerned with issues probably more directly applicable to clinical practice (for example the probability that a person with a positive test result actually has anxiety) they are largely dependent on the characteristics of the population sampled and cannot be universally applied (Altman & Bland, 1994a).

On the other hand, sensitivity and specificity do not necessarily depend on prevalence of anxiety (Altman & Bland, 1994a). For example, sensitivity is concerned with the performance of an identification instrument conditional on a person having anxiety. Therefore the higher false positives often associated with samples of low prevalence will not affect such estimates. The advantage of this approach is that sensitivity and specificity can be applied across populations (Altman & Bland, 1994b). However, the main disadvantage is that clinicians tend to find such estimates more difficult to interpret.

When describing the sensitivity and specificity of the different instruments, the GDG defined values above 0.9 as 'excellent', 0.8 to 0.9 as 'good', 0.5 to 0.7 as 'moderate', 0.3 to 0.4 as 'low' and less than 0.3 as 'poor'.

**Figure 3: Receiver operator characteristic curve**

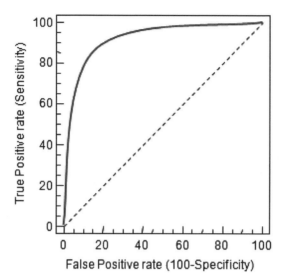

*Receiver operator characteristic curves*

The qualities of a particular tool are summarised in an ROC curve, which plots true positive rate (sensitivity) against the false positive rate (100–specificity) (see Figure 3).

A test with perfect discrimination would have an ROC curve that passed through the top left hand corner; that is, it would have 100% specificity and pick up all true positives with no false positives. While this is never achieved in practice, the area under the curve (AUC) measures how close the tool gets to the theoretical ideal. A perfect test would have an AUC of 1, and a test with AUC above 0.5 is better than chance. As discussed above, because these measures are based on sensitivity and 100-specificity, theoretically these estimates are not affected by prevalence.

*Negative and positive likelihood ratios*

Negative and positive likelihood ratios are thought not to be dependent on prevalence. The positive likelihood ratio is calculated by sensitivity/(1 − specificity) and negative likelihood ratio is (1 − sensitivity)/specificity. A positive likelihood ratio with a value of >5 and a negative likelihood ratio of <0.3 suggests the test is relatively accurate (Fischer et al., 2003).

### 3.5.5    Synthesising the evidence from studies about the experience of care

Themes from the evidence about the experience of care were collated using the matrix of service user experience developed for the service user guidance and quality standards (NCCMH, 2012). The matrix was formed by creating a table with the eight

**Table 5: Matrix of service user experience**

Key points on a pathway of care

Dimensions of person-centred care

dimensions of patient-centred care developed by the Picker Institute Europe[2] (see Appendix 13 for more information) down the vertical axis, and the key points on a pathway of care (as specified by the GDG) across the horizontal axis (see Table 5). With regard to terminology, the service user experience guidance used the term 'person-centred' rather than 'patient-centred', therefore the former is used in the matrix.

The Picker Institute's dimensions of patient-centred care were chosen because they are well established, comprehensive, and based on research. In addition, a variation of these dimensions has been adopted by the US Institute of Medicine (Institute of Medicine, 2001).

Themes evident within the matrix were used during a consultation undertaken with a focus group (User Voice, see Section 4.2.5; see Appendix 14 for a description of the methods used). In addition, the evidence obtained from the reviews was used to inform the process of incorporation and adaptation of existing guideline recommendations where there was insufficient evidence to support the development of recommendations in areas the GDG considered to be important (see Section 4.3; see Section 3.7 for a description of the methods used).

### 3.5.6 Grading the quality of evidence

For questions about interventions, the GRADE approach[3] was used to grade the quality of evidence for each outcome. The technical team produced GRADE evidence profiles (see below) using GRADEprofiler (GRADEpro) software (version 3.6), following advice set out in the GRADE handbook (Schünemann et al., 2009). For questions about the experience of care and the organisation and delivery of care, methodology

---

[2]http:// www.pickereurope.org/patientcentred
[3]For further information about GRADE, see www.gradeworkinggroup.org

checklists were used to assess the risk of bias, and this information was taken into account when interpreting the evidence.

*Evidence profiles*

A GRADE evidence profile was used to summarise both the quality of the evidence and the results of the evidence synthesis for each 'critical' and 'important' outcome (see Table 6 for an example of an evidence profile). The GRADE approach is based on a sequential assessment of the quality of evidence, followed by judgment about the balance between desirable and undesirable effects, and subsequent decision about the strength of a recommendation.

Within the GRADE approach to grading the quality of evidence, the following is used as a starting point:

● randomised trials without important limitations provide high quality evidence

● observational studies without special strengths or important limitations provide low quality evidence.

For each outcome, quality may be reduced depending on five factors: limitations, inconsistency, indirectness, imprecision and publication bias. For the purposes of the guideline, each factor was evaluated using criteria provided in Table 7.

For observational studies without any reasons for down-grading, the quality may be up-graded if there is a large effect, all plausible confounding would reduce the demonstrated effect (or increase the effect if no effect was observed), or there is evidence of a dose–response gradient (details would be provided under the 'other' column).

Each evidence profile also included a summary of the findings: the number of participants included in each group, an estimate of the magnitude of the effect and the overall quality of the evidence for each outcome. Under the GRADE approach, the overall quality for each outcome is categorised into one of four groups (high, moderate, low, very low).

### 3.5.7    Presenting evidence to the Guideline Development Group

Study characteristics tables and, where appropriate, forest plots generated with Stata, and GRADE 'Summary of findings' tables (see below) were presented to the GDG.

Where meta-analysis was not appropriate and/or possible, the reported results from each primary-level study were included in the study characteristics table. The range of effect estimates were included in the GRADE profile and, where appropriate, described narratively.

*Summary of findings tables*

'Summary of findings' tables generated from GRADEpro were used to summarise the evidence for each outcome and the quality of that evidence (Table 8). The tables provide illustrative comparative risks, especially useful when the baseline risk varies for different groups within the population.

## Table 6: Example of a GRADE evidence profile

| No. of studies | Design | Quality assessment | | | | | No. of patients | | Effect | | Quality | Importance |
|---|---|---|---|---|---|---|---|---|---|---|---|---|
| | | Risk of bias | Inconsistency | Indirectness | Imprecision | Other considerations | Intervention | Control group | Relative (95% CI) | Absolute | | |
| Outcome 1 (measured with: any valid method; better indicated by lower values) | | | | | | | | | | | | |
| 2 | randomised trials | no serious risk of bias | no serious inconsistency | no serious indirectness | serious[1] | none | 47 | 43 | – | SMD 0.20 lower (0.61 lower to 0.21 higher) | ⊕⊕⊕⊖ MODERATE | CRITICAL |
| Outcome 2 (measured with: any valid rating scale; better indicated by lower values) | | | | | | | | | | | | |
| 4 | randomised trials | serious[2] | no serious inconsistency | no serious indirectness | serious[1] | none | 109 | 112 | – | SMD 0.42 lower (0.69 to 0.16 lower) | ⊕⊕⊖⊖ LOW | CRITICAL |
| Outcome 3 (measured with: any valid rating scale; better indicated by lower values) | | | | | | | | | | | | |
| 12 | randomised trials | no serious risk of bias | serious[3] | no serious indirectness | no serious imprecision | none | 320 | 400 | RR 0.80 (0.70 to 0.91) | – | ⊕⊕⊕⊖ MODERATE | CRITICAL |
| Outcome 4 (measured with: any valid rating scale; better indicated by lower values) | | | | | | | | | | | | |
| 11 | randomised trials | no serious risk of bias | no serious inconsistency | no serious indirectness | no serious imprecision | none | 280 | 189 | – | SMD 0.34 lower (0.67 to 0.01 lower) | ⊕⊕⊕⊕ HIGH | CRITICAL |

[1]Optimal information size (OIS) (for dichotomous outcomes, OIS = 300 events; for continuous outcomes, OIS = 400 participants) not met.
[2]Risk of bias across domains was generally high or unclear.
[3]There is evidence of moderate heterogeneity of study effect sizes.

**Table 7: Factors that decrease quality of evidence**

| Factor | Description | Criteria |
|---|---|---|
| Limitations | Methodological quality/risk of bias. | In the studies that reported a particular outcome, serious risks across most studies. The evaluation of risk of bias was made for each study using NICE methodology checklists (see Section 1.1.1). |
| Inconsistency | Unexplained heterogeneity of results. | Moderate or greater heterogeneity (see Section 3.5.1 for further information about how this was evaluated). |
| Indirectness | How closely the outcome measures, interventions and participants match those of interest. | If the comparison was indirect or if the question being addressed by the GDG was substantially different from the available evidence regarding the population, intervention, comparator, or an outcome. |
| Imprecision | Results are imprecise when studies include relatively few patients and few events and thus have wide confidence intervals around the estimate of the effect. | If either of the following two situations were met:<br>• the OIS (for dichotomous outcomes, OIS = 300 events; for continuous outcomes, OIS = 400 participants) was not achieved<br>• the 95% CI around the pooled or best estimate of effect included both (1) no effect and (2) appreciable benefit or appreciable harm. |
| Publication bias | Systematic under-estimate or an overestimate of the underlying beneficial or harmful effect due to the selective publication of studies. | If there was evidence of selective publication. This may be detected during the search for evidence, or through statistical analysis of the available evidence. |

## Table 8: Example of a GRADE 'summary of findings' table

**Patient or population:** children and young people with, or at high risk of, conduct disorders (post-treatment)
**Intervention:** child-focused
**Comparison:** any control

| Outcomes | Illustrative comparative risks* (95% CI) | | Relative effect (95% CI) | No. of participants (studies) | Quality of the evidence (GRADE) |
|---|---|---|---|---|---|
| | Assumed risk | Corresponding risk | | | |
| | Any control group | Intervention group | | | |
| **Outcome 1** Any valid rating scale | – | The mean outcome in the intervention group was **0.20 standard deviations lower** (0.61 lower to 0.21 higher) | – | 90 (2) | ⊕⊕⊕⊖ **moderate**[1] |
| **Outcome 2** Any valid rating scale | – | The mean outcome in the intervention group was **0.42 standard deviations lower** (0.69 to 0.16 lower) | – | 221 (4) | ⊕⊕⊖⊖ **low**[1,2] |
| **Outcome 3** Any valid rating scale | Study population | | **RR 0.80** (0.70 to 0.91) | 720 (12) | ⊕⊕⊕⊖ **moderate**[4] |
| | 62 per 100 | 50 per 1000 (44 to 57) | | | |
| | Moderate[3] | | | | |
| | 70 per 100 | 56 per 100 (49 to 64) | | | |
| **Outcome 4** Any valid rating scale | – | The mean outcome in the intervention group was **0.34 standard deviations lower** (0.67 to 0.01 lower) | – | 469 (11) | ⊕⊕⊕⊕ **high** |

*The basis for the assumed risk (for example the median control group risk across studies) is provided in footnotes. The corresponding risk (and its 95% CI) is based on the assumed risk in the comparison group and the relative effect of the intervention (and its 95% CI).
[1]OIS (for dichotomous outcomes, OIS = 300 events; for continuous outcomes, OIS = 400 participants) not met.
[2]Risk of bias across domains was generally high or unclear.
[3]Median control group risk from the studies included in a meta-analysis.
[4]There is evidence of moderate heterogeneity of study effect sizes.

### 3.5.8    Extrapolation

When answering review questions, it may be necessary to consider extrapolating from another data set where direct evidence from a primary data set[4] is not available. In this situation, the following principles were used to determine when to extrapolate:

- a primary dataset is absent, of low quality or is judged to be not relevant to the review question under consideration
- a review question is deemed by the GDG to be important, such that in the absence of direct evidence other data sources should be considered
- a non-primary data source(s) is in the view of the GDG available which may inform the review question.

   When the decision to extrapolate was made, the following principles were used to inform the choice of the non-primary data set:

- the populations (usually in relation to the specified diagnosis or problem which characterises the population) under consideration share some common characteristic but differ in other ways, such as age, gender or in the nature of the disorder (for example a common behavioural problem; acute versus chronic presentations of the same disorder)
- the interventions under consideration in the view of the GDG have one or more of the following characteristics:
  - share a common mode of action (for example the pharmacodynamics of drug; a common psychological model of change – operant conditioning)
  - be feasible to deliver in both populations (for example in terms of the required skills or the demands of the health care system)
  - share common side effects/harms in both populations
- the context or comparator involved in the evaluation of the different data sets shares some common elements which support extrapolation
- the outcomes involved in the evaluation of the different data sets shares some common elements which support extrapolation (for example improved mood or a reduction in challenging behaviour).

   When the choice of the non-primary data set was made, the following principles were used to guide the application of extrapolation:

- the GDG should first consider the need for extrapolation through a review of the relevant primary data set and be guided in these decisions by the principles for the use of extrapolation
- in all areas of extrapolation data sets should be assessed against the principles for determining the choice of data sets. In general, the criteria in the four principles set out above for determining the choice should be met
- in deciding on the use of extrapolation, the GDG will have to determine if the extrapolation can be held to be reasonable, including ensuring that:
  - the reasoning behind the decision can be justified by the clinical need for a recommendation to be made

---

[4]A primary data set is defined as a data set which contains evidence on the population and intervention under review.

- the absence of other more direct evidence, and by the relevance of the potential data set to the review question can be established
- the reasoning and the method adopted is clearly set out in the relevant section of the guideline.

### 3.5.9 Method used to answer a review question in the absence of appropriately designed, high-quality research

In the absence of appropriately designed, high-quality research, or where the GDG were of the opinion (on the basis of previous searches or their knowledge of the literature) that there were unlikely to be such evidence, an informal consensus process was adopted. The process involved a group discussion of what is known about the issues. The views of GDG were synthesised narratively and circulated after the meeting. Feedback was used to revise the text, which was then included in the appropriate evidence review chapter.

### 3.6 HEALTH ECONOMICS METHODS

The aim of the health economics was to contribute to the guideline's development by providing evidence on the cost effectiveness of interventions for conduct disorders in children and young people covered in the guideline. This was achieved by:

- systematic literature review of existing economic evidence
- economic modelling, where economic evidence was lacking or was considered inadequate to inform decisions.

Systematic reviews of economic literature were conducted in all areas covered in the guideline. Economic modelling was undertaken in areas with likely major resource implications, where the current extent of uncertainty over cost effectiveness was significant and economic analysis was expected to reduce this uncertainty, in accordance with *The Guidelines Manual* (NICE, 2009c). Prioritisation of areas for economic modelling was a joint decision between the health economist and the GDG. The rationale for prioritising review questions for economic modelling was set out in an economic plan agreed between NICE, the GDG, the health economist and the other members of the technical team. The following economic questions were selected as key issues that were addressed by economic modelling:

1. What is the cost-effectiveness of child-focused interventions for children and young people with conduct disorder?
2. What is the cost-effectiveness of parent-focused interventions for children and young people with conduct disorder?
3. What is the cost-effectiveness of multimodal interventions for children and young people with conduct disorder?

In addition, literature on the health-related quality of life of children and young people with a conduct disorder was systematically searched to identify studies reporting appropriate utility scores that could be utilised in a cost–utility analysis.

The rest of this section describes the methods adopted in the systematic literature review of economic studies. Methods employed in economic modelling are described in the respective sections of the guideline.

### 3.6.1    Search strategy for economic evidence

*Scoping searches*

A broad preliminary search of the literature was undertaken in November 2010 to obtain an overview of the issues likely to be covered by the scope, and help define key areas. Searches were restricted to economic studies and health technology assessment reports, and conducted in the following databases:

- Embase
- MEDLINE/MEDLINE In-Process
- HTA database (technology assessments)
- NHS Economic Evaluation Database.

Any relevant economic evidence arising from the clinical scoping searches was also made available to the health economist during the same period.

*Systematic literature searches*

After the scope was finalised, a systematic search strategy was developed to locate all the relevant evidence. The balance between sensitivity (the power to identify all studies on a particular topic) and specificity (the ability to exclude irrelevant studies from the results) was carefully considered, and a decision made to utilise a broad approach to searching to maximise retrieval of evidence to all parts of the guideline. Searches were restricted to economic studies and health technology assessment reports, and conducted in the following databases:

- the American Economic Association's electronic bibliography (EconLit)
- Embase
- HTA database (technology assessments)
- MEDLINE/MEDLINE In-Process
- NHS Economic Evaluation Database
- PsycINFO.

Any relevant economic evidence arising from the clinical searches was also made available to the health economist during the same period.

The search strategies were initially developed for MEDLINE before being translated for use in other databases/interfaces. Strategies were built up through a number of trial searches, and discussions of the results of the searches with the review team and GDG to ensure that all possible relevant search terms were covered. In order to ensure comprehensive coverage, search terms for the main population were kept purposely broad to help counter dissimilarities in database indexing practices and imprecise reporting of study populations by authors in the titles and abstracts of records. For standard mainstream bibliographic databases (Embase, MEDLINE, PreMEDLINE and PsycINFO), search terms for the main population were combined with the intervention(s), together with a study design filter for health economic research. For smaller, topic-specific databases (for example EconLit, HTA and NHS Economic Evaluation Database), a broad search was conducted for the main population only. The search terms are set out in full in Appendix 10.

*EndNote*

Citations from each search were downloaded into EndNote and duplicates removed. Records were then screened against the inclusion criteria of the reviews before being quality appraised. The unfiltered search results were saved and retained for future potential re-analysis to help keep the process both replicable and transparent.

*Search filters*

The search filter for health economics is an adaptation of a pre-tested strategy designed by Centre for Reviews and Dissemination (2007). The search filter is designed to retrieve records of economic evidence (including full and partial economic evaluations) from the vast amount of literature indexed to major medical databases such as MEDLINE. The filter, which comprises a combination of controlled vocabulary and free-text retrieval methods, maximises sensitivity (or recall) to ensure that as many potentially relevant records as possible are retrieved from a search. Full details of the filter is provided in Appendix 10.

*Date and language restrictions*

Systematic database searches were initially conducted in June 2011 up to the most recent searchable date. Search updates were generated on a 6-monthly basis, with the final re-runs carried out in July 2012 ahead of the guideline consultation. After this point, studies were included only if they were judged by the GDG to be exceptional (for example the evidence was likely to change a recommendation).

Although no language restrictions were applied at the searching stage, foreign language papers were not requested or reviewed unless they were of particular importance to an area under review. All of the searches were restricted to research published from 1995 onwards in order to obtain data relevant to current healthcare settings and costs.

*Other search methods*

Other search methods involved scanning the reference lists of all eligible publications (systematic reviews, stakeholder evidence and included studies from the economic and clinical reviews) to identify further studies for consideration.

Full details of the search strategies and filter used for the systematic review of health economic evidence are provided in Appendix 10.

### 3.6.2    Inclusion criteria for economic studies

The following inclusion criteria were applied to select studies identified by the economic searches for further consideration:

● Only studies from Organisation for Economic Co-operation and Development countries were included, as the aim of the review was to identify economic information transferable to the UK context.

- Selection criteria based on types of clinical conditions and service users as well as interventions assessed were identical to the clinical literature review.
- Studies were included provided that sufficient details regarding methods and results were available to enable the methodological quality of the study to be assessed, and provided that the study's data and results were extractable. Poster presentations of abstracts were excluded.
- Full economic evaluations that compared two or more relevant options and considered costs and consequences as well as costing analyses that compared only costs between two or more interventions were included in the review.
- Economic studies were included if they used clinical effectiveness data from an RCT, a prospective cohort study, or a systematic review and meta-analysis of clinical studies. Studies that had a mirror-image or other retrospective design were excluded from the review.
- Studies were included only if the examined interventions were clearly described. This involved the dosage and route of administration, and the duration of treatment in the case of pharmacological therapies, and the types of health professionals involved as well as the frequency and duration of treatment in the case of psychological interventions. Evaluations in which medications were treated as a class were excluded from further consideration.
- Studies that adopted a very narrow perspective, ignoring major categories of costs to the NHS, were excluded; for example studies that estimated exclusively drug acquisition costs or hospitalisation costs were considered non-informative to the guideline development process.

### 3.6.3 Applicability and quality criteria for economic studies

All economic papers eligible for inclusion were appraised for their applicability and quality using the methodology checklist for economic evaluations recommended by NICE (2009), which is shown in Appendix 11 of this guideline. The methodology checklist for economic evaluations was also applied to the economic models developed specifically for this guideline. All studies that fully or partially met the applicability and quality criteria described in the methodology checklist were considered during the guideline development process, along with the results of the economic modelling conducted specifically for this guideline. The completed methodology checklists for all economic evaluations considered in the guideline are provided in Appendix 19.

### 3.6.4 Presentation of economic evidence

The economic evidence considered in the guideline is provided in the respective evidence chapters, following presentation of the relevant clinical evidence. The references to included studies and the respective evidence tables with the study characteristics and results are provided in Appendix 20. Methods and results of economic modelling undertaken alongside the guideline development process are presented in the relevant evidence chapters. Characteristics and results of all economic studies considered during the guideline development process (including modelling studies conducted for this guideline) are summarised in economic evidence profiles accompanying respective GRADE clinical evidence profiles in Appendix 18.

### 3.6.5    Results of the systematic search of economic literature

The titles of all studies identified by the systematic search of the literature were screened for their relevance to the topic (that is, economic issues and information on health-related quality of life in children and young people with a conduct disorder). References that were clearly not relevant were excluded first. The abstracts of all potentially relevant studies (381 references) were then assessed against the inclusion criteria for economic evaluations by the health economist. Full texts of the studies potentially meeting the inclusion criteria (including those for which eligibility was not clear from the abstract) were obtained. Studies that did not meet the inclusion criteria, were duplicates, were secondary publications of one study, or had been updated in more recent publications were subsequently excluded. Economic evaluations eligible for inclusion (24 references) were then appraised for their applicability and quality using the methodology checklist for economic evaluations. Finally, 15 economic studies that fully or partially met the applicability and quality criteria were considered at formulation of the guideline recommendations.

### 3.7    THE INCORPORATION AND ADAPTATION OF EXISTING NICE GUIDELINE RECOMMENDATIONS

There are a number of reasons why it might be desirable to reuse recommendations published in NICE guidelines, including to:
1. Increase the efficiency of guideline development and reduce duplication of activity between guidelines.
2. Answer review questions where little evidence exists for the topic under development, but recommendations for a similar topic do exist. For example, if recommendations from an adult guideline are reused for children.
3. Facilitate the understanding or use of other recommendations in a guideline where cross-referral to another guideline might impair the use or comprehension of the guideline under development. For example, if a reader is being constantly referred to another guideline it interrupts the flow of recommendations and undermines the usefulness of the guideline.
4. Avoid possible confusion or contradiction that arises where a pre-existing guideline has addressed a similar question and made different recommendations covering the same or very similar areas of activity.
    In this context, there are two methods of reusing recommendations, that is, *incorporation* and *adaptation*. Incorporation refers to the placement of one

recommendation in a guideline different from that it was originally developed for, where no material changes to wording or structure are made. Recommendations used in this way are referenced appropriately. Adaptation refers to the process by which a recommendation is changed in order to facilitate its placement within a new guideline.

*Incorporation*

In the current guideline, the following criteria were used to determine when a recommendation could be incorporated:

● the recommendation addresses an issue within the scope of the current guideline
● the review question addressed in the current guideline is judged to be sufficiently similar to that associated with the recommendation in the original guideline
● the recommendation can 'standalone' and does not need other recommendations from the original guideline to be relevant or understood within the current guideline
● it is possible in the current guideline to link to or clearly integrate the relevant evidence from the original guideline into the current guideline.

*Adaptation*

When adaptation is used, the meaning and intent of the original recommendation is preserved but the wording and structure of the recommendation may change. Preservation of the original meaning (that is, that the recommendation faithfully represents the assessment and interpretation of the evidence contained in the original guideline evidence reviews) and intent (that is, the intended outcome[s] specified in the original recommendation will be achieved) is an essential element of the process of adaptation.

The precise nature of adaptation may vary, but examples include: when terminology in the NHS has changed, the population has changed (for example young people to adults) or when two recommendations are combined in order to facilitate integration into a new guideline. This is analogous to the practice when creating NICE Pathways whereby some alterations are made to recommendations to make them 'fit' into a pathway structure.

The following criteria were used to determine when a recommendation could be adapted:

● the original recommendation addresses an issue within the scope of the current guideline
● the review question addressed in the current guideline is judged to be sufficiently similar to that associated with the recommendation in the original guideline
● the recommendation can 'standalone' and does not need other recommendations from the original guideline to be relevant
● it is possible in the current guideline to link to or clearly integrate the relevant evidence from the original guideline into the new guideline
● there is no new evidence relevant to the original recommendation that suggests it should be updated
● any new evidence relevant to the recommendation only provides additional contextual evidence, such as background information about how an intervention is

provided in the health care setting(s) that are the focus of the guideline. This may inform the re-drafting or re-structuring of the recommendation but does not alter its meaning or intent (if meaning or intent were altered, a new recommendation should be developed).

In deciding whether to incorporate or adapt existing guideline recommendations, consideration was made about whether the direct evidence obtained from the current guideline dataset was of sufficient quality to allow development of recommendations. It was only where such evidence was not available or insufficient to draw robust conclusions, and drawing on the principles of extrapolation (see Section 3.5.8), that the 'incorporate and adapt' method was used.

*Roles and responsibilities*

The guideline review team, in consultation with the guideline facilitator and GDG Chair, were responsible for identifying existing guideline recommendations that may be appropriate, and deciding if the criteria had been met for incorporation or adaptation. For adapted recommendations, a member of the GDG of the guideline being adapted was consulted to ensure the meaning and intent of the original recommendation was preserved. The GDG confirmed the process had been followed, that there was insufficient evidence to make new recommendations and agreed all adaptations to existing recommendations.

*Drafting of adapted recommendations*

The drafting of adapted recommendations conformed to standard NICE procedures for the drafting of guideline recommendations, preserved the original meaning and intent, and aimed to minimise the degree or re-writing and re-structuring.

In evidence chapters where incorporation and adaptation have been used, tables are provided that set out the original recommendation, the new recommendation and the reasons for adaptation.

## 3.8    FROM EVIDENCE TO RECOMMENDATIONS

Once the clinical and health economic evidence was summarised, the GDG drafted the recommendations. In making recommendations, the GDG took into account the trade-off between the benefits and harms of the intervention/instrument, as well as other important factors, such as economic considerations, values of the development group and society, the requirements to prevent discrimination and to promote equality[5], and the group's awareness of practical issues (Eccles et al., 1998; NICE, 2009c).

Finally, to show clearly how the GDG moved from the evidence to the recommendations, each chapter has a section called 'from evidence to recommendations'. Underpinning this section is the concept of the 'strength' of a recommendation (Schünemann et al., 2003). This takes into account the quality of the evidence but is conceptually different. Some recommendations are 'strong' in that the GDG believes

---

[5] See NICE's equality scheme: www.nice.org.uk/aboutnice/howwework/NICEEqualityScheme.jsp

that the vast majority of healthcare professionals and service users would choose a particular intervention if they considered the evidence in the same way that the GDG has. This is generally the case if the benefits clearly outweigh the harms for most people and the intervention is likely to be cost effective. However, there is often a closer balance between benefits and harms, and some service users would not choose an intervention whereas others would. This may happen, for example, if some service users are particularly averse to some side effect and others are not. In these circumstances the recommendation is generally weaker, although it may be possible to make stronger recommendations about specific groups of service users. The strength of each recommendation is reflected in the wording of the recommendation, rather than by using ratings, labels or symbols.

Where the GDG identified areas in which there are uncertainties or where robust evidence was lacking, they developed research recommendations. Those that were identified as 'high-priority' were developed further in the NICE version of the guideline and presented in Appendix 12.


## 3.9 STAKEHOLDER CONTRIBUTIONS

Professionals, service users, and companies have contributed to and commented on the guideline at key stages in its development. Stakeholders for this guideline include:
- service user and carer stakeholders: national service user and carer organisations that represent the interests of people whose care will be covered by the guideline
- local service user and carer organisations: but only if there is no relevant national organisation
- professional stakeholders' national organisations: that represent the healthcare professionals who provide the services described in the guideline
- commercial stakeholders: companies that manufacture drugs or devices used in treatment of the condition covered by the guideline and whose interests may be significantly affected by the guideline
- providers and commissioners of health services in England and Wales
- statutory organisations: including the Department of Health, the Welsh Assembly Government, NHS Quality Improvement Scotland, the Healthcare Commission and the National Patient Safety Agency
- research organisations: that have carried out nationally recognised research in the area.

NICE clinical guidelines are produced for the NHS in England and Wales, so a 'national' organisation is defined as one that represents England and/or Wales, or has a commercial interest in England and/or Wales.

Stakeholders have been involved in the guideline's development at the following points:
- commenting on the initial scope of the guideline and attending a scoping workshop held by NICE
- contributing possible review questions and lists of evidence to the GDG
- commenting on the draft of the guideline.

## 3.10 VALIDATION OF THE GUIDELINE

Registered stakeholders had an opportunity to comment on the draft guideline, which was posted on the NICE website during the consultation period. Following the consultation, all comments from stakeholders and others were responded to, and the guideline updated as appropriate. NICE also reviewed the guideline and checked that stakeholders' comments had been addressed.

Following the consultation period, the GDG finalised the recommendations and the NCCMH produced the final documents. These were then submitted and the guideline was formally approved by NICE and issued as guidance to the NHS in England and Wales.

# 4    ACCESS TO AND DELIVERY OF SERVICES, AND THE EXPERIENCE OF CARE

## 4.1    INTRODUCTION

As described in Chapter 2, conduct disorders are the most common mental health disorders of childhood and adolescence, and a high proportion of those with a conduct disorder grow up to be antisocial adults with impoverished and destructive lifestyles, impinging negatively on the lives of their families and wider society in many different ways. However, many children and young people with a conduct disorder do not access services and appropriate interventions are not always available. While resource limitations play a part in limited access, a whole range of other factors including personal, familial and societal attitudes to the nature of the problem also impact on access to services and the nature of the care provided. This chapter aims to provide a review of the experience of care of children and young people with, or at risk of, a conduct disorder and their parents and carers, by exploring their experience of access to services and the nature of the care provided.

While health and social care services aim to ensure that people receive treatments that are effective and safe, this is only one part of a service user's experience of the healthcare. High-quality care should be provided in a way that ensures service users have the best possible experience of care (NICE, 2011c). By reviewing service users' experience of care, important information can be obtained about problems with the way that services are delivered and used to assess the impact of efforts to improve the quality of care provided. The way services are accessed, the way that people's problems are assessed, how referrals between different components of health systems are managed, aftercare arrangements, and the process of discharge all play an important part in the service users' overall experience of the care they receive. Misunderstandings and fears about mental health problems and mental health services, and lack of knowledge of the resources available (for example by general practitioners [GPs] or service users) can act as barriers to people receiving effective treatments. The ability of services to understand and respond to such concerns can improve people's experience of services and help make sure that they make best use of available treatments.

Section 4.2 of this chapter contains a review of studies exploring service user experience relating to the barriers to accessing services for children and young people at risk of, or diagnosed with, a conduct disorder, and what might be done to improve the experience of the disorder and the experience of care. This includes exploring the experience of assessment and diagnosis, the relationship between individual service users and professionals, and the way that services and systems are organised and delivered. The second part of Section 4.2 summarises findings from a focus group of young people with conduct problems and experience of the criminal justice system, which was commissioned to inform this guideline. The aim of the focus group was to ascertain children and young people's views on access to and delivery of care and experience of interventions (including parent training programmes and school-based interventions).

Section 4.3 of this chapter is concerned with the application of the evidence reviewed in Section 4.2 in support of the incorporation and adaptation of recommendations developed in other guidelines, namely those on the experience of care in *Service User Experience in Adult Mental Health* (NICE, 2011a) and on improving access to services and developing care pathways in *Common Mental Health Disorders* (NICE, 2011b).

## 4.2    EVIDENCE REVIEW

### 4.2.1    Introduction

Despite being the most common of childhood mental health disorders, children and young people with a conduct disorder are under-represented in those in receipt of care from CAMHS and related services (Vostanis et al., 2003). A number of factors have been considered important in improving access to and uptake of services, some of which, such as improved methods for case identification and assessment, are dealt with in Chapter 6. However, improved case identification and assessment will be of more limited value if children and young people and their parents or carers do not seek help. This review specifically addresses this issue and looks at the barriers that prevent children and young people with a conduct disorder from accessing both effective assessment and treatment interventions. It also considers studies that have sought to overcome these barriers and improve access.

Improved access to care will only bring real benefit if children and young people with a conduct disorder and their parents or carers properly engage with services and receive effective interventions (Kazdin, 1996). As set out in the introduction to this chapter, the experience of the setting, the flexibility and adaptation of interventions to individual needs and a consideration of the family, educational and cultural environment can all play a part in ensuring a positive experience of care and improved retention in treatment with consequential improved outcomes. Both positive and negative experiences of care, and studies aimed at improving the experience for children and young people with a conduct disorder and their parents or carers, are also reviewed.

The scope of these reviews was not limited to children and young people with a conduct disorder because initial scoping searches had suggested that the literature was very limited in this area. Therefore, a number of reviews combined studies from across the range of childhood mental disorders. As a consequence, considerable caution is required when interpreting the results of these reviews.

In addition, the reviews were supplemented in two other ways. First, a consultation on emerging themes from the reviews was undertaken with a focus group (User Voice, see Section 4.2.5). Second, the evidence obtained from the reviews was used to inform the process of incorporation and adaptation of existing guideline recommendations where there was insufficient evidence to support the development of recommendations in areas the GDG considered to be important (see Section 4.3; see Chapter 3 for a description of the methods used). In these areas the reviews and the focus group consultation were used to both inform the need for recommendations and to provide important contextual information to guide the process of incorporation and adaptation.

### 4.2.2    Review protocol

A summary of the review protocol, including the review questions, information about the databases searched, and the eligibility criteria used for this section of the guideline, can be found in Table 9 (a complete list of review questions [RQs] can be found in Appendix 5; further information about the search strategy can be found in Appendix 7; the full review protocols can be found in Appendix 15).

The review strategy involved narratively synthesising the following evidence using a matrix of service user experience (see Appendix 15):

● systematic reviews of qualitative research
● a qualitative analysis of transcripts of people with or at risk of conduct disorders from resources found online (primarily Healthtalkonline and/or Youthhealthtalk)
● user experience surveys.

The synthesised evidence was used to support the incorporation and adaptation of recommendations developed in other guidelines (Section 4.3).

In addition, a focus group was used to explore the experience of young people who have had involvement with the criminal justice system (see Appendix 14 for further information about the methods used).

### 4.2.3    Studies considered[6]

Eighteen studies providing relevant evidence met the eligibility criteria for this review. Of these, four were unpublished and 14 were published in peer-reviewed journals between 2005 and 2010. A further two studies were excluded from the analysis. No relevant surveys or transcripts of people with or at risk of conduct disorders were found.

Of the 18 included studies, there were two reviews of the experience of care, CEFAI2010 (Cefai & Cooper, 2010) and DAVIES2008 (Davies & Wright, 2008) (see Table 10), and 11 primary level studies of the experience of care: ADAMSHICK2010 (Adamshick, 2010), ASHKAR2008 (Ashkar & Kenny, 2008), BARBER2006 (Barber et al., 2006), BROOKMAN-FRAZEE2009 (Brookman-Frazee et al., 2009), CHILDREN1ST2007 (Aldgate et al., 2007), DEMOS2010 (Hannon et al., 2010),

---

[6] Here and elsewhere in the guideline, each study considered for review is referred to by a study ID in capital letters (primary author and date of study publication, except where a study is in press or only submitted for publication, then a date is not used).

**Table 9:  Review protocol for the review of access to and delivery of services and the experience of care**

| Component | Description |
|---|---|
| Review questions* | *Access to and delivery of services:*<br>• What are the barriers to access that prevent children and young people at risk of, or diagnosed with, conduct disorders from accessing services? (RQ-B1)<br>• Do methods designed to remove barriers to services increase the proportion and diversity of children and young people accessing treatment? (RQ-B2)<br>• What are the essential elements that assist in the transition into adulthood services for young people with conduct disorders? (RQ-G2)<br>• What are the effective ways of monitoring progress in conduct disorders? (RQ-G3)<br>• What components of an intervention, or the way in which it is implemented, and by whom are associated with successful outcomes? (RQ-G4)<br>*Experience of care:*<br>• For children and young people with conduct disorders, what can be done to improve the experience of the disorder, and the experience of care? (RQ-F1) |
| Objectives | *Access to and delivery of services:*<br>• To identify barriers relating to the individual child/parents/family/carers, the practitioner, the healthcare/social care and other service systems that prevent an individual from accessing services.<br>• To evaluate any methods and models designed to improve access for children and young people, and/or their parents/family/carers requiring services.<br>*Experience of care:*<br>• To identify the experiences of having the disorder, access to services, and treatment on children and young people.<br>• To identify the experiences of support that parents and carers of children and young people with conduct disorders receive. |

| Population | • Children and young people (aged 18 years and younger) with a diagnosed or suspected conduct disorder, including looked-after children and those in contact with the criminal justice system.<br>• Children and young people identified as being at significant risk of developing conduct disorders.<br>• Consideration will be given to the specific needs of:<br>  – children and young people with conduct disorders and coexisting conditions (such as ADHD, depression, anxiety disorders and attachment insecurity)<br>  – children and young people from particular black or minority ethnic groups<br>  – girls with a diagnosis of, or at risk of developing conduct disorders<br>  – looked-after children and young people children and young people in contact with the criminal justice system. |
|---|---|
| Interventions | *Access to and delivery of services (RQ–B2):*<br>• Service developments or changes which are specifically designed to promote access.<br>• Specific models of service delivery (for example community-based outreach clinics, clinics or services in non-health settings).<br>• Methods designed to remove barriers to access (including stigma (both cultural and self and stigmatisation), misinformation or cultural beliefs about the nature of mental disorder). |
| Comparison | *Access to and delivery of services (RQ–B2):*<br>• Treatment as usual. |
| Critical outcomes | *Access to and delivery of services:*<br>• Proportion of people from the target group who access services.<br>• Uptake of services.<br>• Data on the diversity of the group who access or are retained in services/interventions. |
| Electronic databases | *Mainstream databases:*<br>• Embase, MEDLINE, PreMEDLINE, PsycINFO.<br>Topic specific databases and grey literature databases (see search strategy in Appendix 7). |
| Date searched | Systematic reviews: 1995 to June 2012; other evidence: inception to June 2012. |
| Study design | • Systematic reviews and qualitative reviews.<br>• Qualitative and quantitative studies (for example surveys and observational studies). |

\* Under 'Review questions', the review question reference (for example RQ-A1) can be used to cross-reference against the full review protocol in Appendix 15.

**Table 10:  Study information table for reviews of the experience of care**

| Study ID | DAVIES2008 | CEFAI2010 |
|---|---|---|
| Method used to synthesise evidence | Narrative | Narrative |
| Design of included studies | Qualitative studies | Qualitative: semi-structured interviews, unstructured interviews, participation observation and focus groups. |
| Dates searched | Not stated; included studies were published between 1996 and 2006. | Not specified. Search conducted was for 'local [Maltese] studies on the voice of students with SEBD [social, emotional and behavioural difficulties]'; included studies were published between 1997 and 2009. |
| No. of included studies | 14 | 8 |
| Model/method evaluated | Not applicable | Not applicable |
| Comparison | Not applicable | Not applicable |
| Outcomes | Thematic analysis sought to identify children's views of mental health services, with particular focus on views of looked-after children. | Thematic analysis sought to identify 'school-related themes... in relation to the students' difficulties, disaffection and disengagement'. |
| Participant characteristics | Children using NHS mental health services (UK). | Students with social, emotional and behavioural difficulties in Maltese schools (although lack of explicit detail on diagnostic criteria provided). Study participants range from 11 to 16+ years old. |

JRF2005 (Millie et al., 2005), JRF2007 (Frankham et al., 2007), SODERLUND1995 (Soderlund et al., 1995), TIGHE2012 (Tighe et al., 2012) and WILLIAMS2007 (Williams et al., 2007) (see Table 11). For the review of access to and delivery of services, there were three published reviews evaluating targeted interventions for children and young people: LANDSVERK2009 (Landsverk et al., 2009), LOCHMAN2000 (Lochman, 2000) and SHEPARD2009 (Shepard & Dickstein, 2009) (see Table 12); and two reviews addressing factors affecting service availability and access: FLANZER2005 (Flanzer, 2005) and OLIVER2008 (Oliver et al., 2008) (see Table 13).

### 4.2.4    Evidence from the review of access to services and the experience of care

Evidence extracted from the reviews and primary studies of access to and delivery of services and the experience of care (see Appendix 21) were combined using a matrix of service user experience (see Appendix 13).

The matrix of service user experience is structured so that for each key point on the pathway of care (access to services, assessment and diagnosis, treatment including prevention, and educational settings), evidence is summarised using eight dimensions of person-centred care. These dimensions are subdivided into two groups: (1) the relationship between individual service users and professionals (involvement in decisions and respect for preferences; clear, comprehensible information and support for self-care; emotional support, empathy and respect); and (2) the way that services and systems work (fast access to reliable health advice; effective treatment delivered by trusted professionals; attention to physical and environmental needs; involvement of, and support for, family and carers; continuity of care and smooth transitions).

Where evidence was found that was relevant to each dimension, it is presented in narrative form below.

*Access to services*
**Involvement in decisions and respect for preferences**

A UK study identifying children's views of CAMHS found that it was important to consult with looked-after children in service provision discussions (DAVIES2008).

**Clear, comprehensible information and support for self-care**

Parents and carers from a US study of families with a child with serious emotional and behavioural disorders reported that they would like more information about community services, and available transitional or vocational services. This may be achieved through providing a centrally located office (for example at school) that distributes comprehensive information on all community services; or, by distributing information via intensive case management or community-based agencies. In terms of transitional services, school personnel could work closely with parents to develop a comprehensive plan for each child, addressing both child and family needs (SODERLUND1995).

**Table 11: Study information table for primary research of the experience of care**

| Study ID | ADAMSHICK2010 | ASHKAR2008 | BARBER2006 |
|---|---|---|---|
| Sampling strategy | Sample drawn from an alternative school (in a medium-sized city in the Northeastern US) for young people in Grades 7 to 12 displaying behaviour problems. A purposive sampling method was used with the following inclusion criteria for participants: girls aged between 13 and 17 years referred to the school because of physically aggressive behaviour. | Sample drawn from a population of incarcerated male offenders in a New South Wales, Australia, maximum security detention facility. Staff proposed a list of possible participants to clinical staff who excluded those with:<br>• untreated psychosis<br>• substance withdrawal (excluding nicotine and cannabis)<br>• recent history of self-harming or suicidal behaviour. | Cross-sectional sample taken from English CAMHS outpatients department.<br>*Eligibility criteria:*<br>• English-speaking<br>• child or young person aged 4+ years accompanied by parent or carer<br>• 'attending a routine, non-emergency appointment' (UK). |
| Design/method | Unstructured, in-depth qualitative interview design; data analysed using an interpretive phenomenological approach. | Semi-structured, qualitative interview design; data analysed using phenomenological descriptive methodology. | Mixed-method survey design: qualitative and quantitative<br><br>Self-report data gathered:<br>• parent or carer-completed Experience of Service Questionnaire (Commission for Health Improvement, 2002)<br>• child or young person over 9 years old completed either the Experience of Service Questionnaire (if aged 9 to 10 years or 16+ years) or the Experience of Service Questionnaire and the SDQ. |

| Model/method evaluated | Not applicable | Not applicable | Not applicable |
|---|---|---|---|
| Comparison | Not applicable | Not applicable | Not applicable |
| Outcomes | Lived experience of girl-to-girl aggression. | Self-reported experience of incarceration. | Self-reported satisfaction with CAMHS:<br>• child or young person's satisfaction<br>• parent or carer's satisfaction<br>• relationship between satisfaction and self-reported conduct problems. |
| Participant characteristics | • Interviews were completed with six girls (mean age 15 years; range 13 to 17 years).<br>• One African American origin; two American Caucasian origin; one African/Native American origin; two American Caucasian/Native American origin.<br>• All referred to the school because of physically aggressive behaviour. | • Interviews were completed with 16 male detainees (mean age 17.95 years; range 16 to 19 years).<br>• Eight Australian/Caucasian origin; four Indigenous Australian origin; two Middle Eastern origin; one Pacific Islander origin; one Asian origin. | • 73 parents or carers and 45 children or young people responded.<br>• Median age of children and young people was 13 years (range 4 to 20 years).<br>• To preserve respondent confidentiality and anonymity, no diagnostic detail was sought. |

*Continued*

**Table 11:** *(Continued)*

| Study ID | ADAMSHICK2010 | ASHKAR2008 | BARBER2006 |
|---|---|---|---|
| | | • All convicted of serious offences; 'nearly all had committed offences during their school years'. <br> • 12 met 'criteria for moderate or severe conduct disorder'. | |

| Study IDs | BROOKMAN-FRAZEE2009 | CHILDREN1ST2007 | DEMOS2010 |
|---|---|---|---|
| Sampling strategy | Sample drawn from population of therapists attending staff meetings across 'six community-based outpatient mental health clinics primarily or exclusively serving publicly-funded children and adolescents in San Diego County'. | Study of three community-based projects set up to help children 'try to "turn the curve"' and find a more positive pathway forward'. <br><br> This was an evaluation study of the work of the projects and not a research study – the study does not evaluate the progress of all children who have attended the Directions Projects, but takes a sequential sample from the three sites during 2005 and an intensive sample. <br><br> Total sample: 'between 2003 and July 2007, the three Directions Projects have recorded working with a total of 1010 children and adults.' | Not specified in detail. <br><br> Interviews were conducted with 'a number of policy and academic experts' on the topic and 'projects and services' for case studies were identified 'based on ... scoping work and discussions with experts'. <br><br> The policy seminar was attended by 'a number of policy experts and practitioners in the field, including representatives from local government, academia, and community and voluntary sector organisations that represent the views of looked-after children, care leavers and foster carers'. |

*Continued*

| Design/method | Quantitative survey design: the Therapeutic Strategies Survey (a modified version of the Therapy Process Observational Coding System for Child Psychotherapy was administered 'as part of a larger study (The 'Practice and Research: Advancing Collaboration' study of care provided, and outcomes for children with disruptive behavioural problems). | Quantitative: <br>• the SDQ <br>• the Parenting Daily Hassles Scale. <br>Qualitative: <br>• site visits (periodically throughout the four years of the evaluation) <br>• parents' evaluation of the Webster-Stratton programme (view on Dinosaur School Programme for their child; views on the Parents/Carers Support Programme) <br>• children's evaluation of the Webster-Stratton programme <br>• focus groups with parents in each of the projects <br>• small intensive sample of 17 children and their parents. | Literature review: <br>• 'literature reviews of domestic and international evidence' about looked-after children. <br>In-depth qualitative work: <br>• qualitative interviews with 'policy and academic experts' <br>• focus groups with looked-after children, care leavers and foster carers. <br>Quantitative work: <br>• design of two costed 'exemplar care journeys which represented the two extremes of experiences within the system'. |
|---|---|---|---|
| Model/method evaluated | Not applicable | Aim of the projects were: <br>• to provide individual and group work for children aged 7 to 12 years who had challenging antisocial behaviour | The study focused on children looked after away from home (including in foster care and residential care homes). |

**Table 11:** *(Continued)*

| Study IDs | BROOKMAN-FRAZEE2009 | CHILDREN1ST2007 | DEMOS2010 |
|---|---|---|---|
| | | • to support, assist and advise parents who had difficulty in providing appropriate parental care and control<br>• to provide support in the classroom and school setting to address the needs of children in difficulty and at risk of exclusion.<br><br>Two discrete but inter-related aspects to the evaluation:<br>• exploring process aspects of the projects, such as the environment of the projects, staffing and management and other issues influencing the projects' development, in order to assess the contribution these factors have made to the effectiveness of the interventions<br>• evaluating the impact of the projects' interventions, especially the effectiveness of the Webster-Stratton group work | |

*Continued*

| Comparison | | | |
|---|---|---|---|
| programme chosen by one of the projects as their core group work programme to help children and parents change their behaviour. | Not applicable | Not applicable | Quantitative work involved comparing estimated costs of possible care pathways for:<br>• Child A (looked after but not adopted from 3 to 18 years old; two stable placements'), whose pathway was designed to be 'an aspirational care journey' that was also realistic ('representing the current experience of between 5 per cent and 10 per cent of looked after children') and also one which is likely to result in 'good' outcomes<br>• Child B (looked after but not adopted from 11 to 16.5 years old; 'three periods in care and ten placements', which included: 'a flawed and poor quality care journey'), whose pathway was realistic 'representing the current experience of around |

79

**Table 11:** *(Continued)*

| Study IDs | BROOKMAN-FRAZEE2009 | CHILDRENIST2007 | DEMOS2010 |
|---|---|---|---|
| | | | 10 per cent of looked-after children') and also one likely to result in 'poor' outcomes.<br><br>The study also makes some comparison between England, Scotland and Northern Ireland 'but do[es] not seek to address those nations as separate systems'. |
| Outcomes | Self-reported rating of perceived value of different care strategies.<br><br>Respondents rated both strategies directed to children and those directed to caregivers (separate strategy lists). | Intervention:<br>• children's behaviour and emotional problems at home and at school<br>• parents' skills to manage the behaviour of their children<br>• parents' stress<br>• programme attendance<br>• engagement in programme<br>• community's views of effectiveness of programme.<br><br>Structure and process:<br>• appropriate and welcoming setting<br>• approach that works in partnership with parents | Looked-after children's, care-leavers', carers', practitioners' and experts' views on: the 'purpose and impact' of care; 'what works for children in care', 'areas in need of reform' and recommendations for the future.<br><br>Some data provided on outcomes for looked-after children in respect of, for example: engagement in criminal activity; drug/alcohol misuse; health and mental health from the literature review. |

| | | |
|---|---|---|
| | • referral, assessment and review process<br>• rigorous delivery of projects<br>• flexibility of projects<br>• skilled project staff group<br>• multi-agency relationships in the community<br>• advisory group which has helped the development of the project<br>• management infrastructure. | • In-depth qualitative work.<br>• Expert interviews (n = 16 interviewees) including representatives from: SCIE; Institute of Education; British Association for Adoption and Fostering; Catch 22; National Care Advisory Service; Fostering Network; Action for Children; Care Matters Partnership; Centrepoint, Social Policy Research Unit; Merton Council Children, Schools and Families Department; Health and Social Care Northern Ireland.<br>• Focus groups with foster carers (n = 26 carers in total). |
| Participant characteristics | • 88 therapists; mean therapist age 36 years (range 23 to 64 years).<br>• Therapists' caseloads comprised 'children ages 4–13 with disruptive behaviour problems'.<br>• 53% of respondents provided 'marriage and family therapy; 21% social work; 17% psychology; 8% psychiatry; 1% other'. | • Children and young people with challenging behaviour and their parents/carers.<br>• N = 1,010 children and adults. 77% boys; 23% girls.<br>• The projects set out to work with children likely to be in primary school, aged 7 to 12 years. However, children have been accepted younger than 7 years as part of a deliberate policy of earlier intervention.<br>• Parents/carers – more women than men attended. Sixty per cent of parents were in their 30s. |

*Continued*

81

**Table 11:** *(Continued)*

| Study ID | JRF2005 | JRF2007 | SODERLUND1995 |
|---|---|---|---|
| | | | • Semi-structured interviews with looked-after children and care leavers (n = 37 in total, of which 23 were looked-after children, 14 were care leavers; age range 7 to 21 years; interviews conducted across five local authority areas). |
| Sampling strategy | For survey:<br>• 'Seventeen questions on ASB [antisocial behaviour]' were asked as part of monthly Office for National Statistics omnibus survey which 'offers a true probability sample of the population aged 16 or over'.<br><br>For interviews:<br>• Original selection criteria for the three case studies identified that:<br> – they should be located in different regions;<br> – each should have features, such as relatively high crime levels and levels of deprivation, that are commonly associated with anti-social behaviour problems; | Sample drawn from two institutions: a pupil referral unit (Sparks) and an organisation in the voluntary sector that works with children/young people who have been excluded from school (St John's).<br><br>'Hard to reach' children, young people and parents.<br><br>Special consideration: poverty, multiple disadvantage, black and dual-heritage children/young people. | Sample drawn from five special education cooperatives in DuPage County (Chicago, IL). Children and youths with serious emotional and behavioural disorders, currently in a restrictive living or school environment, and with service needs requiring the coordination of two or more agencies; and their families, were chosen for inclusion in the study. |

| Design/method | | | |
|---|---|---|---|
| Survey:<br>• In-depth qualitative research comprising (in each case study area):<br>– three to four focus groups with residents<br>– 'semi-structured interviews with representatives of local community associations, who were also local residents' | – each should have distinctive and contrasting antisocial behaviour strategies<br>– Conducting in-depth work revealed that 'the three neighbourhoods' ASB [antisocial behaviour] strategies were more similar than we had originally judged' thereby not fulfilling the full criterion'.<br>Authors note that 'there were, nevertheless, some differences in the emphasis and tactics deployed'. | Case study methods; interviews and observation<br>• six case studies of children/ young people and their families<br>• extended observation at both sites.<br><br>Interviews with all key personnel and 19 parents of current or ex-pupils of Sparks and St John's. | Mixed-method survey design: quantitative and qualitative self-report data gathered. Parents completed The Survey of Parents' System of Care Experiences. |

*Continued*

**Table 11:** *(Continued)*

| Study ID | JRF2005 | JRF2007 | SODERLUND1995 |
|---|---|---|---|
| | – 'semi-structured interviews with officers from key agencies, including antisocial behaviour coordinators, police officers, wardens, housing officers, youth offending team (YOT) representatives, community safety officers and Sure Start workers'. Desk research: 'reviews of relevant policy and strategy documents'. | | |
| Model/method evaluated | Models and strategies/initiatives for managing antisocial behaviour. | Practice is a 'product of inter-individual relationships' not a precursor to them – that is, practice is developed in response to individual needs and concerns that are identified over time, and takes into account previous history and experiences | Not applicable |

| | | | | |
|---|---|---|---|---|
| Comparison | Not applicable | Not applicable | Not applicable | Not applicable |
| Outcomes | Public and service providers' perceptions and experiences of antisocial behaviour, and views on its causes and possible solutions. | Relationships between staff and parents. Relationships between staff and children/young people. | Parents – encounters with schools are almost always part of a bigger picture that involves other economic, social and emotional challenges that the parents face. Supporting parents is the key to making progress with their children. | • Perceptions of existing services.<br>• Service needs.<br>• Barriers to services.<br>• Priorities for delivering comprehensive services. |
| Participant characteristics | • Survey (n = 1,678).<br>• Focus groups (n = 85, across ten groups).<br>• Interviews (n = 73).<br>**Case study area characteristics 'Southcity':**<br>• London borough; high deprivation; high crime.<br>• Southcity taking 'tough enforcement strategies'. | • Children and young people who have been permanently excluded from school, and their families.<br>• Adults who work with these children/young people and their families. | | • 121 out of 347 parents responded (35% response rate). |

*Continued*

**Table 11:** *(Continued)*

| Study ID | JRF2005 | JRF2007 | SODERLUND1995 |
|---|---|---|---|
|  | • 'By June 2004, over 80 ASBOs [Anti-Social Behaviour Orders] had been issued.... By April 2004, 60% of its ASBOs related to drug use or dealers, of which only 3% were for borough residents' (citing two Borough Anti-Social Behaviour Scrutiny Panel reports).<br><br>• 'Ethnically mixed (26% [black and minority ethnic])'.<br><br>• Initiatives in Southcity include:<br>  – 'Neighbourhood Management Pathfinder' work in which agencies collaborate with local residents to tackle problem behaviour including that 'associated with drug use, chaotic lifestyles and gangs' |  |  |

*Continued*

- a 'Safer Neighbourhoods Team', a Metropolitan Police initiative aimed at '[providing] a more visible police presence'
- a 'Youth Inclusion Support Panel' which works with the YOT to provide targeted interventions for 'individual 'troublemakers' in the area'
- 'environmental work' for example street cleaning and 'Noise Patrols'.

'Westerncity':
- Outer suburban city in South Wales; high deprivation; high unemployment; predominantly White communities although 'a few [black and minority ethnic] asylum seekers living in the area'.
- Severe antisocial behaviour problems among children and young people
- Westerncity taking a '"softly-softly" approach to antisocial behaviour enforcement'.

**Table 11:** *(Continued)*

| Study ID | JRF2005 | JRF2007 | SODERLUND1995 |
|---|---|---|---|
| | • Initiatives in Westerncity include:<br>  — 'Communities that Care' (based on a model developed in the US) which involves local service providers and residents identifying 'risk' and 'protective' factors for antisocial behaviour and community-based activities that can address them.<br>  — 'Communities First' funding which aims to increase 'community engagement and regeneration'<br>  — 'crime and disorder reduction partnerships (CDRP) anti-social behaviour structure', a model which identifies ASBOs 'as the last resort' in a 'graduated' model of intervention | | |

- a 'community house' which all local residents can use, 'two early intervention programmes', one at pre-school and one at primary school.

'Midcity':
- Outer suburban city in East Midlands; high deprivation; high unemployment; 15% black and minority ethnic.
- Youth antisocial behaviour problems including joyriding and drug use.
- Midcity's approach to antisocial behaviour 'becoming more enforcement focused'.
- Initiatives in Midcity include:
  - 'Area Team and Community Safety Panel' work aims 'improve the health, well-being and education' of residents and 'feeds into the city-wide 'Respect' campaign'

*Continued*

**Table 11:** *(Continued)*

| Study ID | JRF2005 | JRF2007 | SODERLUND1995 |
|---|---|---|---|
| | – 'Respect' aims to reduce antisocial behaviour and at the time of writing, was focused on 'prostitution and street begging'<br>– 'Local housing office antiso-cial behaviour "Task Force" teams' are situated in each of the four local housing areas and comprise officers from the local authority and police force | | |

| Study ID | TIGHE2012 | | WILLIAMS2007 |
|---|---|---|---|
| Sampling strategy | Sample of families drawn from the multisystemic therapy arm of an RCT conducted in the UK for reducing offending behaviour.<br><br>All families who participated in the multisystemic therapy arm were invited to take part in the qualitative study. Of the 28 families, 21 (75%) agreed to participate. | | Sample drawn from population of teachers at 'two elementary schools in the urban core of a moderate-sized Midwestern city' (US). |
| Design/method | Semi-structured interviews were conducted for the parent and young person. | | Qualitative: focus groups; phenomenological approach to analysis. |

| Model/method evaluated | Multisystemic therapy | Not applicable |
|---|---|---|
| Comparison | Comprehensive and targeted usual services delivered by YOTs. | Not applicable |
| Outcomes | • Expectations of multisystemic therapy.<br>• Experience of working with therapist.<br>• What was helpful and unhelpful about treatment.<br>• Whether life had changed since multisystemic therapy, and what facilitated or hindered change. | • Self-reported teacher experience of identifying and responding to children's mental health problems. |
| Participant characteristics | • Twenty-one families (21 parent interviews, 16 young people).<br>• The young people were mainly boys (n = 17, 81%); mean age of 15.3 years; nine (43%) were black, eight were white (38%), three were (14%) of mixed ethnicity and one (5%) was Asian.<br>• The young people had been convicted for a range of violent and non-violent offences, most had poor school attendance and lived in families with high rates of socioeconomic disadvantage.<br>• Fifteen (76%) lived in single parent households, 15 of these with their mother.<br>• The majority of parents had minimal or no educational qualifications, and more than half (n = 12, 57%) were unemployed. | • Nineteen teachers from two schools (ten from one school, nine from the other); mean age 39.65 years (range 30 to 60 years).<br>• Eighteen female, one male.<br>• Thirteen African American, six Caucasian.<br>• Teacher mean class size of 23 pupils (range ten to 32 pupils). |

**Table 12: Study information table for reviews of access to services which evaluate targeted interventions for children and young people**

| Study ID | LANDSVERK2009 | LOCHMAN2000 | SHEPARD2009 |
|---|---|---|---|
| Method used to synthesise evidence | Narrative | Narrative | Narrative |
| Design of included studies | 'Empirical studies carried out across several states plus one nationally representative survey'. | Controlled experimental designs and non-experimental time series designs. | RCTs, case studies |
| Dates searched | Not stated | Not stated | Not stated |
| No. of included studies | Not stated | 25 | Not stated |
| Model/method evaluated | Interventions addressing:<br>• PTSD and abuse-related trauma<br>• disruptive behaviour disorders<br>• depression<br>• substance abuse<br>• children's needs via intensive home- and community-based support. | Parent training programmes that:<br>• are aimed at parents only<br>• have separate parent-focused and child-focused elements (citing 'Coping Power' specifically)<br>• take a 'family focus' as well as providing parent training). | Participants of evidence-based parent management training programmes for children aged 3 to 8 years 'referred for oppositionality and early onset conduct problems'.<br><br>Participant nationality and/or place of residence not specified. |

| | | | |
|---|---|---|---|
| Comparison | Not stated | Not stated | Treatment versus control; prevention versus control. |
| Outcomes | Not specified in detail: broadly, the study summarises the impact of interventions on 'behavioural and social-emotional problems warranting mental health care' in children with specific reference made to PTSD and abuse-related trauma, disruptive behaviour disorders, depression and substance abuse. | Levels of problem behaviours demonstrated by at-risk children as evidenced, for example by assessment of aggressive behaviour, time spent in correctional facilities and referral rates to special classes at school. Ratings of positive and negative parenting behaviour including, for example, assessment of parental response to child's negative behaviour, parent–child communication, parental 'warmth' to child and self-reported parent satisfaction with parenting. Improvements in 'family functioning'. | Children's observed and reported problem behaviours. Observed parent–child interactions. Self-reported parent involvement. |
| Participant characteristics (focus of review) | Children in foster care in the US, with a particular focus on those in receipt of interventions for behavioural or socio-emotional problems. | Participants (parents and families) in preventative interventions programmes targeting 'high risk' children, that is, those at risk of developing 'a later negative outcome', for example substance misuse. Participant nationality and/or place of residence not specified. | Participants of evidence-based parent management training programmes for children aged 3 to 8 years 'referred for oppositionality and early onset conduct problems'. |

**Table 13: Study information table for reviews of factors affecting service availability and access**

| Study ID | FLANZER2005 | OLIVER2008 |
|---|---|---|
| Method used to synthesise evidence | Narrative | Systematic review followed by three-stage narrative synthesis: effectiveness synthesis, views synthesis and cross-study synthesis. |
| Design of included studies | Not stated explicitly. Reference made to qualitative and quantitative: surveys, empirical studies. | Qualitative and quantitative: interventions studies (trials and systematic reviews) and non-intervention studies of young people's views. |
| Dates searched | Not stated | ~1990 to 1999 |
| No. of included studies | Not stated | 33 |
| Outcomes | 'Effectiveness of delivering treatment services; the organization, management and financing of services; and adoption of best practices (technology transfer)'. | 'Barriers to, and facilitators of, good mental health amongst young people'. |
| Participant characteristics | US-based adolescent drug users, with a particular focus on those who are adjudicated. | Children and young people (11 to 21 years). Included outcome evaluations and systematic reviews could be from anywhere in the world while only UK-specific process evaluations and non-intervention studies were included. |

A review of parents participating in parent management training asserted the importance of addressing unmet need in contexts of limited capacity. This may require services to deliver interventions innovatively, for example using 'self-administered programming' and taking advantage of media technology (SHEPARD2009).

**Fast access to reliable health advice**

Children and young people and parents or carers attending UK CAMHS reported that accessibility could be improved (BARBER2006).

Incarcerated male adolescents from an Australian sample reported the limited availability of services tackling criminogenic need, and educational and vocational services. However, those who were able to access these services reported positive experiences of them (ASHKAR2008).

Inconveniently located services are seen, in one study, as the most prominent barrier to services. Meetings conducted at a location designated by the parent, or at home, or a school-linked services approach, could be helpful (SODERLUND1995). Another barrier to access of services, identified by parents involved in parent management training, is that need exceeds capacity (SHEPARD2009).

A review of preventative interventions targeting 'high risk' children reported that there may also be multi-level barriers (community, organisational, individual) to implementing such interventions, including: lack of agency or professional 'ownership' of the programme, lack of training and support for staff, and parents' 'disinterest, resistance and lack of involvement' (LOCHMAN2000).

For US-based adolescent drug users, one study reported the accessibility of treatment and 'the organizational and economic context of service delivery' were critical to treatment effectiveness (FLANZER2005). The lack of available support for adolescent drug users was costly both in terms of the financial impact on other services, and on outcomes for the individual (FLANZER2005).

**Continuity of care and smooth transitions**

A UK study exploring the views of policy and academic experts, looked-after children and foster carers, reported that for children and young people in care, unnecessary delays at entry to care may result in an increased risk of mental health problems (DEMOS2010). Similar points are raised in a study of children in foster care in the US, where it is noted that staff working with looked-after children need to understand the range of mental health services and support available in the locality and how to access and make referrals to them (LANDSVERK2009).

*Assessment and diagnosis*
**Continuity of care and smooth transitions**

Services could consider standardising mental health assessment for children and young people entering care (LANDSVERK2009).

## Treatment (including prevention)

*Involvement in decisions and respect for preferences*
It is important to consult with looked-after children and young people in their individual discussions regarding treatment (DAVIES2008).

A study of community-based projects for children and young people with challenging behaviour and their parents or carers in Scotland, which included the Webster-Stratton parent training programme, reported a sense of cultural dissonance in the programme for some families (CHILDREN1ST2007). The study also reported that there were feelings that the Webster-Stratton programmes take a simplistic and idealistic approach and may not be related to the complexity or the severity of what parents and carers are experiencing, for example not addressing 'bad behaviour' outside the home and so on. Parents and carers therefore expressed a desire for the programmes to be modified to their needs and circumstances, and not run by the book (CHILDREN1ST2007). Another review also reported the needs of parent/family intervention programmes to be culturally appropriate (LOCHMAN2000).

## Clear, comprehensible information and support for self-care

Children and young people like to know what is going to happen to them when they are referred to services, for example through provision of an information leaflet (CHILDREN1ST2007).

## Emotional support, empathy and respect

A narrative review of UK CAMHS reported that building relationships (which includes the sense of something being done, respect for confidentiality and staff interactions) may be just as important to children and young people as the intervention type, techniques and theories used (DAVIES2008). The review also reported that although children and young people have a desire to talk, they have difficulty doing so, and they value non-verbal communication in helping engagement in the therapy process (DAVIES2008).

Children and young people and their parents or carers attending CAMHS are reported as appreciating: having relationships with staff; support, help and advice given; being listened to and given time; and being able to talk and express feelings. However, they reported that attention to initial concerns and worries could be improved (BARBER2006).

One review reported that effective interventions address children and young people's concerns about family conflict, bereavement and/or peer group rejection (OLIVER2008). Another found that an authoritarian management style to treatment is not appreciated by prison detainees (ASHKAR2008).

A qualitative study of the experience of care for multisystemic therapy found that parents strongly valued the sense of having someone there for them to 'share what you're going through' feeling that '[multisystemic therapy] becomes a support and a friend', besides the skills and practical help offered (TIGHE2012).

## The way that services and systems work

For looked-after children in the US, it has been suggested that intensive, longer-term, evidence-based interventions could benefit children and 'prevent further movement away from family and community' (LANDSVERK2009).

Interventions targeting the broader issues that have an impact on mental health, for example housing, finance and so on, may help to improve access to services, and may be particularly useful for reaching marginalised children and young people (OLIVER2008).

## Effective treatment delivered by trusted health professionals

It has been suggested that services might look to capitalise on incarcerated young people's readiness for positive change by developing rehabilitative programming (offence-specific treatment, psychological treatment, counselling, education, vocational training, social skills training, anger management and problem solving) during incarceration (ASHKAR2008).

Another study found that children and young people and their parents or carers attending CAMHS appreciated crisis care. However, the specifics of treatment could be improved. Children and young people with conduct problems were less likely to be satisfied with services, suggesting it is important to work with this group more in the future so that their needs are better understood and expectations met (BARBER2006).

A US-based quantitative study reported how therapists value a wide range of treatment strategies when working with children and young people with disruptive behavioural problems and their parents or carers. It was suggested that understanding the service users' attitudes towards treatment techniques and content may improve how interventions are implemented. It was found that interventions most valued for children are those that focus on the parent/child/family relationship and problem solving/social skills. Interventions most valued for older young people are those that focus on problem solving/social skills and improved communication. For the parents or carers, interventions that were most valued were those that identified strengths and modelling or psychoeducation (the latter for parents or carers of older young people) (BROOKMAN-FRAZEE2009).

Child welfare services staff need to understand 'the importance of early intervention and treatment', reports one US-based study (LANDSVERK2009).

Staff morale and expertise was found to be critical to drug treatment programme success; professionals need expertise in both navigating the criminal justice system and in providing treatment/therapy to young people (FLANZER2005). It is also reported that the accessibility of treatment, and 'the organizational and economic context of … service delivery' are critical to treatment effectiveness (FLANZER2005).

In the multisystemic therapy study, families reported trusting the therapist, feeling 'heard and understood', and indicated that the non-blaming approach, in which the therapist was 'working together with me as opposed to against me' was crucial to their engagement (TIGHE2012).

## Attention to physical and environmental needs

Practical arrangements and physical surroundings are an important therapeutic feature for children and young people (DAVIES2008). For children and young people and parents/carers attending CAMHS, it was reported that facilities could be improved (BARBER2006).

Two reviews also reported that parents may be more likely to engage with family-focused interventions that fit in with their schedules, for example those which are delivered in community settings and have meals, childcare and/or transport provided (LOCHMAN2000, SHEPARD2009).

Families undergoing multisystemic therapy appreciated the flexibility of the multisystemic therapy model around their schedule, and being located in the family home (TIGHE2012).

## Involvement of, and support for, family and carers

Services that did not address family needs were recognised as a barrier. A US-based study suggested that educational programmes for learning effective methods for managing children's behaviour, and recreational/respite programmes providing help in finding recreational activities for children and tips for finding personal time for parents, may be beneficial to families (SODERLUND1995).

It is also reported that parents or carers enjoy being with other adults who share similar difficulties, allowing their sense of isolation to decrease. Incorporating regular support groups and the opportunity to address their lack of confidence or self-esteem in treatment has been welcomed in the Scottish evaluation of community-based projects (CHILDREN1ST2007). Another study reported parents may be more likely to engage with family-focused interventions that enable them to share experiences and bond with other parents (LOCHMAN2000).

It is reported that continuous positive reinforcement may be needed to engage and retain parents or carers in treatment (CHILDREN1ST2007). A study of UK children who have been permanently excluded from school, and their families and adults who work with them, reported that treatment is more difficult with children whose parents or carers cannot engage (JRF2007). A non-judgemental and individualised approach where parents/carers are given the chance to work out their own strategies is appreciated (JRF2007).

In multisystemic therapy, high value is placed on the therapists' ability to connect with different family members, showing empathy, understanding and genuine care (TIGHE2012).

**Continuity of care and smooth transitions**

One study found that children and young people and parents or carers attending UK CAMHS appreciate the flexibility of the service. However, they also found that waiting times for a first appointment could be improved (BARBER2006).

Another study suggests that liaison with schools of the young people is important to the success of the programmes, so that teachers can reinforce new learning and behaviour (CHILDREN1ST2007).

For children and young people in care, placement stability can help mitigate emotional difficulties and challenging behaviour. Training carers to deal with emotional problems and mental health support can minimise the likelihood of placement breakdown. Adequate attention also needs to be given to support for children and young people when they are on the verge of leaving care and living independently (DEMOS2010).

In terms of a community-level approach to antisocial behaviour, it has been suggested in a UK qualitative study that there needs to be better coordination between projects and better integration of antisocial behaviour work within neighbourhood renewal strategies (JRF2005). It may be beneficial to incorporate parent programme delivery into existing community structures to encourage attendance from those unlikely to attend programmes in traditional mental health settings (SHEPARD2009). Case management approaches also, for example, can help deliver integrated, coordinated, coherent care by 'establishing linkages across programmes and systems' (FLANZER2005). In addition, families undergoing multisystemic therapy found the ecological systems approach to understanding and resolving difficulties very helpful because the focus was not solely on the young person, but on links with extended family and other professionals. Families also identified that 'extratherapeutic factors', such as the influence of other professionals and agencies (for example school and Youth Offending Service), and the role of the criminal justice system as deterrents to future offending (TIGHE2012).

It was also noted in the study of multisystemic therapy families that some had struggled after the intervention had ended, and they said they would have preferred a more tapered approach to ending (a 'weaning process') (TIGHE2012).

*Educational settings*
**Involvement in decisions and respect for preferences**

One review reported that effective school-based mental health interventions 'addressed student concerns about teachers' (OLIVER2008).

**Emotional support, empathy and respect**

A qualitative study of children and young people with social, emotional and behavioural difficulties in Maltese schools reported that students experienced animosity from teachers, and that teachers needed to see pupil engagement as a collaborative process rather than something threatening. It was important to cater to holistic needs and engage students in alternative ways of learning (CEFAI2010).

Another study found that separating the child from the behaviour, and conveying this to parents and carers, was important (JRF2007).

## The way that services and systems work

One study reported that teachers believe behaviour management takes precedence over identifying mental health problems. Teachers perceived parents to be significant barriers to mental health services for children in that they often did not act on teachers' referrals or recommendations, as the parents believed the teachers should be the ones to resolve their child's problems. Other barriers to identification and access included: lack of resources in the school, large class sizes, no zero-tolerance policy for certain behaviours, a lack of parenting classes and too much bureaucracy (WILLIAMS2007).

It is also reported that some parents or carers resent the attitude that teachers take, that parents or carers should be expected to help sort out a problem without understanding all the other problems they are facing (JRF2007).

## Effective treatment delivered by trusted health professionals

Interventions for girls with aggression need to be designed along the lines of preventing escalation of aggression (aggression in girls tends to begin as non-physical and leads to physical). Interventions that help girls use aggressive behaviours in positive ways can be useful. Girls' friendships are very much tied up in their aggression, so mentoring programmes that emphasise this affinity for attachment could be helpful (ADAMSHICK2010).

## Attention to physical and environmental needs

The study conducted in Malta reported that there may be challenges for children and young people with social, emotional and behavioural difficulties to adapt to a rigid school environment; and such students may need support and encouragement to have a voice at school (CEFAI2010).

## Involvement of and support for family and carers

It is important for local authorities to consult parents or carers and children and young people in relation to their preferred choices for educational provision after a permanent exclusion from school (JRF2007).

## 4.2.5    The User Voice focus group

The GDG commissioned the views of children and young people with a conduct disorder to inform the development of the guideline via an organisation called User Voice[7]. User Voice is focused on the needs of young offenders. It is led by ex-offenders and aims to enable practitioners and policy makers to listen directly to service users, allowing previously unheard voices to have an impact on policy and the delivery of services for young offenders. The group has considerable experience in collaborating with local and national bodies in supporting the development of policy and practice documents in the area of youth offending.

The purpose and method for the consultation with User Voice was discussed with the GDG and an initial meeting was held with senior staff from the organisation to determine the most effective means of consultation. After this initial meeting and further discussion with the GDG it was agreed that a focus group would be facilitated by User Voice, on behalf of the GDG, to explore the experience of young people who have had involvement with youth justice services to inform the development of the guideline. The full method and report of the findings is described in Appendix 14.

A focus group of seven young people aged between 15 and 18 years old was convened; the group (five males and two females) had significant experience of the criminal justice system and related agencies including youth offending services, health and social services, and youth services. The individuals had all had previous involvement in User Voice work, and their personal histories were consistent with a diagnosis of conduct disorder.

The focus group explored three topics that were determined by the GDG:
● Access to care – including the location of services.
● Interventions – including parent training programmes and family-based support.
● Delivery and coordination of care – including the involvement of schools, confidentiality and the influence of peers.

*Summary of the young people's views*
**Access to care**

When the young people were encouraged to think about who or where they would turn to when they needed help, most cited family and friends. They also identified the internet as a safe and trusted source of information to help them when they, or people they knew, had problems. For some, this was often their first port of call when seeking help, using a search engine such as Google. Some of the young people indicated they would not trust public service websites, however, such as the Youth Offending Service website, because they *'are all connected to the government, which is different'*.

A few young people did identify professionals they would approach if they needed help. One young person said,

---

[7] www.uservoice.org

> *I would go to my YOT worker. Yes most people don't get along with their YOT worker but me and my YOT worker has got a good relationship.*

Mistrust of professionals, based on previously negative experiences of public services, was, however, commonly cited as a barrier to young people seeking out or engaging with professional help. One young person said,

> *It just takes one bad experience with, like, a person, like someone who is professional, like one bad experience with the police, to think that I am never talking to the police again.*

Often this mistrust was linked to confidentiality, an issue that generated a lot of discussion in the group. The young people reported that professionals shared information about them, without informing them, even after being told that it would be kept confidential. One young person described their experience of confidentiality being breached by a counsellor they had seen at a CAMHS service, which led to their withdrawal from the service,

> *Cos I said something to my counsellor, and she has told, and like the next week my youth offending worker has told me, and I am thinking what the hell you are not supposed to, and I did actually say to the woman I don't want my youth worker to know. And she actually betrayed me which was like ... and told her, and I would not go back there again after that.*

Two young people did acknowledge the need for multi-agency working, but emphasised the importance of transparency if information was to be shared between professionals. Not knowing what information would be shared with which professional or agency and in which circumstances led to the young people being reluctant to talk to professionals about their problems.

When the location of services was discussed, in relation to access, this appeared a less significant consideration for the young people compared with issues of professional mistrust. However, some suggested that a community centre or a café may provide a more informal and hence acceptable setting for talking to a professional, rather than their own home.

## Interventions

When discussing the services that the young people had experienced in the past, the importance of establishing a relationship of trust with the service-provider emerged as the most significant consideration. This included developing a sense that the professional concerned genuinely cared for them, for example through maintaining informal contact beyond the remit of their professional role and the interpersonal style of the professional, as well as consistency in the professional involvement, such as an identified professional or worker who remained constant in their lives over time. On talking about social workers, one young person said,

> *They don't give a shit because I had about, like, eight social workers from last year. They come and go.*

Another young person said how important a relationship with their support officer from prison had been, which continued after they left prison: '*The fact that she still makes time to support me, when she doesn't have to... makes me feel happy to know that there is someone who is not my family and is a professional that does care*'. The young person then described how this relationship had helped them think about their actions, as '*I don't want to let her down because she has faith in me*'.

The interpersonal style of the professional, cited as important by many of the young people, included the worker's capacity to demonstrate an understanding of the young person's world and to enable the young person to feel at ease. This included the workers having '*been there themselves*' and thus able to relate to the situation, as well as their style of clothing. Suits were identified as '*uniforms that symbolised authority, control, and professional detachment, in a negative way, for the young people*'.

When the young people were asked about parenting programmes and family-based support services, some expressed concerns about their parents feeling judged or undermined by parenting programmes. One young person said,

> *[T]his person here could not come to my house and tell my mum what to do. She would just – she would look at him and tell him to walk out the door.*

Others, however, felt this approach could work,

> *I think that can work though cos it just comes down to your parents and obviously the young person has to be open minded. You have to see eye to eye. On this thing here you have to not forget that it is your child, you have to forget that in a way that you are not telling them off. You need to see some sort of eye-to-eye level, like, we are not going 'Look...' and shout – we are not going to interrupt, I am going see where you are coming from, see why you are upset, why they are giving me trouble. If that is the case and obviously the young person is going to have to listen to them.*

The young people made some suggestions of how parenting and family-based interventions could be more helpful:
- The worker acting as a mediator between child and parent.
- Offering one-to-one work with the young person in the first instance, to engage the parent in the process by noticing successful change.
- Videoing the individual meeting with the young person and showing this to the parent.

When discussing education and school-based interventions, many young people said they had considerable problems at school, and a sense of disappointment that their potential had not been recognised or supported by teaching staff. The young people frequently referred to feeling that they had been labelled as difficult or problematic from an early age, and that this label had stuck throughout their time in the education system.

Some young people were able to describe positive experiences of teachers and school-based behaviour intervention programmes, and it was discussed what had been different about teachers which the young people had found helpful. One young man identified how *'behaviour officers'* had helped:

> [T]hey used to joke around with us, understand… There would always be kids in our school that would get into trouble just to go and talk to them about something.

One young person spoke of how a teacher who let the class listen to music had *'no problems'* as *'she used to let us listen to music, we do like half an hour of work and half an hour on the computer'*. Most of the young people in the focus group agreed that being allowed to listen to music with their headphones on had improved, or would be likely to improve, their concentration within the classroom.

The young people also described how teachers who had been helpful had been effective in creating a more relaxed atmosphere within the classroom. Teachers who were inflexible and uncompromising were seen as being less helpful, especially when they excluded young people from the class when it was in their view *'unjustified'*.

## Delivery and organisation of care

The young people were asked to think about what had been most useful about the services they had received in the past and what could be changed to make them more likely to use services if they needed help in the future. Themes that emerged were: again, professional mistrust and confidentiality concerns; negative experiences of assessments; the significance of help being offered at times of crisis and change; the importance of feeling listened to and understood by those trying to help them (for example through mentoring); and having choices about who they see and when (for example self-referrals being seen as more helpful than professional/agency referrals).

Professional assessments had been found *'unhelpful and intrusive'* by some young people. In particular, young people did not like that these were carried out by a number of professionals who they had not yet formed a trusting relationship with, and where the young person could see no obvious benefit to engaging in the assessment process. The young people's views were based on previous negative experiences of assessments, feeling that what they had told professionals had been misunderstood or misinterpreted – for example one young person described how professionals had asked about not eating breakfast, and *'bam – they tried to take me off my mum'*.

The importance of professionals explaining what was what was happening and what the problems might be, rather than trying to 'catch people out', was identified, particularly when child safeguarding was the case. Feeling listened to and understood by professionals also frequently emerged as a theme during the focus group discussion, by professionals taking the time and interest to establish the reasons for the young person's difficulties or problematic behaviour.

The young people also spoke of the importance of being given choices about the support offered to them, including choices of which worker they would be referred to, when they saw them, and in identifying personal goals of the intervention.

The young people again noted the significance of engaging with workers who had some understanding of their situation, such as mentors who may have previously experienced similar problems in the past.

Some of the young people described how they had been most receptive to help at times of significant change and crisis in their lives; one young person said the '*most helpful thing for me was going to prison*', and another added, '*Prison, it changed me. It changed my way of thinking…*'. Another person said it was '*falling out with my mum, because I ended up living nowhere… And I realised that I was going to end up being put into care if I didn't go back. So that's what I did.*'

### 4.2.6    Evidence summary

The evidence search identified a limited evidence base even though it was widened to include the experience of children and young people with a broader range of problems than just conduct disorder. This limited evidence supported the decision to conduct the focus group, and to incorporate and adapt recommendations from other guidelines (see Section 4.3). Despite these significant limitations, there was considerable overlap of themes concerning access to and the organisation of care that emerged from the broadly-based evidence review and the more narrowly-focused work with User Voice. This provides some increased confidence when summarising and interpreting the findings.

One theme to emerge from both the evidence review and the focus group was that young people were aware of the negative impact on their lives, and those of their families, due to the lack of access to services. Factors that may be associated with improved access and uptake of services included eliciting young people's preferences and facilitating their involvement in decisions about the treatment available to them, including the location of services. Lack of awareness of the options for help by staff with whom young people were in contact was also cited as a barrier to effective care. Greater flexibility in the venues in which services were provided was also identified as being potentially helpful. Young people and their families also wanted to be provided with clear, comprehensive information about services and cited the internet and other media as important sources of information.

Assessments were often seen as too cursory, with a preference expressed for one thorough, standardised assessment preferably provided or led by a single professional with whom it was possible to build a trusting relationship. The importance of tailoring services to individual families' needs, including exploring safe ways that the young person can communicate their needs and wishes to their parents, was also identified as a key factor. Respect for confidentiality and greater clarity about the sharing of information was also a recurring theme.

For the provision of treatment and the organisation and delivery of services, the importance of tailoring services to individual needs and respecting parents, not blaming or stigmatising them, also emerged. A lack of respect was seen as a key reason for children and young people and their parents or carers withdrawing from treatment. Flexibility in the means of delivery of interventions and a recognition of the practical difficulties families face in accessing treatment was also seen as a way of improving access to treatment and promoting continuing engagement. Finally, the review suggested that young peoples' relationships with their teachers is critical to managing their behaviour at school or college. Creative ways to engage young people in the school environment, such as flexibility in lessons, emerged as a theme.

## 4.3    REVIEW OF EXISTING GUIDANCE

Given the limited evidence identified on the experience of access to, and delivery and organisation of, care, the GDG made the decision to use the evidence in Section 4.2 to inform and provide a context for a review of existing NICE guidelines with the aim of incorporating or adapting recommendations from them. The GDG followed the methods outlined in Chapter 3 and reviewed NICE mental health guidelines, and identified the following as containing recommendations based on review questions that were of most relevance to the concerns raised in Section 4.2:
● *Service User Experience in Adult Mental Health* (NICE, 2011c)
● *Common Mental Health Disorders* (NICE, 2011b).

### 4.3.1    Service User Experience in Adult Mental Health

The *Service User Experience in Adult Mental Health* guidance addressed several questions that were applicable to the current guideline:
● For people who use adult NHS mental health services, what are the key problems associated with their experience of care?
● For people who use adult NHS mental health services, what would help improve the experience of care?

   After a careful review of the evidence considered in Section 4.2, the GDG judged that although the *Service User Experience in Adult Mental Health* guidance was for adult service users, a number of areas applied to the experience of care of children and young people with a conduct disorder, including: relationships and communication; providing information; avoiding stigma and promoting social inclusion; decisions, capacity and safeguarding; and involving families and carers. Some recommendations required only limited adaptation. Several other recommendations required more extensive adaptation to be relevant to the current context. The GDG adapted the recommendations based on the methodological principles outlined in Chapter 3 and in all cases the adaptation retained the original meaning and intent of the recommendations (confirmed by the Chair of the existing guidance).

   Table 14 contains the original recommendations from *Service User Experience in Adult Mental Health* in column one, the original evidence base in column two, and the adapted recommendations in column three. Where recommendations required adaptation, the rationale is provided in column four. In column one, the numbers refer to the recommendations in the *Service User Experience in Adult Mental Health* NICE guideline. In column three, the numbers in brackets following the recommendation refer to Section 4.5 in this guideline.

These recommendations reflect the expert opinion of the GDG in combination with the evidence presented in Section 4.2, including the need to give clear, comprehensible information to children and young people with a conduct disorder, and their parents and carers. They also emphasise the importance of health and social care professionals being transparent with children and young people, and building a relationship with them based on trust and respect, as well as an increased respect for parents and carers and greater care in the management of confidentiality.

### 4.3.2    Common Mental Health Disorders

The *Common Mental Health Disorders* guideline addressed several review questions that were applicable to the current guideline:
● In adults (18 years and older) at risk of depression or anxiety disorders[8] (in particular black and minority ethnic groups and older people), what factors prevent people accessing mental healthcare services?
● In adults (18 years and older) at risk of depression or anxiety disorders[9] (in particular older people and people from ethnic minorities), do changes to specific models of service delivery (that is, community based outreach clinics, clinics or services in non-health settings), increase the proportion of people from the target group who access treatment, when compared with standard care?
● In adults (18 years and older) at risk of depression or anxiety disorders[10] (in particular, black and minority ethnic groups and older people), do service developments and interventions that are specifically designed to promote access increase the proportion of people from the target group who access treatment, when compared with standard care?
● In adults (18 years and older) with depression (including subthreshold disorders) or an anxiety disorder[11], what are the aspects of a clinical care pathway that are associated with better individual or organisations outcomes?
● In adults (18 years and older) identified with depression (including subthreshold disorders) or an anxiety disorder[12], should routine outcome monitoring be used, and if so, what systems are effective for the delivery of routine outcome monitoring and use within clinical decision making?

---

[8] Including generalised anxiety disorder (GAD), panic disorder, social anxiety disorder, obsessive-compulsive disorder (OCD), specific phobias and PTSD.
[9] Including GAD, panic disorder, social anxiety disorder, OCD, specific phobias and PTSD.
[10] Including GAD, panic disorder, social anxiety disorder, OCD, specific phobias and PTSD.
[11] Including GAD, panic disorder, social anxiety disorder, OCD, specific phobias and PTSD.
[12] Including GAD, panic disorder, social anxiety disorder, OCD, specific phobias and PTSD.

**Table 14: Recommendations from *Service User Experience in Adult Mental Health* (NICE, 2011c) for inclusion**

| Original recommendation from *Service User Experience in Adult Mental Health* | Evidence base of existing recommendation | Recommendation following adaptation for this guideline | Reasons for adaptation |
|---|---|---|---|
| 1.4.7    Health and social care providers should ensure that service users:<br>• can routinely receive care and treatment from a single multidisciplinary community team<br>• are not passed from one team to another unnecessarily<br>• do not undergo multiple assessments unnecessarily. | Key problems associated with service user experience (based on review of 133 qualitative studies or reviews of qualitative studies and three surveys); key requirements for high-quality service user experience (based on GDG expert opinion). See Chapter 7 (NCCMH, 2012). | Health and social care providers should ensure that children and young people:<br>• can routinely receive care and treatment from a single team or professional<br>• are not passed from one team to another unnecessarily<br>• do not undergo multiple assessments unnecessarily. [4.5.1.2] | This recommendation was adapted to be suitable for the service context of children and young people with a conduct disorder and to address the issue of the need for continuity of professional care to help build a trusting relationship. |
| 1.1.13    Consider service users for assessment according to local safeguarding procedures for vulnerable adults if there are concerns regarding exploitation or self-care, or if they have been in contact with the criminal justice system. | Key problems associated with service user experience (based on review of 133 qualitative studies or reviews of qualitative studies and three surveys); key requirements for high-quality service user experience (based on GDG expert opinion). See Chapter 6 (NCCMH, 2012). | Consider children and young people for assessment according to local safeguarding procedures if there are concerns regarding exploitation or self-care, or if they have been in contact with the criminal justice system. [4.5.1.4] | The original recommendation was adapted to refer to children and young people; no further adaptation was required. |

| | | |
|---|---|---|
| | Key problems associated with service user experience (based on review of 133 qualitative studies or reviews of qualitative studies and three surveys); key requirements for high-quality service user experience (based on GDG expert opinion). See Chapter 7 (NCCMH, 2012). | The original recommendation was considered relevant because young people who are mature enough to make informed decisions might wish to negotiate how their parents or carers are involved with their care. Therefore the recommendation was adapted to make it clear that the young person should be of an 'appropriate developmental level, emotional maturity and cognitive capacity'. The GDG, however, wished to make it clear that as this was a guideline for children and young people it would be assumed that parents or carers would be involved where possible and therefore added 'Where parents or carers are involved in the treatment of young people with a conduct disorder'. |
| 1.1.14 Discuss with the person using mental health services if and how they want their family or carers to be involved in their care. Such discussions should take place at intervals to take account of any changes in circumstances, and should not happen only once. As the involvement of families and carers can be quite complex, staff should receive training in the skills needed to negotiate and work with families and carers, and also in managing issues relating to information sharing and confidentiality. | If parents or carers are involved in the treatment of young people with a conduct disorder, discuss with young people of an appropriate developmental level, emotional maturity and cognitive capacity how they want their parents or carers to be involved in their care. Such discussions should take place at intervals to take account of any changes in circumstances, including developmental level, and should not happen only once. [4.5.1.11] | |

*Continued*

**Table 14:** *(Continued)*

| Original recommendation from *Service User Experience in Adult Mental Health* | Evidence base of existing recommendation | Recommendation following adaptation for this guideline | Reasons for adaptation |
|---|---|---|---|
| | | | The last sentence of the original recommendation was removed because it had been covered by another recommendation developed by the GDG. [4.5.1.17] |
| 1.1.4 When working with people using mental health services:<br>• make sure that discussions take place in settings in which confidentiality, privacy and dignity are respected<br>• be clear with service users about limits of confidentiality (that is, which health and social care professionals have access to information about their diagnosis and its | Key problems associated with service user experience (based on review of 133 qualitative studies or reviews of qualitative studies and three surveys); key requirements for high-quality service user experience (based on GDG expert opinion). See Chapter 9 (NCCMH, 2012). | When working with children and young people with a conduct disorder and their parents or carers:<br>• make sure that discussions take place in settings in which confidentiality, privacy and dignity are respected<br>• be clear with the child or young person and their parents or carers about limits of confidentiality (that is, which health and social care professionals | The original recommendation was adapted to refer to children and young people; no further adaptation was required. |

| | | | |
|---|---|---|---|
| treatment and in what circumstances this may be shared with others). | | have access to information about their diagnosis and its treatment and in what circumstances this may be shared with others). [4.5.1.9] | |
| 1.1.6  Ensure that you are:<br>• familiar with local and national sources (organisations and websites) of information and/or support for people using mental health services<br>• able to discuss and advise how to access these resources<br>• able to discuss and actively support service users to engage with these resources. | Key problems associated with service user experience (based on review of 133 qualitative studies or reviews of qualitative studies and three surveys); key requirements for high-quality service user experience (based on GDG expert opinion). See Chapter 7 (NCCMH, 2012). | When giving information to children and young people with a conduct disorder and their parents or carers, ensure that you are:<br>• familiar with local and national sources (organisations and websites) of information and/or support for children and young people with a conduct disorder and their parents or carers<br>• able to discuss and advise how to access these resources<br>• able to discuss and actively support children and young people and their parents or carers to engage with these resources. [4.5.1.15] | The original recommendation was adapted to refer to children and young people and to clarify the context in which information and support organisations are discussed; no further adaptation was required. |

*Continued*

111

**Table 14:** (*Continued*)

| Original recommendation from *Service User Experience in Adult Mental Health* | Evidence base of existing recommendation | Recommendation following adaptation for this guideline | Reasons for adaptation |
|---|---|---|---|
| 1.4.1 When communicating with service users use diverse media, including letters, phone calls, emails or text messages, according to the service user's preference. | Key problems associated with service user experience (based on review of 133 qualitative studies or reviews of qualitative studies and three surveys); key requirements for high-quality service user experience (based on GDG expert opinion). See Chapter 7 (NCCMH, 2012). | When communicating with a child or young person use diverse media, including letters, phone calls, emails or text messages, according to their preference. [4.5.1.16] | The original recommendation was adapted to refer to children and young people; no further adaptation was required. |
| 1.1.7 When working with people using mental health services<br>• take into account that stigma and discrimination are often associated with using mental health services<br>• be respectful of and sensitive to service users' | Key problems associated with service user experience (based on review of 133 qualitative studies or reviews of qualitative studies and three surveys); key requirements for high-quality service user experience (based on GDG expert | When working with children and young people with a conduct disorder and their parents or carers:<br>• take into account that stigma and discrimination are often associated with using mental health services | The original recommendation was adapted to refer to children and young people; no further adaptation was required. |

*Continued*

| | | |
|---|---|---|
| • be respectful of and sensitive to children and young people's gender, sexual orientation, socioeconomic status, age, background (including cultural, ethnic and religious background) and any disability<br>• be aware of possible variations in the presentation of mental health problems in children and young people of different genders, ages, cultural, ethnic, religious or other diverse backgrounds. [4.5.1.17] | Health and social care professionals working with children and young people with a conduct disorder and their parents or carers should have competence in:<br>• assessment skills and using explanatory models of | This recommendation was considered relevant by the GDG because of the evidence of inadequate explanations of the nature of the problems faced by children and young people identified in Section 4.2. The original |
| opinion). See Chapter 6 (NCCMH, 2012). | Key problems associated with service user experience (based on review of 133 qualitative studies or reviews of qualitative studies and three surveys); key requirements for high-quality service user experience | |
| gender, sexual orientation, socioeconomic status, age, background (including cultural, ethnic and religious background) and any disability<br>• be aware of possible variations in the presentation of mental health problems in service users of different genders, ages, cultural, ethnic, religious or other diverse backgrounds.<br><br>1.1.8    Health and social care professionals working with people using mental health services should have competence in:<br>• assessment skills and using explanatory models of illness for people from | | |

113

**Table 14:** *(Continued)*

| Original recommendation from *Service User Experience in Adult Mental Health* | Evidence base of existing recommendation | Recommendation following adaptation for this guideline | Reasons for adaptation |
|---|---|---|---|
| different cultural, ethnic, religious or other diverse backgrounds<br>• explaining the possible causes of different mental health problems, and care, treatment and support options<br>• addressing cultural, ethnic, religious or other differences in treatment expectations and adherence<br>• addressing cultural, ethnic, religious or other beliefs about biological, social and familial influences on the possible causes of mental health problems<br>• conflict management and conflict resolution. | (based on GDG expert opinion). See Chapter 6 (NCCMH, 2012). | conduct disorder for people from different cultural, ethnic, religious or other diverse backgrounds<br>• explaining the possible causes of different mental health problems, and care, treatment and support options<br>• addressing cultural, ethnic, religious or other differences in treatment expectations and adherence<br>• addressing cultural, ethnic, religious or other beliefs about biological, social and familial influences on the possible causes of mental health problems<br>• conflict management and conflict resolution. [4.5.1.19] | recommendation was adapted to refer to children and young people; no further adaptation was required. |

| 1.7.1    Anticipate that withdrawal and ending of treatments or services, and transition from one service to another, may evoke strong emotions and reactions in people using mental health services. Ensure that:<br>• such changes, especially discharge, are discussed and planned carefully beforehand with the service user and are structured and phased<br>• the care plan supports effective collaboration with social care and other care providers during endings and transitions, and includes details of how to access services in times of crisis<br>• when referring a service user for an assessment in other services (including for psychological treatment), they are supported during the referral period and arrangements for support are agreed beforehand with them. | Key problems associated with service user experience (based on review of 133 qualitative studies or reviews of qualitative studies and three surveys); key requirements for high-quality service user experience (based on GDG expert opinion) (Full guideline 136, Chapter 10). | Anticipate that withdrawal and ending of treatments or services, and transition from one service to another, may evoke strong emotions and reactions in children and young people with a conduct disorder and their parents or carers. Ensure that:<br>• such changes, especially discharge and transfer from CAMHS to adult services, are discussed and planned carefully beforehand with the child or young person and their parents or carers, and are structured and phased<br>• children and young people and their parents or carers are given comprehensive information about the way adult services work and the nature of any potential interventions provided<br>• any care plan supports effective collaboration with social care and other care providers during endings | This recommendation was adapted because the GDG wished to emphasise that transfer from CAMHS to adult mental health services was a particular problem for children and young people with a conduct disorder, and that they, and their parents or carers, should be given information about adult services and any potential interventions. |

*Continued*

Table 14: *(Continued)*

| Original recommendation from *Service User Experience in Adult Mental Health* | Evidence base of existing recommendation | Recommendation following adaptation for this guideline | Reasons for adaptation |
|---|---|---|---|
| | | and transitions, and includes details of how to access services in times of crisis<br>• when referring a child or young person for an assessment in other services (including for psychological interventions), they are supported during the referral period and arrangements for support are agreed beforehand with them. [4.5.1.20] | |

It was apparent to the GDG based on their own experience of the evaluation and provision of services, from the evidence reviewed in Section 4.2 and from the consultation with User Voice that not only were there problems with accessing care but there were also considerable problems throughout the care pathway. Fortunately, a number of potential solutions to these problems also emerged from the review and consultation in Section 4.2. These included: the provision of greater information, better coordination and strengthening of the assessment process; flexibility in the venues were services are provided; practical support in maintaining engagement with services; increased knowledge on the part of staff concerned with the delivery of service; and improved continuity of service provision. After considering these factors, the GDG made the decision to incorporate or adapt certain recommendations from existing guidance. The GDG followed the methods outlined in Chapter 3 and reviewed the *Common Mental Health Disorders* (NICE, 2011b) guidance which, as with the other guidelines reviewed in this section, had been initially developed for adult service users. The GDG carefully scrutinised the relevant sections of the *Common Mental Health Disorders* guideline for recommendations, which, in the expert opinion of the GDG, addressed the concerns identified in the evidence reviews in Section 4.2. A number of areas concerned with improving access and the delivery/organisation of care for children and young people with a conduct disorder were identified which required limited adaptation to address the issues identified above. A number of recommendations were also identified as being particularly important for improving access to and the delivery and organisation of care, but required some more extensive adaptation to be relevant to the current context. The GDG then adapted the recommendations based on the methodological principles outlined in Chapter 3, in all cases the adaptation retained the original meaning and intent of the recommendations (confirmed by the GDG Chair of the existing guidance).

Table 15 contains the original recommendations from *Common Mental Health Disorders* in column one, the original evidence base in column two, and the adapted recommendations in column three. Where recommendations required adaptation, the rationale is provided in column four. In column one the numbers refer to the recommendations in the *Common Mental Health Disorders* NICE guideline. In column three the numbers in brackets following the recommendation refer to Section 4.5 in this guideline.

## 4.4    FROM EVIDENCE TO RECOMMENDATIONS

*Relative value placed on the outcomes considered*

For the review questions concerning barriers to services, the proportion of people from the target group who access services, uptake of services and data on the diversity of the group who access or are retained in services/interventions were considered to be most important. Satisfaction, preference, anxiety about treatment, experience of care and the number of participants leaving the study early were also considered important. For all other questions, themes that emerged from the qualitative evidence and focus group were considered to be the most important.

**Table 15:  Recommendations from *Common Mental Health Disorders* (NICE, 2011b) for inclusion**

| Original recommendation from *Common Mental Health Disorders* | Evidence base of existing recommendation | Recommendation following adaptation for this guideline | Reasons for adaptation |
|---|---|---|---|
| 1.1.1.1  Primary and secondary care clinicians, managers and commissioners should collaborate to develop local care pathways (see also section 1.5) that promote access to services for people with common mental health disorders by:<br>• supporting the integrated delivery of services across primary and secondary care<br>• having clear and explicit criteria for entry to the service<br>• focusing on entry and not exclusion criteria<br>• having multiple means (including self-referral) to access the service<br>• providing multiple points of access that facilitate | Review* of existing systematic reviews (k = 22) and GDG expert opinion. See Chapter 4 (NCCMH, 2011).<br><br>*It included reviews of populations with a range of physical and mental disorders with severe mental illness (in some cases also including common mental health disorders), and populations where the only disorder was a common mental health disorder. | Health and social care professionals, managers and commissioners should collaborate with colleagues in educational settings to develop local care pathways [see also recommendations 4.5.1.30–4.5.1.39] that promote access to services for children and young people with a conduct disorder and their parents and carers by:<br>• supporting the integrated delivery of services across all care settings<br>• having clear and explicit criteria for entry to the service<br>• focusing on entry and not exclusion criteria<br>• having multiple means (including self-referral) of access to the service | This recommendation was adapted on the advice of the GDG to take account of the range of services and settings with which the child or young person may come into contact. |

| | | | |
|---|---|---|---|
| links with the wider healthcare system and community in which the service is located. | | • providing multiple points of access that facilitate links with the wider care system, including educational and social care services and the community in which the service is located. [4.5.1.22] | No adaptation required – incorporated. |
| 1.1.1.2 Provide information about the services and interventions that constitute the local care pathway, including the: <br>• range and nature of the interventions provided <br>• settings in which services are delivered <br>• processes by which a person moves through the pathway <br>• means by which progress and outcomes are assessed <br>• delivery of care in related health and social care services. | Review* of existing systematic reviews (k = 22) and GDG expert opinion. See Chapter 4 (NCCMH, 2011). <br><br>*It included reviews of populations with a range of physical and mental disorders with severe mental illness (in some cases also including common mental health disorders), and populations where the only disorder was a common mental health disorder. | Provide information about the services and interventions that constitute the local care pathway, including the: <br>• range and nature of the interventions provided <br>• settings in which services are delivered <br>• processes by which a child or young person moves through the pathway <br>• means by which progress and outcomes are assessed <br>• delivery of care in related health and social care services. <br>• delivery of care in related health and social care services. [4.5.1.23] | |

*Continued*

**Table 15:** *(Continued)*

| Original recommendation from *Common Mental Health Disorders* | Evidence base of existing recommendation | Recommendation following adaptation for this guideline | Reasons for adaptation |
|---|---|---|---|
| 1.1.1.3 When providing information about local care pathways to people with common mental health disorders and their families and carers, all healthcare professionals should:<br>• take into account the person's knowledge and understanding of mental health disorders and their treatment<br>• ensure that such information is appropriate to the communities using the pathway. | Review* of existing systematic reviews (k = 22) and GDG expert opinion. See Chapter 4 (NCCMH, 2011).<br><br>*It included reviews of populations with a range of physical and mental disorders with severe mental illness (in some cases also including common mental health disorders), and populations where the only disorder was a common mental health disorder. | When providing information about local care pathways for children and young people with a conduct disorder and their parents and carers:<br>• take into account the person's knowledge and understanding of conduct disorders and their care and treatment<br>• ensure that such information is appropriate to the communities using the pathway. [4.5.1.24] | The original recommendation was adapted to refer to children and young people with a conduct disorder; no further adaptation was required. |
| 1.1.1.4 Provide all information about services in a range of languages and formats (visual, verbal and aural) and ensure that it is available from a range of settings throughout the whole | Review* of existing systematic reviews (k = 22) and GDG expert opinion. See Chapter 4 (NCCMH, 2011).<br><br>*It included reviews of populations with a range of | Provide all information about services in a range of languages and formats (visual, verbal and aural) and ensure that it is available in a range of settings throughout the whole community to | No adaptation required – incorporated. |

| | | |
|---|---|---|
| community to which the service is responsible. | physical and mental disorders with severe mental illness (in some cases also including common mental health disorders), and populations where the only disorder was a common mental health disorder. | which the service is responsible. [4.5.1.25] |
| 1.1.1.5 Primary and secondary care clinicians, managers and commissioners should collaborate to develop local care pathways (see also section 1.5) that promote access to services for people with common mental health disorders from a range of socially excluded groups including:<br>• black and minority ethnic groups<br>• older people<br>• those in prison or in contact with the criminal justice system<br>• ex-service personnel. | Review* of existing systematic reviews (k = 22) and GDG expert opinion. See Chapter 4 (NCCMH, 2011).<br><br>*It included reviews of populations with a range of physical and mental disorders with severe mental illness (in some cases also including common mental health disorders), and populations where the only disorder was a common mental health disorder. | Health and social care professionals, managers and commissioners should collaborate with colleagues in educational settings to develop local care pathways [see also recommendations 4.5.1.30–4.5.1.39] that promote access for a range of groups at risk of under-utilising services, including:<br>• girls and young women<br>• black and minority ethnic groups<br>• people with a coexisting condition (such as ADHD or autism). [4.5.1.26]<br><br>This recommendation was adapted on the advice of the GDG to reflect the fact that other groups from those specified in the original recommendation (girls and young women, and children and young people with a coexisting condition) do not present to services as often as other people with a conduct disorder. The inclusion of girls and young women in the adapted recommendation necessitated a change to the stem of the recommendation, to indicate that girls and young women do not constitute an 'excluded' group. |

*Continued*

121

**Table 15:** *(Continued)*

| Original recommendation from *Common Mental Health Disorders* | Evidence base of existing recommendation | Recommendation following adaptation for this guideline | Reasons for adaptation |
|---|---|---|---|
| 1.1.1.6  Support access to services and increase the uptake of interventions by:<br>• ensuring systems are in place to provide for the overall coordination and continuity of care of people with common mental health disorders<br>• designating a healthcare professional to oversee the whole period of care (usually a GP in primary care settings). | Review* of existing systematic reviews (k = 22) and GDG expert opinion. See Chapter 4 (NCCMH, 2011).<br><br>*It included reviews of populations with a range of physical and mental disorders with severe mental illness (in some cases also including common mental health disorders), and populations where the only disorder was a common mental health disorder. | Support access to services and increase the uptake of interventions by:<br>• ensuring systems are in place to provide for the overall coordination and continuity of care<br>• designating a professional to oversee the whole period of care (for example a staff member in a CAMHS or social care setting). [4.5.1.27] | This recommendation was adapted on the basis of expert GDG opinion to make it relevant to the particular services that children and young people receive. |
| 1.1.1.7  Support access to services and increase the uptake of interventions by providing services for people with common mental health disorders in a variety of settings. Use an assessment of | Review* of existing systematic reviews (k = 22) and GDG expert opinion. See Chapter 4 (NCCMH, 2011).<br><br>*It included reviews of populations with a range of | Support access to services and increase the uptake of interventions by providing services for children and young people with a conduct disorder and their parents and carers, in a variety of | This recommendation was adapted on the basis of expert GDG opinion to make it relevant to children and young people's settings, for example the emphasis on schools and colleges. |

*Continued*

physical and mental disorders with severe mental illness (in some cases also including common mental health disorders), and populations where the only disorder was a common mental health disorder.

settings. Use an assessment of local needs as a basis for the structure and distribution of services, which should typically include delivery of:

- assessment and interventions outside normal working hours
- assessment and interventions in the person's home or other residential settings
- specialist assessment and interventions in accessible community-based settings (for example community centres, schools and colleges and social centres) and if appropriate, in conjunction with staff from those settings
- both generalist and specialist assessment and intervention services in primary care settings.
[4.5.1.28]

local needs as a basis for the structure and distribution of services, which should typically include delivery of:

- assessment and interventions outside normal working hours
- interventions in the person's home or other residential settings
- specialist assessment and interventions in non-traditional community-based settings (for example community centres and social centres) and where appropriate, in conjunction with staff from those settings
- both generalist and specialist assessment and intervention services in primary care settings.

**Table 15:** *(Continued)*

| Original recommendation from *Common Mental Health Disorders* | Evidence base of existing recommendation | Recommendation following adaptation for this guideline | Reasons for adaptation |
|---|---|---|---|
| 1.1.1.8  Primary and secondary care clinicians, managers and commissioners should consider a range of support services to facilitate access and uptake of services. These may include providing:<br>• crèche facilities<br>• assistance with travel<br>• advocacy services. | Review* of existing systematic reviews (k = 22) and GDG expert opinion. See Chapter 4 (NCCMH, 2011).<br><br>*It included reviews of populations with a range of physical and mental disorders with severe mental illness (in some cases also including common mental health disorders), and populations where the only disorder was a common mental health disorder. | Health and social care professionals, managers and commissioners should collaborate with colleagues in educational settings to look at a range of services to support access to and uptake of services. These could include:<br>• crèche facilities<br>• assistance with travel<br>• advocacy services.<br>[4.5.1.29] | This recommendation was adapted on the basis of expert GDG opinion to make it relevant to the structures in children and young people's services and to increase understanding by those working in the field. |
| 1.5.1.1  Local care pathways should be developed to promote implementation of key principles of good care. Pathways should be:<br>• negotiable, workable and understandable for people with common mental | Review of existing systematic reviews (k = 21) and GDG expert opinion. See Chapter 7 (NCCMH, 2011). | Local care pathways should be developed to promote implementation of key principles of good care. Pathways should be:<br>• negotiable, workable and understandable for children and young people with a | The original recommendation was adapted to refer to children and young people; no further adaptation was required. |

| | | |
|---|---|---|
| health disorders, their families and carers, and professionals<br>• accessible and acceptable to all people in need of the services served by the pathway<br>• responsive to the needs of people with common mental health disorders and their families and carers<br>• integrated so that there are no barriers to movement between different levels of the pathway<br>• outcomes focused (including measures of quality, service-user experience and harm). | conduct disorder and their parents and carers as well as professionals<br>• accessible and acceptable to all people in need of the services served by the pathway<br>• responsive to the needs of children and young people with a conduct disorder and their parents and carers<br>• integrated so that there are no barriers to movement between different levels of the pathway<br>• focused on outcomes (including measures of quality, service user experience and harm). [4.5.1.30] | This recommendation was adapted on the basis of expert GDG opinion to make it relevant to the structures in children and young people's services and to increase understanding by those working in the field. |
| 1.5.1.2 Responsibility for the development, management and evaluation of local care pathways should lie with a designated leadership team, which should include primary and secondary care clinicians, | Review of existing systematic reviews (k = 21) and GDG expert opinion. See Chapter 7 (NCCMH, 2011). | Responsibility for the development, management and evaluation of local care pathways should lie with a designated leadership team, which should include health and social care professionals, managers and commissioners. |

*Continued*

**Table 15:** *(Continued)*

| Original recommendation from *Common Mental Health Disorders* | Evidence base of existing recommendation | Recommendation following adaptation for this guideline | Reasons for adaptation |
|---|---|---|---|
| managers and commissioners. The leadership team should have particular responsibility for:<br>• developing clear policy and protocols for the operation of the pathway<br>• providing training and support on the operation of the pathway<br>• auditing and reviewing the performance of the pathway. | | The leadership team should work in collaboration with colleagues in educational settings and take particular responsibility for:<br>• developing clear policy and protocols for the operation of the pathway<br>• providing training and support on the operation of the pathway<br>• auditing and reviewing the performance of the pathway. [4.5.1.31] | |
| 1.5.1.3   Primary and secondary care clinicians, managers and commissioners should work together to design local care pathways that promote a stepped-care model of service delivery that: | Review of existing systematic reviews (k = 21) and GDG expert opinion. See Chapter 7 (NCCMH, 2011). | Health and social care professionals, managers and commissioners should work with colleagues in educational settings to design local care pathways that promote a model of service delivery that: | This recommendation was adapted to make it relevant to children and young people's services. In particular it addresses the lack of clarity in identifying and providing clear information on the access to and the nature of the treatment |

| | | | |
|---|---|---|---|
| • provides the least intrusive, most effective intervention first<br>• has clear and explicit criteria for the thresholds determining access to and movement between the different levels of the pathway<br>• does not use single criteria such as symptom severity to determine movement between steps<br>• monitors progress and outcomes to ensure the most effective interventions are delivered and the person moves to a higher step if needed. | | • has clear and explicit criteria for the thresholds determining access to and movement between the different levels of the pathway<br>• does not use single criteria such as symptom severity or functional impairment to determine movement within the pathway<br>• monitors progress and outcomes to ensure the most effective interventions are delivered. [4.5.1.32] | options available in Section 4.2. In addition, the adapted recommendation does not refer to a 'stepped-care model' of service delivery because although CAMHS use a tiered model of care which is essentially a stepped care model, the term 'stepped care' is not used in CAMHS so the GDG decided to remove it as it might be seen to suggest the adoption of an adult approach to care. |
| 1.5.1.4 Primary and secondary care clinicians, managers and commissioners should work together to design local care pathways that promote a range of evidence-based interventions at each step in the pathway | Review of existing systematic reviews (k = 21) and GDG expert opinion. See Chapter 7 (NCCMH, 2011). | Health and social care professionals, managers and commissioners should work with colleagues in educational settings to design local care pathways that promote a range of evidence-based interventions in the | This recommendation was adapted on the basis of expert GDG opinion to make it relevant to children and young people's services. |

*Continued*

**Table 15:** *(Continued)*

| Original recommendation from *Common Mental Health Disorders* | Evidence base of existing recommendation | Recommendation following adaptation for this guideline | Reasons for adaptation |
|---|---|---|---|
| and support people with common mental health disorders in their choice of interventions. | | pathway and support children and young people with a conduct disorder and their parents and carers in their choice of interventions. [4.5.1.33] | |
| 1.5.1.5    All staff should ensure effective engagement with families and carers, where appropriate, to: <br>• inform and improve the care of the person with a common mental health disorder <br>• meet the identified needs of the families and carers. | Review of existing systematic reviews (k = 21) and GDG expert opinion. See Chapter 7 (NCCMH, 2011). | All staff should ensure effective engagement with parents and carers, if appropriate, to: <br>• inform and improve the care of the child or young person with a conduct disorder <br>• meet the needs of parents and carers. [4.5.1.34] | No significant adaptation required. |
| 1.5.1.6    Primary and secondary care clinicians, managers and commissioners should work together to design local care pathways | Review of existing systematic reviews (k = 21) and GDG expert opinion. See Chapter 7 (NCCMH, 2011). | Health and social care professionals, managers and commissioners should work with colleagues in educational settings to design | This recommendation was adapted on the basis of expert GDG opinion to make it relevant to children and young people's services and settings. |

| | | | |
|---|---|---|---|
| that promote the active engagement of all populations served by the pathway. Pathways should: <br>• offer prompt assessments and interventions that are appropriately adapted to the cultural, gender, age and communication needs of people with common mental health disorders <br>• keep to a minimum the number of assessments needed to access interventions. | local care pathways that promote the active engagement of all populations served by the pathway. Pathways should: <br>• offer prompt assessments and interventions that are appropriately adapted to the cultural, gender, age and communication needs of children and young people with a conduct disorder and their parents and carers <br>• keep to a minimum the number of assessments needed to access interventions. [4.5.1.35] | | In particular it addresses the concerns identified in Section 4.2 to provide clear and structured assessments. |
| 1.5.1.7 Primary and secondary care clinicians, managers and commissioners should work together to design local care pathways that respond promptly and effectively to the changing | Health and social care professionals, managers and commissioners should work with colleagues in educational settings to design local care pathways that respond promptly and | Review of existing systematic reviews (k = 21) and GDG expert opinion. See Chapter 7 (NCCMH, 2011). | This recommendation was adapted on the basis of expert GDG opinion to make it relevant to children and young people's services and settings. It addresses concerns about lack of clarity and purpose to |

*Continued*

129

**Table 15:** *(Continued)*

| Original recommendation from *Common Mental Health Disorders* | Evidence base of existing recommendation | Recommendation following adaptation for this guideline | Reasons for adaptation |
|---|---|---|---|
| needs of all populations served by the pathways. Pathways should have in place:<br>• clear and agreed goals for the services offered to a person with a common mental health disorder<br>• robust and effective means for measuring and evaluating the outcomes associated with the agreed goals<br>• clear and agreed mechanisms for responding promptly to identified changes to the person's needs. | | effectively to the changing needs of all populations served by the pathways. Pathways should have in place:<br>• clear and agreed goals for the services offered to children and young people with a conduct disorder and their parents and carers<br>• robust and effective means for measuring and evaluating the outcomes associated with the agreed goals<br>• clear and agreed mechanisms for responding promptly to changes in individual needs. [4.5.1.36] | interventions, and the need for clarity when explaining the nature and purpose of the interventions. |
| 1.5.1.8 Primary and secondary care clinicians, managers and commissioners should work together to | Review of existing systematic reviews (k = 21) and GDG expert opinion. See Chapter 7 (NCCMH, 2011). | Health and social care professionals, managers and commissioners should work with colleagues in educational | This recommendation was adapted on the basis of expert GDG opinion and the evidence review in Section 4.2 to make |

| | | |
|---|---|---|
| design local care pathways that provide an integrated programme of care across both primary and secondary care services. Pathways should:<br><br>• minimise the need for transition between different services or providers<br>• allow services to be built around the pathway and not the pathway around the services<br>• establish clear links (including access and entry points) to other care pathways (including those for physical healthcare needs)<br>• have designated staff who are responsible for the coordination of people's engagement with the pathway. | settings to design local care pathways that provide an integrated programme of care across all care settings. Pathways should:<br><br>• minimise the need for transition between different services or providers<br>• allow services to be built around the pathway and not the pathway around the services<br>• establish clear links (including access and entry points) to other care pathways (including those for physical healthcare needs)<br>• have designated staff who are responsible for the coordination of people's engagement with the pathway. [4.5.1.37] | it relevant to children and young people's services and settings, in particular to address the need for continuity and trusting relationships. |

*Continued*

131

**Table 15:** *(Continued)*

| Original recommendation from *Common Mental Health Disorders* | Evidence base of existing recommendation | Recommendation following adaptation for this guideline | Reasons for adaptation |
|---|---|---|---|
| 1.5.1.9 Primary and secondary care clinicians, managers and commissioners should work together to ensure effective communication about the functioning of the local care pathway. There should be protocols for:<br>• sharing and communicating information with people with common mental health disorders, and where appropriate families and carers, about their care<br>• sharing and communicating information about the care of service users with other professionals (including GPs)<br>• communicating information between the services provided within the pathway | Review of existing systematic reviews (k = 21) and GDG expert opinion. See Chapter 7 (NCCMH, 2011). | Health and social care professionals, managers and commissioners should work with colleagues in educational settings to ensure effective communication about the functioning of the local care pathway. There should be protocols for:<br>• sharing information with children and young people with a conduct disorder, and their parents and carers, about their care<br>• sharing and communicating information about the care of children and young people with other professionals (including GPs)<br>• communicating information between the services provided within the pathway | This recommendation was adapted on the basis of expert GDG opinion and the evidence reviews in Section 4.2 to make it relevant to children and young people's services and settings. In particular it addresses the issue of confidentiality and the sharing of information. |

| | | | |
|---|---|---|---|
| • communicating information to services outside the pathway. | | • communicating information to services outside the pathway. [4.5.1.38] | This recommendation was adapted on the basis of expert GDG opinion to make it relevant to children and young people's services and settings. This was viewed by the GDG as important in order to set the same standards for evaluation and monitoring as apply to other childhood mental disorders. |
| 1.5.1.10  Primary and secondary care clinicians, managers and commissioners should work together to design local care pathways that have robust systems for outcome measurement in place, which should be used to inform all involved in a pathway about its effectiveness. This should include providing: • individual routine outcome measurement systems • effective electronic systems for the routine reporting and aggregation of outcome measures • effective systems for the audit and review of the overall clinical and cost-effectiveness of the pathway. | Review of one systematic review and one meta-analysis, and GDG expert opinion. See Chapter 6 (NCCMH, 2011). | Health and social care professionals, managers and commissioners should work with colleagues in educational settings to design local care pathways that have robust systems for outcome measurement in place, which should be used to inform all involved in a pathway about its effectiveness. This should include providing: • individual routine outcome measurement systems • effective electronic systems for the routine reporting and aggregation of outcome measures • effective systems for the audit and review of the overall clinical and cost effectiveness of the pathway. [4.5.1.39] | |

*Trade-off between clinical benefits and harms*

Little quantitative data were found that could be used to address the review questions; therefore, the themes from the qualitative reviews and focus group became the primary source of evidence.

Despite the limitations of the evidence review conducted in Section 4.2, several themes emerged concerning access to care and the delivery and organisation of services for children and young people with a conduct disorder. Eliciting children and young people's preferences and facilitating their involvement in decisions about the treatment available to them, including the location of services, was one such theme. Children and young people and their parents or carers also wanted to be provided with clear, comprehensive information about services and cited the internet and other media as important sources of information. The importance of tailoring services to individual families' needs, including exploring safe ways in which the child or young person could communicate their needs and wishes to their parents, as well as respect for confidentiality and greater clarity about the sharing of information were also recurring themes. These views fed into the GDG discussion about assessment and ultimately into the development of the recommendations.

For the provision of treatment and the organisation and delivery of services, the importance of respecting (and not blaming or stigmatising) parents also emerged. A lack of respect was seen as a key reason for children and young people and their parents or carers withdrawing from treatment. Flexibility in the means of delivery of interventions and a recognition of the practical difficulties families face in accessing treatment was also seen as a way of improving access to treatment and promoting continuing engagement. Finally, the review suggested that young peoples' relationships with their teachers is critical to managing their behaviour at school or college. Creative ways to engage young people in the school environment, such as flexibility in lessons, was reiterated.

Due to the paucity of evidence, the technical team reviewed existing NICE mental health guidelines and found that many of the themes emerging from the evidence review and the focus group were articulated in *Service User Experience in Adult Mental Health* and *Common Mental Health Disorders*. After the technical team checked that the scope and review questions were appropriate, the GDG agreed that various degrees of adaptation were necessary (see Section 4.3). Regarding the evidence base that underpinned the existing guidelines, as can be seen in Table 14 and Table 15, a large number of published reviews were utilised. However, it should be noted that not all evidence was directly relevant and considerable expert opinion was needed for interpretation and development of recommendations. Because of the nature of the evidence utilised in the two existing guidelines, and the fact that both were published relatively recently, it was agreed by the GDG that any new evidence was unlikely to change the existing recommendations and, therefore, adaptation was appropriate.

In addition to the adapted recommendations, the GDG developed a further ten recommendations based on the evidence review, the focus group and their expert opinion, using the consensus methods outlined in Chapter 3. To address the negative perception and stigmatisation of children and young people with a conduct disorder identified by the evidence review and the focus group, the GDG wished to remind health and social care professionals that many children and young people with a conduct disorder may have had substandard or punitive experiences of care from family members and/or statutory services and therefore may be mistrustful or dismissive of offers of help. Hope and optimism should be fostered, and a positive, caring and trusting relationship established to ensure the engagement with services of all involved (see recommendation 4.5.1.5). The evidence review and the focus group both highlighted the importance of confidentiality and information sharing for young people with a conduct disorder; therefore, the GDG saw the value in advising health and social care professionals to make sure that the right to confidentiality is respected, but that children and young people and their parents or carers understand why information about their care might need to be shared (see recommendations 4.5.1.7, 4.5.1.8 and 4.5.1.10). Linked to this, they should also be able to assess capacity and competence, and understand how to apply all relevant legislation including the Children Act (HMSO, 1989) (amended 2004), the Mental Health Act (HMSO, 1983) (amended 1995 and 2007) and the Mental Capacity Act (HMSO, 2005) (see recommendation 4.5.1.1). Related to the issue of competence is informed consent and the need to ensure that children and young people can understand what is being communicated to them. The GDG therefore wished to emphasise that professionals should use simple, jargon-free language, explain any clinical language, and employ communication aids if needed (see recommendation 4.5.1.14). This was an important issue raised in the evidence review in Section 4.2.

Discussing issues of stigma and discrimination, the GDG wished to advise that interpreters should be provided if needed and that a list of local education providers offering English language teaching should be supplied to those who have difficulties speaking and understanding English (see recommendation 4.5.1.18). Mindful of the feelings of blame that parents of children with a conduct disorder can experience, the GDG wished to draw health and social care professionals' attention to this and advise them to address any concerns that parents may have, as well as explain the reasons for offering them interventions such as parent training programmes and how the programmes might help them (see recommendation 4.5.1.12). Related to the needs of parents and carers, the GDG was concerned that they should be offered an assessment of their needs, including personal, social, emotional and practical support (see recommendation 4.5.1.13).

Finally, when considering the adapted recommendation on transfer and discharge (see recommendation 4.5.1.20), the GDG wished to make a further recommendation, in particular for vulnerable young people, who had reached their 18th birthday and were continuing to exhibit antisocial behaviour (see recommendation 4.5.1.21).

## 4.5    RECOMMENDATIONS

### 4.5.1    Clinical practice recommendations

*Working safely and effectively with children and young people*
4.5.1.1    Health and social care professionals should ensure that they:
- can assess capacity and competence, including 'Gillick competence', in children and young people of all ages **and**

● understand how to apply legislation, including the Children Act (1989), the Mental Health Act (1983; amended 1995 and 2007) and the Mental Capacity Act (2005), in the care and treatment of children and young people.

4.5.1.2  Health and social care providers should ensure that children and young people:

● can routinely receive care and treatment from a single team or professional

● are not passed from one team to another unnecessarily

● do not undergo multiple assessments unnecessarily[13].

4.5.1.3  When providing assessment or treatment interventions for children and young people, ensure that the nature and content of the intervention is suitable for the child or young person's developmental level.

4.5.1.4  Consider children and young people for assessment according to local safeguarding procedures if there are concerns regarding exploitation or self-care, or if they have been in contact with the criminal justice system[14].

*Establishing relationships with children and young people and their parents or carers*

4.5.1.5  Be aware that many children and young people with a conduct disorder may have had poor or punitive experiences of care and be mistrustful or dismissive of offers of help as a result.

4.5.1.6  Develop a positive, caring and trusting relationship with the child or young person and their parents or carers to encourage their engagement with services.

4.5.1.7  Health and social care professionals working with children and young people should be trained and skilled in:

● negotiating and working with parents and carers **and**

● managing issues relating to information sharing and confidentiality as these apply to children and young people.

4.5.1.8  If a young person is 'Gillick competent' ask them what information can be shared before discussing their condition with their parents or carers.

4.5.1.9  When working with children and young people with a conduct disorder and their parents or carers:

● make sure that discussions take place in settings in which confidentiality, privacy and dignity are respected

● be clear with the child or young person and their parents or carers about limits of confidentiality (that is, which health and social care professionals have access to information about their diagnosis and its treatment and in what circumstances this may be shared with others)[15].

---

[13]Adapted from *Service User Experience in Adult Mental Health* (NICE clinical guidance 136).
[14]Adapted from *Service User Experience in Adult Mental Health* (NICE clinical guidance 136).
[15]Adapted from *Service User Experience in Adult Mental Health* (NICE clinical guidance 136).

4.5.1.10    When coordinating care and discussing treatment decisions with children and young people and their parents or carers, ensure that:
● everyone involved understands the purpose of any meetings and why information might need to be shared between services **and**
● the right to confidentiality is respected throughout the process.

*Working with parents and carers*

4.5.1.11    If parents or carers are involved in the treatment of young people with a conduct disorder, discuss with young people of an appropriate developmental level, emotional maturity and cognitive capacity how they want them to be involved. Such discussions should take place at intervals to take account of any changes in circumstances, including developmental level, and should not happen only once[16].

4.5.1.12    Be aware that parents and carers of children and young people with a conduct disorder might feel blamed for their child's problems or stigmatised by their contact with services. When offering or providing interventions such as parent training programmes, directly address any concerns they have and set out the reasons for and purpose of the intervention.

4.5.1.13    Offer parents and carers an assessment of their own needs including:
● personal, social and emotional support **and**
● support in their caring role, including emergency plans **and**
● advice on practical matters such as childcare, housing and finances, and help to obtain support.

*Communication and information*

4.5.1.14    When communicating with children and young people with a conduct disorder and their parents or carers:
● take into account the child or young person's developmental level, emotional maturity and cognitive capacity, including any learning disabilities, sight or hearing problems, or delays in language development or social communication difficulties
● use plain language if possible and clearly explain any clinical language; adjust strategies to the person's language ability, for example, breaking up information, checking back, summarising and recapping
● check that the child or young person and their parents or carers understand what is being said
● use communication aids (such as pictures, symbols, large print, braille, different languages or sign language) if needed.

4.5.1.15    When giving information to children and young people with a conduct disorder and their parents or carer, ensure you are:
● familiar with local and national sources (organisations and websites) of information and/or support for children and young people with a conduct disorder and their parents or carers

---

[16]Adapted from *Service User Experience in Adult Mental Health* (NICE clinical guidance 136).

*Access to and delivery of services, and the experience of care*

- able to discuss and advise how to access these resources
- able to discuss and actively support children and young people and their parents or carers to engage with these resources[17].

4.5.1.16 When communicating with a child or young person use diverse media, including letters, phone calls, emails or text messages, according to their preference[18].

*Culture, ethnicity and social inclusion*

4.5.1.17 When working with children and young people with a conduct disorder and their parents or carers:
- take into account that stigma and discrimination are often associated with using mental health services
- be respectful of and sensitive to children and young people's gender, sexual orientation, socioeconomic status, age, background (including cultural, ethnic and religious background) and any disability
- be aware of possible variations in the presentation of mental health problems in children and young people of different genders, ages, cultural, ethnic, religious or other diverse backgrounds[19].

4.5.1.18 When working with children and young people and their parents or carers who have difficulties speaking English:
- provide and work proficiently with interpreters if needed
- offer a list of local education providers who can provide English language teaching.

4.5.1.19 Health and social care professionals working with children and young people with a conduct disorder and their parents or carers should have competence in:
- assessment skills and using explanatory models of conduct disorder for people from different cultural, ethnic, religious or other diverse backgrounds
- explaining the possible causes of different mental health problems, and care, treatment and support options
- addressing cultural, ethnic, religious or other differences in treatment expectations and adherence
- addressing cultural, ethnic, religious or other beliefs about biological, social and familial influences on the possible causes of mental health problems
- conflict management and conflict resolution[20].

---

[17]Adapted from *Service User Experience in Adult Mental Health* (NICE clinical guidance 136).
[18]Adapted from *Service User Experience in Adult Mental Health* (NICE clinical guidance 136).
[19]Adapted from *Service User Experience in Adult Mental Health* (NICE clinical guidance 136).
[20] Adapted from *Service User Experience in Adult Mental Health* (NICE clinical guidance 136).

*Transfer and discharge*

4.5.1.20    Anticipate that withdrawal and ending of treatments or services, and transition from one service to another, may evoke strong emotions and reactions in children and young people with a conduct disorder and their parents or carers. Ensure that:
- such changes, especially discharge and transfer from CAMHS to adult services, are discussed and planned carefully beforehand with the child or young person and their parents or carers, and are structured and phased
- children and young people and their parents or carers are given comprehensive information about the way adult services work and the nature of any potential interventions provided
- any care plan supports effective collaboration with social care and other care providers during endings and transitions, and includes details of how to access services in times of crisis
- when referring a child or young person for an assessment in other services (including for psychological interventions), they are supported during the referral period and arrangements for support are agreed beforehand with them[21].

4.5.1.21    For young people who continue to exhibit antisocial behaviour or meet criteria for a conduct disorder while in transition to adult services (in particular those who are still vulnerable, such as those who have been looked after or who have limited access to care) refer to *Antisocial Personality Disorder* (NICE clinical guideline 77). For those who have other mental health problems refer to other NICE guidance for the specific mental health problem.

*Improving access to services*

4.5.1.22    Health and social care professionals, managers and commissioners should collaborate with colleagues in educational settings to develop local care pathways that promote access to services for children and young people with a conduct disorder and their parents and carers by:
- supporting the integrated delivery of services across all care settings
- having clear and explicit criteria for entry to the service
- focusing on entry and not exclusion criteria
- having multiple means (including self-referral) of access to the service
- providing multiple points of access that facilitate links with the wider care system, including educational and social care services and the community in which the service is located[22].

4.5.1.23    Provide information about the services and interventions that constitute the local care pathway, including the:

---

[21]Adapted from *Service User Experience in Adult Mental Health* (NICE clinical guidance 136).
[22]From *Common Mental Health Disorders* (NICE clinical guideline 123).

● range and nature of the interventions provided
● settings in which services are delivered
● processes by which a child or young person moves through the pathway
● means by which progress and outcomes are assessed
● delivery of care in related health and social care services[23].

4.5.1.24  When providing information about local care pathways for children and young people with a conduct disorder and their parents and carers:
● take into account the person's knowledge and understanding of conduct disorders and their care and treatment
● ensure that such information is appropriate to the communities using the pathway[24].

4.5.1.25  Provide all information about services in a range of languages and formats (visual, verbal and aural) and ensure that it is available in a range of settings throughout the whole community to which the service is responsible[25].

4.5.1.26  Health and social care professionals, managers and commissioners should collaborate with colleagues in educational settings to develop local care pathways that promote access for a range of groups at risk of under-utilising services, including:
● girls and young women
● black and minority ethnic groups
● people with a coexisting condition (such as ADHD or autism)[26].

4.5.1.27  Support access to services and increase the uptake of interventions by:
● ensuring systems are in place to provide for the overall coordination and continuity of care
● designating a professional to oversee the whole period of care (for example, a staff member in a CAMHS or social care setting)[27].

4.5.1.28  Support access to services and increase the uptake of interventions by providing services for children and young people with a conduct disorder and their parents and carers, in a variety of settings. Use an assessment of local needs as a basis for the structure and distribution of services, which should typically include delivery of:
● assessment and interventions outside normal working hours
● assessment and interventions in the person's home or other residential settings
● specialist assessment and interventions in accessible community-based settings (for example, community centres, schools and colleges and social centres) and if appropriate, in conjunction with staff from those settings

---

[23] From *Common Mental Health Disorders* (NICE clinical guideline 123).

[24] Adapted from *Common Mental Health Disorders* (NICE clinical guideline 123).

[25] From *Common Mental Health Disorders* (NICE clinical guideline 123).

[26] Adapted from *Common Mental Health Disorders* (NICE clinical guideline 123).

[27] Adapted from *Common Mental Health Disorders* (NICE clinical guideline 123).

- both generalist and specialist assessment and intervention services in primary care settings[28].

4.5.1.29 Health and social care professionals, managers and commissioners should collaborate with colleagues in educational settings to look at a range of services to support access to and uptake of services. These could include:
- crèche facilities
- assistance with travel
- advocacy services[29].

*Developing local care pathways*

4.5.1.30 Local care pathways should be developed to promote implementation of key principles of good care. Pathways should be:
- negotiable, workable and understandable for children and young people with a conduct disorder and their parents and carers as well as professionals
- accessible and acceptable to all people in need of the services served by the pathway
- responsive to the needs of children and young people with a conduct disorder and their parents and carers
- integrated so that there are no barriers to movement between different levels of the pathway
- focused on outcomes (including measures of quality, service user experience and harm)[30].

4.5.1.31 Responsibility for the development, management and evaluation of local care pathways should lie with a designated leadership team, which should include health and social care professionals, managers and commissioners. The leadership team should work in collaboration with colleagues in educational settings and take particular responsibility for:
- developing clear policy and protocols for the operation of the pathway
- providing training and support on the operation of the pathway
- auditing and reviewing the performance of the pathway[31].

4.5.1.32 Health and social care professionals, managers and commissioners should work with colleagues in educational settings to design local care pathways that promote a model of service delivery that:
- has clear and explicit criteria for the thresholds determining access to and movement between the different levels of the pathway
- does not use single criteria such as symptom severity or functional impairment to determine movement within the pathway

---

[28] Adapted from *Common Mental Health Disorders* (NICE clinical guideline 123).
[29] Adapted from *Common Mental Health Disorders* (NICE clinical guideline 123).
[30] Adapted from *Common Mental Health Disorders* (NICE clinical guideline 123).
[31] Adapted from *Common Mental Health Disorders* (NICE clinical guideline 123).

- monitors progress and outcomes to ensure the most effective interventions are delivered[32].

4.5.1.33  Health and social care professionals, managers and commissioners should work with colleagues in educational settings to design local care pathways that promote a range of evidence-based interventions in the pathway and support children and young people with a conduct disorder and their parents and carers in their choice of interventions[33].

4.5.1.34  All staff should ensure effective engagement with parents and carers, if appropriate, to:
- inform and improve the care of the child or young person with a conduct disorder
- meet the needs of parents and carers[34].

4.5.1.35  Health and social care professionals, managers and commissioners should work with colleagues in educational settings to design local care pathways that promote the active engagement of all populations served by the pathway. Pathways should:
- offer prompt assessments and interventions that are appropriately adapted to the cultural, gender, age and communication needs of children and young people with a conduct disorder and their parents and carers
- keep to a minimum the number of assessments needed to access interventions[35].

4.5.1.36  Health and social care professionals, managers and commissioners should work with colleagues in educational settings to design local care pathways that respond promptly and effectively to the changing needs of all populations served by the pathways. Pathways should have in place:
- clear and agreed goals for the services offered to children and young people with a conduct disorder and their parents and carers
- robust and effective means for measuring and evaluating the outcomes associated with the agreed goals
- clear and agreed mechanisms for responding promptly to changes in individual needs[36].

4.5.1.37  Health and social care professionals, managers and commissioners should work with colleagues in educational settings to design local care pathways that provide an integrated programme of care across all care settings. Pathways should:
- minimise the need for transition between different services or providers
- allow services to be built around the pathway and not the pathway around the services

---

[32] Adapted from *Common Mental Health Disorders* (NICE clinical guideline 123).
[33] Adapted from *Common Mental Health Disorders* (NICE clinical guideline 123).
[34] Adapted from *Common Mental Health Disorders* (NICE clinical guideline 123).
[35] Adapted from *Common Mental Health Disorders* (NICE clinical guideline 123).
[36] Adapted from *Common Mental Health Disorders* (NICE clinical guideline 123).

- establish clear links (including access and entry points) to other care pathways (including those for physical healthcare needs)
- have designated staff who are responsible for the coordination of people's engagement with the pathway[37].

4.5.1.38　Health and social care professionals, managers and commissioners should work with colleagues in educational settings to ensure effective communication about the functioning of the local care pathway. There should be protocols for:

- sharing information with children and young people with a conduct disorder, and their parents and carers, about their care
- sharing and communicating information about the care of children and young people with other professionals (including GPs)
- communicating information between the services provided within the pathway
- communicating information to services outside the pathway[38].

4.5.1.39　Health and social care professionals, managers and commissioners should work with colleagues in educational settings to design local care pathways that have robust systems for outcome measurement in place, which should be used to inform all involved in a pathway about its effectiveness. This should include providing:

- individual routine outcome measurement systems
- effective electronic systems for the routine reporting and aggregation of outcome measures
- effective systems for the audit and review of the overall clinical and cost effectiveness of the pathway[39].

## 4.5.2　Research recommendation

4.5.2.1　What strategies are effective in improving uptake of and engagement with interventions for conduct disorders?

---

[37] Adapted from *Common Mental Health Disorders* (NICE clinical guideline 123).

[38] Adapted from *Common Mental Health Disorders* (NICE clinical guideline 123).

[39] Adapted from *Common Mental Health Disorders* (NICE clinical guideline 123).

# 5    SELECTIVE PREVENTION INTERVENTIONS

## 5.1    INTRODUCTION

It is challenging to classify prevention interventions. The field has grown rapidly, and often neither the goals of prevention nor the population to which the program is addressed define an exclusive and/or exhaustive category. A number of authors have suggested classification schemes. Adelman and Taylor (1994) suggest a four-step continuum where an intervention is offered in relation to problem development: (1) public health promotion, (2) early age-targeted intervention, (3) early-onset correction, and, finally, (4) treatment for chronic problems. At the first level, *primary prevention strategies* are aimed at children with risk factors but no overt symptomatology. At the second and third levels, the child's problems are likely to be at a subclinical level. These are *secondary prevention interventions*. At the fourth level, the aim is to reduce the duration of, and the secondary complications from, established disorders. These have frequently been labelled *tertiary prevention interventions*. The 1994 Institute of Medicine report makes clear that the treatment of chronic problems, even if to some measure preventive, should not be considered under the heading of 'prevention'.

The current framework for prevention is based on the work of Gordon (1983), and promoted by the 1994 Institute of Medicine report (Mrazek et al., 1994). The report outlines three types of strategies of prevention, which target different groups. The first strategies are universal, the second are selective and the third are indicated.

*Universal strategies of prevention* are aimed at the general population. The term 'universal' is to be preferred to the traditional concept of primary prevention because it specifies that the population to which the intervention is applied is not preselected. Most universal prevention strategies do identify high-risk populations, but unlike selected intervention programmes they do not target a specific group that has characteristics that define its members as being at high risk within the population for developing the disorder. Thus, the program is delivered universally. It is the population, and not the individual within the population, that may carry the risk, which is generally relatively low in these interventions.

*Selective prevention interventions* are generally considered to be secondary preventions, although it might be more appropriate to put many of these under the heading of primary prevention. Selective prevention interventions are aimed at individuals who are at high risk of developing the disorder or are showing very early signs or symptoms. Interventions tend to focus on reducing risk and strengthening resilience. Risk is obviously higher in these selected groups and is often the result of a combination of risk factors rather than the intensity of any single factor. Factors such as poverty, unemployment, inadequate transportation, substandard housing, parental mental health problems, and marital conflict, which may affect a particular child, could be addressed by selected prevention programmes.

*Indicated prevention interventions* in part mirror the category of tertiary prevention. These interventions are aimed at specific groups in which prodromal symptoms of a disorder are already evident but the full disorder has not yet developed. It is often difficult to distinguish between selective and indicated prevention interventions in terms of the therapeutic activity that might be involved. Parent training, for example, can be part of both selective and indicated interventions for prevention of conduct problems. Some intervention programmes are complex packages made up of universal, selective and indicated prevention interventions (Conduct Problems Prevention Research Group, 1992).

Two distinctly different approaches have been taken in the prevention of conduct problems in childhood. The universal approach has been directed at a whole population, typically a school, to promote the development of social and emotional competence. Other universal programmes have addressed the behaviour of teachers and the school atmosphere. During the past 10 years there have been a number of good syntheses of universal interventions, primarily those based in school specifically concerned with addressing antisocial and aggressive behaviour (Durlak et al., 2011; Lösel & Beelmann, 2003; Wilson et al., 2003).

The second approach has been to identify young children at risk on the basis of what is known about the developmental pathway of conduct problems (see Chapter 2). Prevention trials have employed both child-focused and parent-training components.

Why should conduct disorder be a target of early preventive intervention? First, it is a serious problem for the individual and wider society. As we have seen, it is the most common reason for the referral of boys to mental health services. It is also strongly developmentally linked to delinquency and adult criminality. Also, the cost to the criminal justice system is extremely high. Second, conduct disorder has been difficult to treat, particularly among chronically dysfunctional adolescents who are least likely to 'grow out' of their problems (Scott, 2007). Third, although the cause of antisocial behaviour is still a topic of debate, regarding, for example, the relative importance of individual and environmental factors, preventive interventions could be theory-driven, directed against either individual characteristics or characteristics of the social environment. Fourth, there is evidence from community-based universal or selective prevention programmes that early interventions aimed at enriching the preschool period and preventing school failures among high-risk populations have had an unexpected impact on delinquency and other related behaviours (Farrington, 1994; Offord & Bennett, 1994). In short, with an understanding of the antecedents of serious antisocial behaviour, early preventive interventions may be effective in modifying trajectories and thus interrupting the course towards chronic antisocial behaviour.

The goal of early identification of conduct disorder has become increasingly realistic. Over the past 20 years a new discipline that integrates epidemiological findings with public health treatment initiatives has emerged, which Kellam and Van Horn (1997) have termed 'developmental epidemiologically based prevention research'. This approach has been strongly influenced by the integration of public health concepts and methods with concepts and methods from other mental health and developmental science disciplines. The basic framework is provided by developmental epidemiology, which suggests paths including individual biological and psychological characteristics, characteristics of the environment, and characteristics of the interaction between individual and environment. This leads to experimental preventive trials that are targeted at specific risk antecedents. The proximal risk antecedents that are targeted tend to be conduct problems, aggression and poor achievement, with a view to influencing distal outcomes such as antisocial behaviour and delinquency.

The most important risk factors that predict conduct disorder and delinquency include impulsiveness, low IQ, low school achievement, poor parental supervision, punitive or erratic parental discipline, cold parental attitude, child physical abuse, parental conflict, disrupted families, antisocial parents, large family size, low family income, antisocial peers, high delinquency rate schools and high-crime neighbourhoods (Murray et al., 2010). However, for many of these factors it is unknown whether they have causal effects or are merely markers of other risk mechanisms (Murray & Farrington, 2010). Genetic studies have reported that unique environmental and genetic factors are responsible for similar proportions of the variability in antisocial behaviour; shared environmental factors, although markedly less significant, nevertheless play a more prominent role in explaining conduct disorder than most other mental disorders of childhood (Maes et al., 2007).

Epidemiological studies have shown that excessive disobedience in relation to adults is a key precursor to the development of full-blown conduct disorder. In a clinical sample of boys assessed between the ages of 7 and 17 years, there was some year-to-year stability, but there were also fluctuations between no diagnosis (37%), oppositional defiant disorder (36%) and conduct disorder (27%) (Rowe et al., 2010). Thus, while oppositional defiant disorder is an important risk factor for conduct disorder, not all children with oppositional defiant disorder develop conduct disorder (Burke et al., 2005). Certain factors, such as low socioeconomic status (Greene et al., 2002) and higher parental hostility (Kolko et al., 2008) increase the likelihood of oppositional defiant disorder turning into conduct disorder. Conduct disorder is more stable than oppositional defiant disorder, with persistence over several years following diagnosis estimated to be around 50 to 60% (Rowe et al., 2010) and even as high as 88% (Lahey et al., 1995).

Aggression is another early sign of risk for conduct disorder (Loeber et al., 2000). Recent evidence suggests that the relationship between autonomic nervous system functioning and aggression/conduct problems may differ between the genders. Beauchaine and colleagues (2008) found that boys with aggression and conduct problems showed reduced autonomic functioning compared with controls, while girls with similar behavioural profiles exhibited greater electrodermal responding than controls, with no differences in cardiovascular reactivity to incentives. There is a strong linear increase from early childhood to the late teenage years in the prevalence of non-aggressive antisocial behaviour (Maughan et al., 2004), with the occurrence of status violations rising especially sharply in adolescence (Maughan et al., 2004; Moffit et al., 2001). A number of longitudinal studies have revealed declining ratings of physical aggression from childhood to adolescence (Campbell et al., 2006; Côté et al., 2002; Lahey et al., 2000). Physical aggression during childhood is a predictor of adjustment problems, particularly in girls (Fontaine et al., 2008).

## 5.2    CURRENT PRACTICE

Professionals working in children's mental health and other agencies in the UK have become increasingly interested in focusing on prevention in their effort to treat emotional and behavioural problems, including conduct disorder and related problems, in children and adolescents. A major initiative, the Sure Start initiative, began in 1998 to address a wide range of childhood emotional problems by targeting at-risk children and their families. According to the current prevailing view, this programme has had only limited success, and this is generally attributed to the fact that insufficient measures have been taken to target the families in greatest need (Belsky et al., 2006). Where targeting has occurred the benefits have been significant, but overall the results have been equivocal (Melhuish et al., 2007).

There has been interest in developing and implementing programmes based on the Nurse-Family model developed by David Olds (Olds et al., 1986). Such programmes, targeting vulnerable parents and children, are currently being evaluated in the UK (Barnes et al., 2008). Programmes in this area have often lacked a clear focus. In the UK, although there is considerable interest in and willingness to define treatment goals more tightly, it is probably fair to say that at present such services lack an overall structure, and are not uniformly directed towards any standard early intervention goal.

In 2010, Frank Field produced an influential report entitled 'The foundation years: preventing poor children becoming poor adults' (Field, 2010). The review concluded that the UK needed to address the issue of child poverty in a fundamental way following early evidence concerning the influence of the first 5 years of life. The dual recommendation of the review highlighted the importance of life chances indicators, which the country could use as a measure of success in ensuring optimal outcomes for its children, and establishing 0 to 5 as the foundation years of later development where interventions may be most cost-effectively made. Although the recommendations were broadly in line with the policies supported in Sure Start, the changes suggested were more specifically targeted and recommended implementation with much sharper definition. Graham Allen's (2011) review covered a similar domain focused on early interventions. These covered selected and targeted early interventions, primarily but not exclusively for conduct problems, with a strong emphasis on evidence-based packages. The report was particularly valuable in including a section on the economic benefits of early intervention, based in part on data from the Nurse–Family Partnership (see below). The report identified the 19 programmes that met the highest criteria for rigorous evaluation, although only those that had conduct disorder as a clearly defined endpoint are relevant to these guidelines. The most recent report by Martin Knapp and his colleagues (Knapp et al., 2011) provided coverage of a similar dataset purely from an economic standpoint. Although conduct problems are only a small part of this review, they provided some of the strongest evidence for a high yield in terms of cost offset.

## 5.3 CLINICAL EVIDENCE REVIEW

### 5.3.1 Categorisation of interventions

For the purposes of the guideline, interventions were categorised as:
- child-focused (delivered to child only)
- parent-focused (delivered to parent only)
- foster carer-focused (delivered to foster carer only)
- parent–child-based (separate interventions delivered to parent and child)
- parent–teacher-based (separate interventions delivered to parent and teacher)
- family-focused (delivered to the family)
- multimodal (integrated approach involving the family and community)
- multi-component (separate interventions delivered to parents, child, and family or school)
- classroom-based – teacher involved (programmes delivered in classrooms and involving a teacher[40])
- classroom-based – other, non-teacher, involved (programmes delivered in classrooms, but involving someone other than a teacher).

Further information about each category can be found in Chapter 7.

### 5.3.2 Prevention and treatment interventions

As described above, a distinction can be made between prevention and treatment interventions; and within prevention interventions, a further distinction can be made between universal, selective and indicated interventions (Muñoz et al., 1996). Separate review questions were initially developed for selective, indicated and treatment interventions (universal interventions were excluded from the scope; further information about each category can be found in the full review protocols presented in Appendix 15).

After the evidence had been synthesised, it became evident that there was considerable overlap between trials of indicated prevention and treatment interventions, both in terms of (a) the sample of participants recruited, as shown by recruitment methods and baseline symptom scores, and (b) by the interventions offered. Although selective prevention interventions show some similarity with indicated and treatment interventions, the sample is by definition very different, because recruitment of children and young people is based on individual risk factors (for example low school achievement), family risk factors (for example antisocial parents) or socioeconomic risk factors (for example low family income) as opposed to essentially clinical characteristics. Therefore, selective prevention interventions are reviewed here, while indicated prevention and treatment interventions are reviewed in Chapter 7.

---

[40] The intervention could be delivered to a group of teachers who were trained to use the intervention in the classroom.

### 5.3.3    Clinical review protocol

A summary of the review protocol including the review questions, information about the databases searched, and the eligibility criteria used for this section of the guideline can be found in Table 16 (a complete list of review questions can be found in Appendix 5; further information about the search strategy can be found in Appendix 7; the full review protocols can be found in Appendix 15).

The primary aim of the review strategy was to evaluate the clinical effectiveness of the interventions using meta-analysis. However, in the absence of adequate data, the available evidence was synthesised using narrative methods. Consideration was given to whether any amendments due to common mental health disorders were needed. Studies of children with subaverage IQ (where the mean of sample was above 60) will be analysed separately. Studies of children with a mean IQ of below 60 were excluded.

**Table 16:  Clinical review protocol for the review of
prevention interventions**

| Component | Description |
|---|---|
| Review question* | What selective prevention interventions for at risk individuals (including children/young people or their parents/families/carers) reduce the likelihood of children and young people developing a conduct disorder? (RQ-A1a) |
| Objectives | To conduct a systematic review of the effectiveness of interventions which aim to prevent 'at risk' children and young people from developing a conduct disorder. |
| Population | Children and young people and their parents/families/carers, including looked-after children, who are considered to be 'at risk' of developing a conduct disorder (conduct disorder and oppositional defiance disorder; characterised by repetitive and persistent patterns of antisocial, aggressive or defiant behaviour that amounts to significant and persistent violations of age-appropriate social expectations). 'At risk' was defined as having an individual, family or socioeconomic risk factor or scoring above the cut-off on a screening instrument based on risk factor research. |

*Continued*

149

**Table 16:** (*Continued*)

| Component | Description |
|---|---|
| Interventions | • **Child-focused** (for example social skills training) <br> • **Parent-focused** (for example Incredible Years Parent Training; Triple P) <br> • **Foster carer-focused** (for example Keeping Foster Parents Trained and Supported) <br> • **Parent–child-based** (for example Incredible Years Parent Training + Incredible Years Dina Dinosaur Child Training) <br> • **Parent–teacher-based** (for example the Early Impact Intervention for parents and for teachers) <br> • **Family-focused** (for example functional family therapy) <br> • **Multimodal** (for example multisystemic therapy) <br> • **Multi-component** (for example Incredible Years – Teacher Classroom Management Program + Incredible Years Parent Training + Incredible Years Dina Dinosaur Child Training) <br> • **Classroom-based** (for example Incredible Years – Teacher Classroom Management Program). |
| Comparison | Treatment as usual, no treatment, waitlist control, attention control. |
| Critical outcomes | Antisocial behaviour (at home, at school, in the community). |
| Electronic databases | Mainstream databases: <br> • Embase, MEDLINE, PreMEDLINE, PsycINFO. <br> Topic specific databases and grey literature databases (see search strategy in Appendix 7). |
| Date searched | Inception to June 2012. |
| Study design | RCT |

*The reference in parentheses after each review question (RQ) can be used to cross-reference these with the full review protocol presented in Appendix 15.

### 5.3.4 Studies considered[41]

Fifty-eight RCTs (N = 24,774) met the eligibility criteria for this review: BANKS1996 (Banks et al., 1996), BOTVIN2006 (Botvin et al., 2006), BRODY2008 (Brody et al., 2008), BRODY2012 (Brody et al., 2012), BROTMAN2003 (Brotman et al., 2003),

---

[41]Here and elsewhere in the guideline, each study considered for review is referred to by a study ID in capital letters (primary author and date of study publication, except where a study is in press or only submitted for publication, then a date is not used).

BROTMAN2005 (Brotman et al., 2005), BRUNK1987 (Brunk et al., 1987), BUTZ2001 (Butz et al., 2001), CHENG2008 (Cheng et al., 2008), COWAN2009 (Cowan et al., 2009), DEROSIER2007 (DeRosier & Gilliom, 2007), DIONNE2009 (Dionne et al., 2009), DOMITROVICH2007 (Domitrovich et al., 2007), DURANT1996 (DuRant et al., 1996), FARRELL2001 (Farrell et al., 2001), FARRELL2003 (Farrell et al., 2003), FLANNERY2003 (Flannery et al., 2003), FLAY2004 (Flay et al., 2004), FORGATCH1999 (Forgatch & DeGarmo, 1999), FRANZ2011 (Franz et al., 2011), GOTTFREDSON2006 (Gottfredson et al., 2006), GROSS2003 (Gross et al., 2003), GROSSMAN1998 (Grossman & Tierney, 1998), HOWARD2008 (Howard, 2008), IRVINE1999 (Irvine et al., 1999), IZARD2008A (Izard & King, 2008), IZARD2008B (Izard & King, 2008), JOHNSON1982 (Johnson & Breckenridge, 1982), KABLE2007 (Kable et al., 2007), KELLY2010 (Kelly et al., 2010), KITZMAN1997 (Kitzman et al., 1997), KLIEWER2011 (Kliewer et al., 2011), KNOX2011 (Knox et al., 2011), KRATOCHWILL2004 (Kratochwill et al., 2004), LANG2009 (Lang et al., 2009), LI2011 (Li et al., 2011), LOWELL2011 (Lowell et al., 2011), MAGUIN1994 (Maguin et al., 1994), MARTINEZ2005 (Martinez & Eddy, 2005), MCDONALD2006 (McDonald et al., 2006), MCFARLANE2005 (McFarlane et al., 2005), MOORE1998 (Moore & Gogerty, 1998), MOSS2011 (Moss et al., 2011), OLDS1986 (Olds et al., 1986), OLDS2002 (Olds et al., 2002), RAO1998 (Rao, 1998), SANDERS2004 (Sanders et al., 2004), SCOTT2005 (Scott, 2005), SHAW2006 (Shaw et al., 2006), STANGER2011 (Stanger et al., 2011), SUKHODOLSKY2005 (Sukhodolsky et al., 2005), TOLAN2004 (Tolan et al., 2004), WEBSTER-S1998 (Webster-Stratton, 1998), WEBSTER-S2001 (Webster-Stratton et al., 2001), WEBSTER-S2008 (Webster-Stratton et al., 2008), WOLCHIK1993 (Wolchik et al., 1993), WOLCHIK2000 (Wolchik et al., 2000) and YOUMANS2001 (Youmans, 2001). Of these, four were unpublished doctoral theses and the remainder were published in peer-reviewed journals between 1982 and 2012. In addition, 74 studies were excluded from the review. Further information about both included and excluded studies can be found in Appendix 16a.

Of the 58 eligible trials, 31 (N = 9,393) included sufficient data to be included in the meta-analysis (selective prevention intervention compared with a control group), and categorised as child-focused (delivered to child only), parent-focused (delivered to parent only), parent–child-based (separate interventions delivered to parent and child), parent–teacher-based (separate interventions delivered to parent and teacher), family-focused (delivered to the family), multi-component (separate interventions delivered to parents, child, and family or school), classroom-based – teacher involved (programmes delivered in classrooms and involving a teacher[42]), and classroom-based – other, non-teacher involved (programmes delivered in classrooms, but involving someone other than a teacher). Table 17, Table 18, Table 19 and Table 20 provide an overview of the trials included in each category. For the trials not included in at least one of the meta-analyses, a brief narrative synthesis is provided to assess whether these support or refute the meta-analyses. One trial (SUKHODOLSKY2005) was eligible, but did not report any critical outcomes, and therefore, is not described further.

---

[42] The intervention could be delivered to a group of teachers, who were trained to use the intervention in the classroom.

**Table 17: Study information table for trials included in the meta-analysis of selective prevention interventions (child-focused and parent-focused) versus any control**

| | Child-focused versus any control | Parent-focused versus any control |
|---|---|---|
| Total no. of trials (N) | 4 RCTs (544) | 15 RCTs (4,251) |
| Study ID | GOTTFREDSON2006<br>HOWARD2008<br>LANG2009<br>YOUMANS2001 | BUTZ2001<br>COWAN2009<br>FORGATCH1999<br>GOTTFREDSON2006<br>IRVINE1999<br>KITZMAN1997<br>LOWELL2011<br>MAGUIN1994<br>MCFARLANE2005<br>MOSS2011<br>OLDS1986<br>OLDS2002<br>RAO1998<br>SHAW2006<br>WOLCHIK2000 |
| Country | US (k = 4) | Canada (k = 1)<br>US (k = 14) |
| Year of publication | 2001 to 2009 (k = 4) | 1986 to 2011 (k = 15) |
| Age of children/young people | 11+ (k = 2)<br><11 (k = 2)<br>Both (k = 0) | 11+ (k = 2)<br><11 (k = 11)<br>Both (k = 2) |

| Gender of children/young people (% female) | 0 to 25% (k = 1)<br>26 to 50% (k = 1)<br>51 to 75% (k = 0)<br>76 to 100% (k = 1)<br>Not reported (k = 1) | 0 to 25% (k = 2)<br>26 to 50% (k = 5)<br>51 to 75% (k = 1)<br>76 to 100% (k = 0)<br>Not reported (k = 7) |
|---|---|---|
| Ethnicity of children/young people (% white) | 0 to 25% (k = 3)<br>26 to 50% (k = 0)<br>51 to 75% (k = 0)<br>76 to 100% (k = 0)<br>Not reported (k = 1) | 0 to 25% (k = 2)<br>26 to 50% (k = 1)<br>51 to 75% (k = 0)<br>76 to 100% (k = 3)<br>Not reported (k = 9) |
| Timepoint (weeks) | Post-treatment: 13 to 25 (k = 4) | Post-treatment: 8 to 204 (k = 15)<br>Follow-up: 25 to 991 (k = 10) |
| Comparisons | Child-focused versus attention control (k = 2)<br>Child-focused versus treatment as usual (k = 1)<br>Child-focused versus waitlist (k = 1) | Parent-focused versus attention control + treatment as usual (k = 1)<br>Parent-focused versus attention control (k = 4)<br>Parent-focused versus no treatment (k = 5)<br>Parent-focused versus treatment as usual (k = 4)<br>Parent-focused versus waitlist control (k = 1) |

**Table 18: Study information table for trials included in the meta-analysis of selective prevention interventions (parent–child-based and parent–teacher-based) versus any control**

| | Parent–child-based versus any control | Parent–teacher-based versus any control |
|---|---|---|
| Total no. of trials (N) | 6 RCTs (1,020) | 3 RCTs (1,007) |
| Study ID | BROTMAN2003<br>BROTMAN2005<br>CHENG2008<br>MOORE1998<br>TOLAN2004<br>WOLCHIK2000 | GROSS2003<br>WEBSTER-S1998<br>WEBSTER-S2001 |
| Country | US (k = 6) | US (k = 3) |
| Year of publication | 1998 to 2008 (k = 6) | 1998 to 2003 (k = 3) |
| Age of children/ young people | 11+ (k = 0)<br><11 (k = 4)<br>Both (k = 2) | 11+ (k = 0)<br><11 (k = 3)<br>Both (k = 0) |
| Gender of children/young people (% female) | 0 to 25% (k = 0)<br>26 to 50% (k = 4)<br>51 to 75% (k = 2)<br>76 to 100% (k = 0)<br>Not reported (k = 0) | 0 to 25% (k = 0)<br>26 to 50% (k = 2)<br>51 to 75% (k = 0)<br>76 to 100% (k = 0)<br>Not reported (k = 1) |
| Ethnicity of children/young people (% white) | 0 to 25% (k = 3)<br>26 to 50% (k = 0)<br>51 to 75% (k = 0)<br>76 to 100% (k = 1)<br>Not reported (k = 2) | 0 to 25% (k = 0)<br>26 to 50% (k = 1)<br>51 to 75% (k = 0)<br>76 to 100% (k = 0)<br>Not reported (k = 2) |
| Timepoint (weeks) | Post-treatment: 26 to 624 (k = 6)<br>Follow-up: 104 to 624 (k = 4) | Post-treatment: 9 to 30 (k = 3)<br>Follow-up: 64 to 82 (k = 2) |
| Comparisons | Parent–child-based versus attention control (k = 1)<br>Parent–child-based versus no treatment (k = 3)<br>Parent–child-based versus treatment as usual (k = 2) | Parent–teacher-based versus treatment as usual (k = 2)<br>Parent–teacher-based versus waitlist control (k = 1) |

**Table 19: Study information table for trials included in the meta-analysis of selective prevention interventions (family-focused and multi-component) versus any control**

| | Family-focused interventions versus any control | Multi-component versus any control |
|---|---|---|
| Total no. of trials (N) | 1 RCT (362) | 2 RCTs (805) |
| Study ID | GOTTFREDSON2006 | FLAY2004 JOHNSON1982 |
| Country | US (k = 1) | US (k = 2) |
| Year of publication | 2006 (k = 1) | 1982 to 2004 |
| Age of children/young people | 11+ (k = 0) <11 (k = 1) Both (k = 0) | 11+ (k = 0) <11 (k = 2) Both (k = 0) |
| Gender of children/ young people (% female) | Not reported (k = 1) | 0 to 25% (k = 0) 26 to 50% (k = 1) 51 to 75% (k = 0) 76 to 100% (k = 0) Not reported (k = 1) |
| Ethnicity of children/ young people (% white) | Not reported (k = 1) | Not reported (k = 2) |
| Timepoint (weeks) | Post-treatment: 14 (k = 1) | Post-treatment: 104 to 204 (k = 2) Follow-up: 365 (k = 2) |
| Comparisons | Family-focused versus attention control (k = 1) | Multi-component versus attention control (k = 1) Multi-component versus waitlist control (k = 1) |

### 5.3.5    Clinical evidence for selective prevention interventions

The critical outcomes of antisocial behaviour, offending behaviour and drug and/ or alcohol use were sub-categorised according to the person who rated the outcome: (a) observer rated, (b) researcher/clinician rated, (c) peer rated, (d) teacher rated and (e) parent rated. The GDG recognised that blinding of outcome raters who received the intervention was not possible; therefore, congruence of the effect between outcome raters was considered to be stronger evidence. Because few trials reported offending behaviour as a continuous outcome, data for this outcome were pooled

155

**Table 20: Study information table for trials included in the
meta-analysis of selective prevention interventions (classroom-based)
versus any control**

| | Classroom-based (teacher involved) versus any control | Classroom-based (other, non-teacher, involved) versus any control |
|---|---|---|
| Total no. of trials (N) | 4 RCTs (689) | 1 RCT (789) |
| Study ID | DOMITROVICH2007 GROSS2003 IZARD2008A SCOTT2005 | FLAY2004 |
| Country | US (k = 4) | US (k = 1) |
| Year of publication | 2003 to 2008 (k = 4) | 2004 (k = 1) |
| Age of children/young people | 11+ (k = 0) <11 (k = 4) Both (k = 0) | 11+ (k = 0) <11 (k = 1) Both (k = 0) |
| Gender of children/ young people (% female) | 0 to 25% (k = 0) 26 to 50% (k = 1) 51 to 75% (k = 1) 76 to 100% (k = 1) | Not reported (k = 1) |
| Ethnicity of children/ young people (% white) | 0 to 25% (k = 2) 26 to 50% (k = 1) 51 to 75% (k = 0) 76 to 100% (k = 0) Not reported (k = 1) | Not reported (k = 1) |
| Timepoint (weeks) | Post-treatment: 12 to 43 (k = 4) Follow-up: 64 (k = 1) | Post-treatment: 204 (k = 1) |
| Comparisons | Classroom-based (teacher involved) versus treatment as usual (k = 2) Classroom-based (teacher involved) versus waitlist control (k = 2) | Classroom-based (other, non-teacher, involved) versus attention control (k = 1) |

with rating scale data in the meta-analyses of antisocial behaviour. No other critical outcomes were reported in adequate numbers to be included in the meta-analysis. It should be noted that harms associated with treatment are possible (for example problems associated with stigmatisation), but the GDG felt the risk was small.

Furthermore, the included trials do not measure harm. Therefore, this issue is not examined further within this section.

In the included trials, the interventions were compared with a variety of control groups that were categorised as: (a) treatment as usual, (b) attention control, (c) wait-list control and (d) no treatment. In the evidence statements below, the control group is named only where all studies used the same control, otherwise it should be assumed that studies included in each analysis used different controls. Further information about the control group used in each trial can be found in the forest plots presented in Appendix 17.

Summary of findings tables are used below to summarise the evidence. The full GRADE evidence profiles can be found in Appendix 18.

*Child-focused interventions*
From the four trials with appropriate data for meta-analysis (see Table 17 for study characteristics), moderate quality evidence from one comparison with 30 participants and one comparison with 47 participants showed that child-focused interventions when compared with an attention control or treatment as usual reduced antisocial behaviour when rated by researchers/clinicians or teachers at post-treatment (Table 21). However, the evidence from parent-rated (two comparisons with 282 participants) and self-rated (one trial with 227 participants) antisocial behaviour was inconclusive. Of the three comparisons, two were conducted with children aged under 11 years and one with children and young people over 11 years old. At follow-up, no comparisons had useable data.

With regard to trials not included in the meta-analyses, one reported statistically significant effects favouring the intervention (KABLE2007), two found treatment effects on some antisocial behaviour outcomes (FARRELL2001, FARRELL2003) and two found no effects on the outcomes of interest (KELLY2010, KLIEWER2011).

*Parent-focused interventions*
From the 15 trials with appropriate data for meta-analysis (see Table 17 for study characteristics), high quality evidence from 14 comparisons with 2,774 participants suggested that parent-focused interventions, when compared with a control group, did not improve antisocial behaviour when rated by parents at post-treatment (Table 22). The majority of trials were conducted with children under 11 years old. Moderate quality evidence from one trial (195 participants) reporting researcher-/clinician-rated offending behaviour, one comparison (40 participants) reporting teacher-rated antisocial behaviour and two comparisons (259 participants) reporting self-rated antisocial behaviour was inconclusive. At follow-up, high quality evidence from eight comparisons with 1,648 participants suggested no benefit with regard to parent-rated antisocial behaviour (Table 23). High quality evidence from two comparisons (807 participants) reporting researcher-rated antisocial/offending behaviour and moderate quality evidence from one comparison (130 participants) reporting teacher-rated antisocial behaviour were inconclusive. In addition, three comparisons had dichotomous outcomes at follow-up (Table 24). Moderate quality evidence from one comparison (613 participants) reporting researcher-rated offending behaviour and one

**Table 21: Summary of findings table for child-focused interventions compared with a control group (post-treatment)**

**Patient or population:** children and young people at risk of a conduct disorder (post-treatment)
**Intervention:** child-focused
**Comparison:** any control group

| Outcomes | Illustrative comparative risks (95% CI) | | No. of participants (studies) | Quality of the evidence (GRADE) |
|---|---|---|---|---|
| | Assumed risk | Corresponding risk | | |
| | Any control group | Child-focused | | |
| **Researcher-/clinician-rated antisocial behaviour** Any valid rating scale | – | The mean researcher-/clinician-rated antisocial behaviour in the intervention groups was **0.82 standard deviations lower** (1.54 to 0.09 lower) | 30 (1) | ⊕⊕⊕⊖ **moderate**[1] |
| **Teacher-rated antisocial behaviour** Any valid rating scale | – | The mean teacher-rated antisocial behaviour in the intervention groups was **1.93 standard deviations lower** (2.61 to 1.24 lower) | 47 (1) | ⊕⊕⊕⊖ **moderate**[1] |
| **Parent-rated antisocial behaviour** Any valid rating scale | – | The mean parent-rated antisocial behaviour in the intervention groups was **0.08 standard deviations lower** (0.31 lower to 0.16 higher) | 282 (2) | ⊕⊕⊕⊖ **moderate**[1] |
| **Self-rated antisocial behaviour** Any valid rating scale | – | The mean self-rated antisocial behaviour in the intervention groups was **0.06 standard deviations lower** (0.32 lower to 0.20 higher) | 227 (1) | ⊕⊕⊕⊖ **moderate**[1] |

[1]OIS (for dichotomous outcomes, OIS = 300 events; for continuous outcomes, OIS = 400 participants) not met.

**Table 22: Summary of findings table for parent-focused interventions compared with a control group (post-treatment)**

**Patient or population:** children and young people at risk of a conduct disorder (post-treatment)
**Intervention:** parent-focused
**Comparison:** any control group

| Outcomes | Illustrative comparative risks (95% CI) | | No. of participants (studies) | Quality of the evidence (GRADE) |
|---|---|---|---|---|
| | **Assumed risk** | **Corresponding risk** | | |
| | **Any control group** | **Parent-focused** | | |
| **Researcher-/clinician-rated offending behaviour** frequency of arrest | – | The mean researcher-/clinician-rated offending behaviour in the intervention groups was **0.08 standard deviations higher** (0.22 lower to 0.37 higher) | 195 (1) | ⊕⊕⊕⊝ **moderate**[1] |
| **Teacher-rated antisocial behaviour** Any valid rating scale | – | The mean teacher-rated antisocial behaviour in the intervention groups was **0.05 standard deviations lower** (0.66 lower to 0.56 higher) | 40 (1) | ⊕⊕⊕⊝ **moderate**[1] |
| **Parent-rated antisocial behaviour** Any valid rating scale | – | The mean parent-rated antisocial behaviour in the intervention groups was **0.09 standard deviations lower** (0.16 to 0.01 lower) | 2,774 (14) | ⊕⊕⊕⊕ **high** |
| **Self-rated antisocial behaviour** Any valid rating scale | – | The mean self-rated antisocial behaviour in the intervention groups was **0.17 standard deviations higher** (0.61 lower to 0.95 higher) | 259 (2) | ⊕⊕⊝⊝ **low**[1,2] |

[1]OIS (for dichotomous outcomes, OIS = 300 events; for continuous outcomes, OIS = 400 participants) not met.
[2]There is evidence of substantial heterogeneity of study effect sizes.

**Table 23: Summary of findings table for parent-focused interventions compared with a control group (follow-up)**

**Patient or population:** children and young people at risk of a conduct disorder (follow-up)
**Intervention:** parent-focused
**Comparison:** any control group

| Outcomes | Illustrative comparative risks (95% CI) | | No. of participants (studies) | Quality of the evidence (GRADE) |
|---|---|---|---|---|
| | Assumed risk | Corresponding risk | | |
| | Any control group | Parent-focused | | |
| **Researcher-/clinician-rated antisocial/offending behaviour** <br> Any valid rating scale/any measure of offending behaviour <br> Follow-up: 663 weeks | – | The mean researcher-/clinician-rated antisocial/offending behaviour in the intervention groups was **0.12 standard deviations lower** (0.27 lower to 0.02 higher) | 807 (2) | ⊕⊕⊕⊕ **high** |
| **Teacher-rated antisocial behaviour** <br> Any valid rating scale <br> Follow-up: 416 weeks | – | The mean teacher-rated antisocial behaviour in the intervention groups was **0.25 standard deviations lower** (0.61 lower to 0.12 higher) | 130 (1) | ⊕⊕⊕⊖ **moderate**[1] |
| **Parent-rated antisocial behaviour** <br> Any valid rating scale <br> Follow-up: 25 to 312 weeks | – | The mean parent-rated antisocial behaviour in the intervention groups was **0.02 standard deviations lower** (0.12 lower to 0.09 higher) | 1,648 (8) | ⊕⊕⊕⊕ **high** |

[1] OIS (for dichotomous outcomes, OIS = 300 events; for continuous outcomes, OIS = 400 participants) not met.

**Table 24:  Summary of findings table for parent-focused interventions compared with a control group (follow-up)**

**Patient or population:** children and young people at risk of a conduct disorder (dichotomous outcomes) (follow-up)
**Intervention:** parent-focused
**Comparison:** any control group

| Outcomes | Relative effect (95% CI) | No. of participants (studies) | Quality of the evidence (GRADE) |
|---|---|---|---|
| **Researcher-/clinician-rated offending behaviour** Follow-up: 663 weeks | RR 1.02 (0.39 to 2.64) | 613 (1) | ⊕⊕⊕⊖ moderate[1] |
| **Parent-rated antisocial behaviour** Any valid rating scale Follow-up: 52 weeks | RR 0.60 (0.3 to 1.2) | 117 (1) | ⊕⊕⊕⊖ moderate[1] |
| **Self-rated offending behaviour conviction, lifetime** Follow-up: 991 weeks | RR 0.43 (0.23 to 0.80) | 231 (1) | ⊕⊕⊕⊖ moderate[1] |

[1]OIS (for dichotomous outcomes, OIS = 300 events; for continuous outcomes, OIS = 400 participants) not met.

comparison (117 participants) reporting parent-rated antisocial behaviour were inconclusive (both compared the intervention with treatment as usual). Finally, moderate quality evidence from one comparison involving prenatal and infancy home visitation by nurses (OLDS1986) found a large benefit in terms of self-rated offending behaviour at 19-year follow-up. It should be noted that 231 of 300 (77%) randomised were included in the follow-up analysis.

With regard to trials not included in the meta-analyses, two reported effects favouring the intervention (FRANZ2011, MARTINEZ2005), one reported mixed findings (WOLCHIK1993) and one reported no promising effects (DIONNE2009).

*Parent–child-based interventions*
From the six trials with appropriate data for meta-analysis (see Table 18 for study characteristics), moderate quality evidence from three comparisons with 242 participants showed that parent-rated antisocial behaviour at post-treatment was inconclusive (Table 25). Similarly, one comparison (99 participants) reporting observer-rated antisocial behaviour and one comparison (370 participants)

**Table 25: Summary of findings table for parent–child-based interventions compared with a control group (post-treatment)**

**Patient or population:** children and young people at risk of a conduct disorder (post-treatment)
**Intervention:** parent–child-based
**Comparison:** any control group

| Outcomes | Illustrative comparative risks (95% CI) | | No. of participants (studies) | Quality of the evidence (GRADE) |
|---|---|---|---|---|
| | **Assumed risk** | **Corresponding risk** | | |
| | **Any control group** | **Parent–child-based** | | |
| **Observer-rated antisocial behaviour** Any valid rating scale | – | The mean observer-rated antisocial behaviour in the intervention groups was **0.1 standard deviations lower** (0.49 lower to 0.29 higher) | 99 (1) | ⊕⊕⊕⊖ **moderate**[1] |
| **Researcher-/clinician-rated antisocial behaviour** Any valid rating scale | – | The mean researcher-/clinician-rated antisocial behaviour in the intervention groups was **0.14 standard deviations higher** (0.07 lower to 0.34) | 370 (1) | ⊕⊕⊕⊖ **moderate**[1] |
| **Parent-rated antisocial behaviour** Any valid rating scale | – | The mean parent-rated antisocial behaviour in the intervention groups was **0.12 standard deviations lower** (0.45 lower to 0.22 higher) | 242 (3) | ⊕⊕⊕⊖ **moderate**[1] |

[1]OIS (for dichotomous outcomes, OIS = 300 events; for continuous outcomes, OIS = 400 participants) not met.

reporting researcher-/clinician-rated antisocial behaviour were both inconclusive (both used a no treatment control group). All but one comparison included children under 11 years old. At follow-up, moderate quality evidence from two comparisons (442 participants) reporting researcher-/clinician-rated antisocial behaviour, and two comparisons (258 participants) reporting parent-rated antisocial behaviour was inconclusive (Table 26). One comparison with 99 participants demonstrated moderate quality evidence favouring the intervention when antisocial behaviour was rated by observers.

*Parent–teacher-based interventions*
From the three trials with appropriate data for meta-analysis (see Table 18 for study characteristics), low to moderate quality evidence from three comparisons with 771 participants (<11 years old) was inconclusive when antisocial behaviour was rated by observers, teachers and parents at post-treatment (Table 27). At follow-up, there were two comparisons reporting low quality evidence in favour of the intervention when rated by observers, teachers and parents. However, wide confidence intervals meant the evidence was inconclusive when rated by teachers and parents (Table 28).

*Family-focused interventions*
One trial had appropriate data for meta-analysis (see Table 18 for study characteristics) and moderate quality evidence (252 participants <11 years old), which compared a family-focused intervention with an attention control, and reported inconclusive parent and self-rated antisocial behaviour at post-treatment (Table 29). No data were reported at follow-up.

There were two trials (BRODY2008, BRODY2012) that could not be included in the meta-analysis. Both reported an effect favouring the intervention using self-reported frequency with which, during the past year, participants engaged in disruptive behaviours involving theft, truancy and suspension from school.

*Multi-component interventions*
From the two trials with appropriate data for meta-analysis (see Table 19 for study characteristics), one trial (JOHNSON1982) with 128 participants (<11 years old) reported data separately for male and female participants, and so was entered into the meta-analysis as two comparisons. Evidence from this trial was of moderate quality and suggested that the intervention when compared with waitlist control improved parent-rated antisocial behaviour (Table 30). In addition, one trial (FLAY2004) with 373 participants reported moderate quality evidence of self-rated antisocial behaviour that was inconclusive (the intervention was compared with an attention control). At follow-up, one trial (JOHNSON1982) reported teacher-rated antisocial behaviour (Table 31). The evidence was of moderate quality and suggested that the intervention improved antisocial behaviour when compared with a waitlist control.

**Table 26: Summary of findings table for parent–child-based interventions compared with a control group (follow-up)**

**Patient or population:** children and young people at risk of a conduct disorder (follow-up)
**Intervention:** parent–child-based
**Comparison:** any control group

| Outcomes | Illustrative comparative risks (95% CI) | | No. of participants (studies) | Quality of the evidence (GRADE) |
|---|---|---|---|---|
| | Assumed risk | Corresponding risk | | |
| | Any control group | Parent–child-based | | |
| **Observer-rated antisocial behaviour** Any valid rating scale Follow-up: 104 weeks | – | The mean observer-rated antisocial behaviour in the intervention groups was **0.41 standard deviations lower** (0.8 to 0.01 lower) | 99 (1) | ⊕⊕⊕⊝ **moderate**[1] |
| **Researcher-/clinician-rated antisocial behaviour** Any valid rating scale Follow-up: 624 weeks | – | The mean researcher-/clinician-rated antisocial behaviour in the intervention groups was **0.09 standard deviations lower** (0.73 lower to 0.54 higher) | 442 (2) | ⊕⊕⊕⊝ **moderate**[2] |
| **Parent-rated antisocial behaviour** Any valid rating scale Follow-up: 104 to 312 weeks | – | The mean parent-rated antisocial behaviour in the intervention groups was **0.08 standard deviations lower** (0.32 lower to 0.16 higher) | 258 (2) | ⊕⊕⊕⊝ **moderate**[1] |

[1] OIS (for dichotomous outcomes, OIS = 300 events; for continuous outcomes, OIS = 400 participants) not met.
[2] CI includes both (1) no effect and (2) appreciable benefit or appreciable harm.

**Table 27: Summary of findings table for parent–teacher-based interventions compared with a control group (post-treatment)**

**Patient or population:** children and young people at risk of a conduct disorder (post-treatment)
**Intervention:** parent–teacher-based
**Comparison:** any control group

| Outcomes | Illustrative comparative risks (95% CI) | | No. of participants (studies) | Quality of the evidence (GRADE) |
| --- | --- | --- | --- | --- |
| | Assumed risk — Any control group | Corresponding risk — Parent–teacher-based | | |
| **Observer-rated antisocial behaviour** — Any valid rating scale | – | The mean observer-rated antisocial behaviour in the intervention groups was **0.22 standard deviations lower** (0.44 lower to 0.01 higher) | 771 (3) | ⊕⊕⊕⊝ **moderate**[1] |
| **Teacher-rated antisocial behaviour** — Any valid rating scale | – | The mean teacher-rated antisocial behaviour in the intervention groups was **0.20 standard deviations lower** (0.85 lower to 0.44 higher) | 771 (3) | ⊕⊕⊝⊝ **low**[1,2] |
| **Parent-rated antisocial behaviour** — Any valid rating scale | – | The mean parent-rated antisocial behaviour in the intervention groups was **0.03 standard deviations lower** (0.22 lower to 0.15 higher) | 771 (3) | ⊕⊕⊕⊝ **moderate**[1] |

[1] Risk of bias across domains was generally high or unclear.
[2] There is evidence of substantial heterogeneity of study effect sizes.

**Table 28: Summary of findings table for parent–teacher-based interventions compared with a control group (follow-up)**

**Patient or population:** children and young people at risk of a conduct disorder (follow-up)
**Intervention:** parent–teacher-based
**Comparison:** any control group

| Outcomes | Illustrative comparative risks (95% CI) | | No. of participants (studies) | Quality of the evidence (GRADE) |
|---|---|---|---|---|
| | Assumed risk | Corresponding risk | | |
| | Any control group | Parent–teacher-based | | |
| **Observer-rated antisocial behaviour** Any valid rating scale Follow-up: 64 to 82 weeks | – | The mean observer-rated antisocial behaviour in the intervention groups was **0.31 standard deviations lower** (0.58 to 0.04 lower) | 320 (2) | ⊕⊕⊝⊝ **low**[1,2] |
| **Teacher-rated antisocial behaviour** Any valid rating scale Follow-up: 64 weeks | – | The mean teacher-rated antisocial behaviour in the intervention groups was **0.39 standard deviations lower** (0.89 lower to 0.11 higher) | 137 (1) | ⊕⊕⊝⊝ **low**[1,2] |
| **Parent-rated antisocial behaviour** Any valid rating scale Follow-up: 64 to 82 weeks | – | The mean parent-rated antisocial behaviour in the intervention groups was **0.15 standard deviations lower** (0.46 lower to 0.17 higher) | 320 (2) | ⊕⊕⊝⊝ **low**[1,2] |

[1]Risk of bias across domains was generally high or unclear.
[2]OIS (for dichotomous outcomes, OIS = 300 events; for continuous outcomes, OIS = 400 participants) not met.

**Table 29: Summary of findings table for family-focused interventions compared with a control group (post-treatment)**

**Patient or population:** children and young people at risk of a conduct disorder (post-treatment)
**Intervention:** family focused
**Comparison:** any control group

| Outcomes | Illustrative comparative risks (95% CI) | | No. of participants (studies) | Quality of the evidence (GRADE) |
|---|---|---|---|---|
| | Assumed risk | Corresponding risk | | |
| | Any control group | Family-focused | | |
| **Parent-rated antisocial behaviour** Any valid rating scale | – | The mean parent-rated antisocial behaviour in the intervention groups was **0.05 standard deviations lower** (0.3 lower to 0.19 higher) | 252 (1) | ⊕⊕⊕⊝ **moderate**[1] |
| **Self-rated antisocial behaviour** Any valid rating scale | – | The mean self-rated antisocial behaviour in the intervention groups was **0.11 standard deviations lower** (0.37 lower to 0.14 higher) | 238 (1) | ⊕⊕⊕⊝ **moderate**[1] |

[1] OIS (for dichotomous outcomes, OIS = 300 events; for continuous outcomes, OIS = 400 participants) not met.

167

Table 30: Summary of findings table for multi-component interventions compared with a control group (post-treatment)

**Patient or population:** children and young people at risk of a conduct disorder (post-treatment)
**Intervention:** multi-component
**Comparison:** any control group

| Outcomes | Illustrative comparative risks (95% CI) | | No. of participants (studies) | Quality of the evidence (GRADE) |
|---|---|---|---|---|
| | Assumed risk | Corresponding risk | | |
| | Any control group | Multi-component | | |
| **Parent-rated antisocial behaviour** Any valid rating scale | – | The mean parent-rated antisocial behaviour in the intervention groups was **0.37 standard deviations lower** (0.72 to 0.02 lower) | 128 (2) | ⊕⊕⊕⊝ **moderate**[1] |
| **Self-rated antisocial behaviour** Any valid rating scale | – | The mean self-rated antisocial behaviour in the intervention groups was **0.02 standard deviations lower** (0.27 lower to 0.24 higher) | 373 (1) | ⊕⊕⊕⊝ **moderate**[1] |

[1]OIS (for dichotomous outcomes, OIS = 300 events; for continuous outcomes, OIS = 400 participants) not met.

**Table 31: Summary of findings table for multi-component interventions compared with a control group (follow-up)**

**Patient or population:** children and young people at risk of conduct disorders (follow-up)
**Intervention:** multi-component
**Comparison:** any control group

| Outcomes | Illustrative comparative risks (95% CI) | | No. of participants (studies) | Quality of the evidence (GRADE) |
|---|---|---|---|---|
| | Assumed risk | Corresponding risk | | |
| | Any control group | Multi-component | | |
| **Teacher-rated antisocial behaviour** Any valid rating scale Follow-up: 104 weeks | – | The mean teacher-rated antisocial behaviour in the intervention groups was **0.48 standard deviations lower** (0.83 to 0.13 lower) | 128 (2) | ⊕⊕⊕⊖ **moderate**[1] |

[1]OIS (for dichotomous outcomes, OIS = 300 events; for continuous outcomes, OIS = 400 participants) not met.

*Classroom-based interventions*

Classroom-based interventions were sub-categorised by whether teachers or others were involved in the intervention (see Table 20 for study characteristics). For interventions involving a teacher, high quality evidence from four comparisons with 507 participants showed that the intervention when compared with any control, reduced teacher-rated antisocial behaviour (Table 32). However, moderate quality evidence from one comparison (111 participants) reporting observer-rated antisocial behaviour and two comparisons (273 participants) reporting parent-rated antisocial behaviour were consistent but inconclusive (all comparisons were against waitlist control). All comparisons were with children under 11 years old. At follow-up, one comparison (111 participants) of the intervention with waitlist control demonstrated moderate quality evidence from observer, teacher and parent-rated antisocial behaviour that was inconclusive (Table 33).

Moderate quality evidence from one large trial with 392 participants (<11 years old), suggested that a classroom-based intervention delivered by someone other than a teacher was not effective when compared with an attention control at post-treatment (Table 34). No follow-up data were reported.

With regard to trials not included in the meta-analyses, two reported that the intervention produced statistically significant improvements in antisocial behaviour compared with a control group (FLANNERY2003, WEBSTER-S2008).

### 5.3.6   Clinical evidence for the review of head-to-head comparisons of interventions

There were relatively few trials that reported relevant direct (head-to-head) comparisons of one category of an intervention with another category, and in all cases there was not more than one trial that could be synthesised using meta-analysis.

GROSS2003 conducted a four-arm trial that compared a parent-focused intervention versus a parent–teacher-based intervention versus a classroom-based intervention versus a waitlist control (264 participants in total). The trial reported no clear intervention effects when antisocial behaviour was rated by observers or parents. However, there was some evidence from the teacher-rated outcome that the combined parent–teacher-based intervention was no more effective than either intervention alone. An additional trial compared a classroom-based intervention delivered by teachers with a child-focused intervention (IZARD2008B), but reported no statistically significant difference between groups using a teacher-rated outcome.

In all other cases neither intervention was shown to be effective when compared with a control group (see Section 5.2.5), and so the GDG did not review the evidence further.

**Table 32: Summary of findings table for classroom-based (teacher involved) interventions compared with a control group (post-treatment)**

**Patient or population:** children and young people at risk of a conduct disorder (post-treatment)
**Intervention:** classroom-based (teacher involved)
**Comparison:** any control group

| Outcomes | Illustrative comparative risks (95% CI) | | No. of participants (studies) | Quality of the evidence (GRADE) |
| | Assumed risk | Corresponding risk | | |
| | Any control group | Classroom-based (teacher involved) | | |
|---|---|---|---|---|
| **Observer-rated antisocial behaviour** Any valid rating scale | – | The mean observer-rated antisocial behaviour in the intervention groups was **0.43 standard deviations lower** (0.96 lower to 0.09 higher) | 111 (1) | ⊕⊕⊕⊖ **moderate**[1] |
| **Teacher-rated antisocial behaviour** Any valid rating scale | – | The mean teacher-rated antisocial behaviour in the intervention groups was **0.43 standard deviations lower** (0.96 to 0.09 lower) | 507 (4) | ⊕⊕⊕⊕ **high** |
| **Parent-rated antisocial behaviour** Any valid rating scale | – | The mean parent-rated antisocial behaviour in the intervention groups was **0.13 standard deviations lower** (0.39 lower to 0.13 higher) | 273 (2) | ⊕⊕⊕⊖ **moderate**[1] |

[1]OIS (for dichotomous outcomes, OIS = 300 events; for continuous outcomes, OIS = 400 participants) not met.

171

**Table 33: Summary of findings table for classroom-based (teacher involved) interventions compared with a control group (follow-up)**

**Patient or population:** children and young people at risk of a conduct disorder (follow-up)
**Intervention:** classroom-based (by teacher)
**Comparison:** any control group

| Outcomes | Illustrative comparative risks (95% CI) | | No. of participants (studies) | Quality of the evidence (GRADE) |
| --- | --- | --- | --- | --- |
| | Assumed risk | Corresponding risk | | |
| | Any control group | Classroom-based (teacher involved) | | |
| **Observer-rated antisocial behaviour** Any valid rating scale Follow-up: 64 weeks | – | The mean observer-rated antisocial behaviour in the intervention groups was **0.07 standard deviations lower** (0.59 lower to 0.45 higher) | 111 (1) | ⊕⊕⊕⊝ **moderate**[1] |
| **Teacher-rated antisocial behaviour** Any valid rating scale Follow-up: 64 weeks | – | The mean teacher-rated antisocial behaviour in the intervention groups was **0.40 standard deviations lower** (0.92 lower to 0.13 higher) | 111 (1) | ⊕⊕⊕⊝ **moderate**[1] |
| **Parent-rated antisocial behaviour** Any valid rating scale Follow-up: 64 weeks | – | The mean parent-rated antisocial behaviour in the intervention groups was **0.24 standard deviations lower** (0.76 lower to 0.28 higher) | 111 (1) | ⊕⊕⊕⊝ **moderate**[1] |

[1]OIS (for dichotomous outcomes, OIS = 300 events; for continuous outcomes, OIS = 400 participants) not met.

**Table 34: Summary of findings table for classroom-based (other, non–teacher involved) interventions compared with a control group (post-treatment)**

**Patient or population:** children and young people at risk of a conduct disorder (post-treatment)
**Intervention:** classroom-based (other, non-teacher, involved)
**Comparison:** any control group

| Outcomes | Illustrative comparative risks (95% CI) | | No. of participants (studies) | Quality of the evidence (GRADE) |
|---|---|---|---|---|
| | **Assumed risk** | **Corresponding risk** | | |
| | **Any control group** | **Classroom-based (other, non-teacher involved)** | | |
| **Self-rated antisocial behaviour** Any valid rating scale | – | The mean self-rated antisocial behaviour in the intervention groups was **0.04 standard deviations higher** (0.22 lower to 0.29 higher) | 392 (1) | ⊕⊕⊕⊝ **moderate**[1] |

[1]OIS (for dichotomous outcomes, OIS = 300 events; for continuous outcomes, OIS = 400 participants) not met.

### 5.3.7 Clinical evidence summary

Overall there is limited moderate-to-high quality evidence to show that, for younger children (<11 years old) at risk of a conduct disorder, classroom-based interventions involving teachers may be effective in reducing antisocial behaviour. In addition, moderate quality evidence suggests that a parent-focused intervention involving prenatal and infancy home visitation by nurses (known in the UK as Family Nurse Partnership) may reduce the risk of serious offending behaviour over the long term. Based on comparisons with a control group, there was insufficient evidence to determine if any other intervention is effective. There is limited evidence from head-to-head comparisons of two different interventions that supports the conclusion that the use of a multi-component intervention is not more effective than a classroom-based intervention.

## 5.4 HEALTH ECONOMIC EVIDENCE

### 5.4.1 Economic evidence on selective prevention interventions for children and young people at risk of conduct disorder

*Systematic literature review*

No studies assessing the cost effectiveness of selective prevention programmes for children and young people at risk of conduct disorder were identified by the systematic search of the economic literature undertaken for this guideline. Details on the methods used for the systematic search of the economic literature are described in Chapter 3.

## 5.5 FROM EVIDENCE TO RECOMMENDATIONS

### 5.5.1 Relative value placed on the outcomes considered

The GDG considered antisocial behaviour (at home, at school, in the community) to be the most important outcome. Diagnosis of conduct disorder and a defined reduction in conduct problems were also considered important, although no trials reported these outcomes in a way that could be included in the meta-analysis.

### 5.5.2 Trade-off between clinical benefits and harms

In children 'at risk'[43] of a conduct disorder, there was some evidence that the benefits of classroom-based selective prevention interventions outweighed the possible risk of harm (for example problems associated with stigmatisation). Although the size of the evidence base was limited, the GDG felt that the potential for benefit across a large proportion of the population justified making a recommendation. Based on the trials included in the review and the GDG's expert opinion, it was agreed that programmes based in classrooms should be considered for children aged between 3 and 7 years old, and aim

---

[43]In this context, 'at risk' was defined as having an individual, family or socioeconomic risk factor, or scoring above the cut-off on a screening instrument based on risk factor research.

to increase children's awareness of their own and others' emotions, teach self-control of arousal and behaviour, promote a positive self-concept and good peer relations, and develop children's problem solving skills. The GDG concluded that programmes should consist of up to 30 sessions over the course of the school year. The GDG agreed that schools with a high proportion of children with individual, family or socioeconomic risk factors should be the target for classroom-based prevention programmes. In particular, the following risk factors were considered most important: low socioeconomic status, low school achievement, child abuse or abused mothers, divorced parents, parental mental health or drug problems and parental contact with the criminal justice system. Finally, the limited evidence base did not allow a conclusion to be made about the involvement of teachers in delivering classroom-based prevention programmes.

The evidence for parent-focused interventions is largely inconclusive with regard to antisocial behaviour outcomes, although nurse home visitation (known as Family Nurse Partnership in the UK) has shown long-term benefits in self-reported offending behaviour. It should be noted that no selective prevention trials included in the meta-analysis were conducted in the UK and, although a trial[44] examining the Family Nurse Partnership is underway, it is a universal prevention programme with no outcomes of relevance to this particular guideline. The aim of the current review was to examine the effect of interventions on antisocial behaviour and, therefore it is possible that some interventions have benefits that have not been captured here. It should be noted that in the NICE clinical practice guideline on antisocial personality disorder (NCCMH, 2010), early interventions targeted at parents were recommended. However, since 2009 when the search for evidence was conducted, the number of relevant trials has doubled and, therefore, the GDG felt there was good justification for not continuing to recommend interventions for parents.

### 5.5.3    Trade-off between net health benefits and resource use

The systematic review did not identify any evidence that examined the cost-effectiveness of classroom-based selective prevention interventions.

### 5.5.4    Quality of the evidence

Evidence for classroom-based interventions was graded moderate to high quality, although at most only four trials reported a critical outcome that could be pooled using meta-analysis.

## 5.6    RECOMMENDATIONS

### 5.6.1    Clinical practice recommendations

In this guideline, selective prevention refers to interventions targeted to individuals or to a subgroup of the population whose risk of developing a conduct disorder is

---

[44]www.controlled-trials.com/ISRCTN23019866

significantly higher than average, as evidenced by individual, family and social risk factors. Individual risk factors include low school achievement and impulsiveness; family risk factors include parental contact with the criminal justice system and child abuse; social risk factors include low family income and little education.

5.6.1.1 Offer classroom-based emotional learning and problem-solving programmes for children aged typically between 3 and 7 years in schools where classroom populations have a high proportion of children identified to be at risk of developing oppositional defiant disorder or conduct disorder as a result of the following factors:
- low socioeconomic status
- low school achievement
- child abuse or parental conflict
- separated or divorced parents
- parental mental health or substance misuse problems
- parental contact with the criminal justice system.

5.6.1.2 Classroom-based emotional learning and problem-solving programmes should be provided in a positive atmosphere and consist of interventions intended to:
- increase children's awareness of their own and others' emotions
- teach self-control of arousal and behaviour
- promote a positive self-concept and good peer relations
- develop children's problem solving skills.

Typically the programmes should consist of up to 30 classroom-based sessions over the course of 1 school year.

## 5.6.2    Research recommendations

5.6.2.1 What is the efficacy of classroom-based interventions for conduct disorders?

# 6    CASE IDENTIFICATION AND ASSESSMENT

## 6.1    INTRODUCTION

The prevalence of conduct disorder ranges from 4 to 13% in children and young people aged under 18 years, and from 3 to 16% for oppositional defiant disorder (American Psychiatric Association, 1994). More than half of the referrals to mental health clinics are children with conduct problems (Kazdin et al., 1990; Schuhmann et al., 1996). In the UK, reports indicate that around 10% of children and young people have emotional, behaviour disorder or social impairment (Goodman et al., 2002; Meltzer et al., 2000) and that only about 20% of these children are in contact with CAMHS (Garralda et al., 2000; Leaf et al., 1996; Meltzer et al., 2000).

The early identification of children and young people with a conduct disorder is crucial because increasing evidence suggests that untreated disruptive behaviour persists and is associated with significant consequences for the child or young person and other family members and impaired functioning later in life (Campbell & Ewing, 1990). In addition there is considerable impact on the child or young person's education, which incurs wider costs to society (Koot, 1995).

Preventing children who show early signs of behavioural problems from developing a conduct disorder should be a priority. With the resources in place, primary care professionals may be able to identify conduct disorders earlier (Sharp et al., 2005), which in turn, will ease the access to CAMHS, making the service more effective (Heywood et al., 2003).

Accurate identification alone will not ensure that effective interventions are offered – this requires a thorough assessment of need and one that takes into account the complex family environments in which many young people with a conduct disorder live and the comorbid disorders that can often complicate both assessment and treatment.

## 6.2    CLINICAL EVIDENCE REVIEW

### 6.2.1    Introduction

The use of questionnaires and scales in the assessment of psychopathological symptoms in children and young people is important for three reasons. First, they can help to identify children at high risk of developing behavioural and emotional disorders; second, they can be used as part of a clinical assessment to screen for type and severity of psychiatric disorder; and third, they can also be employed as a measure to monitor the effects of treatment (Achenbach, 1998).

Although there are limitations in the use of rating scales, such as bias due to halo effects and subjective perceptions, there are also several advantages. The most important is their low cost and ease of administration for clinicians and teachers because rating scales require less time to complete than assessment methods involving structured interviews or classroom behavioural observation (Querido & Eyberg, 2003).

The early identification of children and young people with, or at risk of developing, a conduct disorder is crucial in order to be able to refer the child to appropriate care and treatment. The diagnosis of a disorder is important for the referral of children to the appropriate services to receive further assessment or access to appropriate treatment. It is also important to consider the context in which behavioural problems occurred and how they interact with family, educational and social environments.

A non-specialist screening tool may also be useful in the identification of children and young people with a conduct disorder. Professionals in different settings such as primary care, social care, residential, educational and criminal justice settings might not be familiar with conduct disorders, and this may affect the access to appropriate care and effective treatment.

Any assessment should be focused on the child and young person's needs. For example, when dealing with less complex problems, a brief assessment might be sufficient to support a referral to interventions such as parent training programmes. However, the presence of associated features or suspicion of comorbid conditions in more complex cases would almost certainly require a full comprehensive assessment.

The assessment of disruptive behaviour is context dependent and varies across settings (Achenbach et al., 1987); therefore, to achieve a comprehensive understanding of the child or young person's problem the involvement of multiple informants can be important. The combination of parent and teacher reports can be helpful because teachers observe the behaviour of children in situations different from their parents and are less personally involved. Ratings from multiple informants are also particularly important for children and young people with several care placements and/or carers, such as those who have been looked after by local authorities (Callaghan et al., 2004; Goodman et al., 2004) or who are cared for in residential settings (Muris & Maas, 2004).

Early in the guideline development process, the GDG agreed that the review should prioritise those review questions concerning the evaluation of case identification instruments; questions relating to assessment would be addressed through informal consensus (using the method set out in Chapter 3) because both expert opinion and early scoping reviews had confirmed that there was no or very limited evidence of the effectiveness of different assessment methods.

*Definition of case identification instruments*
For the purposes of the guideline, case identification instruments were defined as validated psychometric measures that are used to identify children and young people with a suspected conduct disorder. The inclusion criteria applied to the instruments are described below.

## 6.2.2 Methodological approach

When evaluating case identification instruments, the following criteria were used to decide whether an instrument was eligible for inclusion in the review.

*Primary aim of the instrument:* the identification of children and young people with a suspected conduct disorder.

*Clinical utility:* the criterion required the primary use of the case identification instrument to be feasible and implementable in a routine clinical care. The instrument should contribute to the identification of further assessment needs and therefore be potentially useful for care planning and for referral to treatment.

*Tool characteristics and administrative properties:* the case identification tool should have validated cut-offs in the patient population of interest. Furthermore, and dependent on the practitioner skill set and the setting, instruments were evaluated for the time needed to administer and score them as well as the nature of the training (if any) required for administration or scoring. A case identification instrument should be brief (no more than 5 minutes), easy to administer and score (preferably no more than 5 minutes), and be able to be interpreted without extensive and specialist training. Non-experts from a variety of care settings (for example primary care, general medical services, educational, residential or criminal justice settings) should be able to complete the instrument with relative ease. Lastly, the availability of the tool, its cost and copyright issues were also considered.

*Population:* the population being assessed reflects the scope of this guideline. The instrument should have been validated in a population younger than 18 years old and preferably be applicable to children and young people in the UK, for example by being validated in a UK population or a population that is similar to UK demographics. It will also be assessed whether the instrument can be completed by different informants including parents, teachers and the children and young people themselves.

*Psychometric data:* the instrument should have established reliability and validity (although these data will not be reviewed at this stage). It should have been validated against a gold standard diagnostic instrument such as DSM-IV-TR or ICD-10 in the diagnosis of conduct disorder or oppositional defiant disorder (American Psychiatric Association, 1994; World Health Organization, 1992) and report sensitivity and specificity. Reported data for sensitivity, specificity in addition to AUC, positive predictive value and negative predictive value were considered. See Chapter 3 for a description of these diagnostic test accuracy terms.

### 6.2.3    Review protocol

A summary of the review protocol, including the review questions, information about the databases searched, and the eligibility criteria used for this section of the guideline, is presented in Table 35. A complete list of review questions can be found in Appendix 5; further information about the search strategy can be found in Appendix 7; the full review protocols can be found in Appendix 15.

**Table 35: Review protocol for the review of case identification
instruments and assessment of conduct disorder**

| Component | Description |
|---|---|
| Review questions* | • What are the most appropriate methods/instruments for case identification of conduct disorders in children and young people? (RQ-C2)<br>• In children and young people with possible conduct disorders, what are the key components of, and the most appropriate structure for, a diagnostic assessment? (RQ-D1)<br>To answer this question, consideration should be given to:<br>• the nature and content of the interview and observation, which should both include an early developmental history where possible<br>• formal diagnostic methods/psychological instruments for the assessment of core features of conduct disorders<br>• the assessment of risk<br>• the assessment of need<br>• the setting(s) in which the assessment takes place<br>• the role of the any informants<br>• gathering of independent and accurate information from informants.<br>When making a diagnosis of conduct disorders in children and young people, what amendments (if any) need to be made to take into account coexisting conditions (such as ADHD, depression, anxiety disorders and attachment insecurity)? (RQ-D2)<br>What amendments, if any, need to be made to take into account particular cultural or minority ethnic groups or gender? (RQ-D3) |
| Objectives | To identify and evaluate the most effective instruments for case identification of conduct disorders in children and young people. |
| Population | Children and young people (aged 18 years and younger) with a suspected conduct disorder, including looked-after children and those in contact with the criminal justice system. |
| Intervention(s) | Any assessment types except general screening that meet eligibility criteria. |
| Comparison | Gold standard: DSM-IV or ICD-10 diagnosis of conduct disorder<br>Other assessment instruments or strategies. |

*Continued*

**Table 35:** (*Continued*)

| Component | Description |
|---|---|
| Critical outcomes | Sensitivity, specificity, positive predictive value, negative predictive value, AUC. |
| Electronic databases | Mainstream databases:<br>• Embase, MEDLINE, PreMEDLINE, PsycINFO.<br><br>Topic specific databases and grey literature databases (see search strategy in Appendix 7). |
| Date searched | Inception to June 2012. |
| Study design | RCTs, cross-sectional studies. |

*The reference in parentheses after each review question (RQ) can be used to cross-reference these with the full review protocol presented in Appendix 15.

The review strategy was to conduct a pooled test accuracy meta-analysis on the sensitivity and specificity of eligible case identification instruments.

**6.2.4    Case identification instruments included in the review**

The instruments that met the inclusion criteria and are included in the review are the SDQ (Goodman, 1997), the Eyberg Child Behavior Inventory (ECBI) (Eyberg & Pincus, 1999) and the Sutter–Eyberg Student Behavior Inventory (SESBI-R) (Eyberg & Pincus, 1999). See Table 36 for a summary of characteristics of these instruments.

*Strengths and Difficulties Questionnaire*
The SDQ is a screening instrument for child and young people with mental health problems, which covers emotional, behavioural and social functioning in children and young people.

The instrument allows for a multi-informant assessment with the development of different versions. An informant version is administered to both parents and teachers of children and young people between the ages of 4 and 16 years (Goodman et al., 1998), and a self-reported version is completed by children and young people between the ages of 11 and 16 years. The authors have also recently included a version for children of 3 to 4 years to be completed by parents and preschool professionals.

The scale consists of 25 items arranged in five subscales, which assess five behavioural traits. Four of them relate to difficulties (conduct problems, emotional symptoms, hyperactivity/inattention and peer relationship problems) and one to strengths (pro-social behaviour) (Goodman, 1997). The items are almost identical in the different versions except for grammatical changes from third to first person, depending on who is to complete the form. The conduct problems scale includes five items: 'I get

**Table 36: Summary of characteristics of the three case identification instruments included in the review**

| Instrument | Screen for | Age group | Scale information: number items, subscales, scores, cut-offs, source of information and format | Time to administer; Time to score (training and by whom) | Availability | Other information |
|---|---|---|---|---|---|---|
| **Strengths and Difficulties Questionnaire (SDQ)** | Conduct-oppositional disorders | 4 to 16 years | **Scale:** 25 items. **Subscales:** conduct problems, emotional symptoms, hyperactivity/inattention, peer relationship problems, pro-social behaviour (five items in each subscale). **Score:** whole scale: 0 to 40 as pro-social behaviour subscale not included; subscales: 0 to 10. **Cut-off:** 0 to 3 normal, 4 borderline, 5 to 10 abnormal. **Source of information:** parent and teachers (4 to 16 years), self-report (11 to 16 years). **Format:** pen and paper. | **Administer:** 5 minutes (no training needed). **Score:** 5 minutes (no training needed). | **Freely available** at authors webpage, www.sdqinfo.org | Translated into over 70 languages. |

| | | | | **Administer:** 5 minutes (administered by parents, teachers or professionals). **Score:** 5 minutes (training required). | **Not freely available** Copyright: Psychological Assessment Resources, permission required to use. | Available in English and Spanish. |
|---|---|---|---|---|---|---|
| **Eyberg Child Behavior Inventory (ECBI)** | Disruptive behaviour | 2 to 16 years | **Scale:** 36 items. **Score:** intensity score: 36 to 252, problem score: 0 to 36. **Cut-off:** score above 90th percentile or intensity score: > 131, problem score: >15. **Source of information:** parent. **Format:** pen and paper. | | | |
| **Sutter–Eyberg Student Behavior Inventory-Revised (SESBI-R)** | Disruptive behaviour | 2 to 16 years | **Scale:** 38 items. **Score:** intensity score: 38 to 266, problem score: 0 to 38. **Cut off:** score above 90th percentile or intensity score: >131, problem score >15. **Source of information:** teacher. **Format:** pen and paper. | | | |

very angry and often lose my temper', 'I usually do as I am told', 'I fight a lot', 'I can make other people do what I want', 'I am often accused of lying or cheating', 'I take things that are not mine from home, school or elsewhere'. Each item is scored on a three-point response scale ('not true', 'somewhat true' and 'certainly true') and scored zero, one and two, respectively.

Administering this instrument only takes 5 minutes and scoring is straight-forward. A total difficulty score ranges from 0 to 40 and is computed by combining the four difficulties subscales (which each range from 0 to 10) and omitting the pro-social subscale. When the total score is above the 90th percentile, this has been found to increase the probability of an independently assessed psychiatric diagnostic by an odds ratio of 15.7 (Goodman, 2001). The cut off score is 3/4 for each subscale whereby scores of 0 to 2 are considered as 'normal', 3 as 'borderline' and 4 to 10 as 'abnormal' (Goodman, 1997).

The SDQ also includes an impact supplement that assesses the overall severity and chronicity of the problem, burden to others, child distress and interference in everyday life. The impact score is based on five items rated on a four-point scale ('no', 'minor', 'definite' or 'severe') (for example 'Do you think the young person has difficulties in one or more of the following areas: emotions, concentration, behaviour or being able to get on with other people?', 'Do the difficulties upset or distress your child?') (Goodman, 1999). These five questions ask about different domains such as home, life, friendship, classroom learning and leisure activities (Ford et al., 2003), which are the areas that the World Health Organization recommends assessing in the multi-axial classification of child and adolescent psychiatric disorders (World Health Organization, 1992).

The authors also developed a computerised diagnostic algorithm to calculate the probability of psychiatric disorders. It is based on the impact scores and the parent and teacher SDQ symptom scales together. The algorithm generates three levels of prediction (unlikely, possible or probable) of the existence of a psychiatric disorder generating different diagnoses (for example conduct problems and emotional problems).

The SDQ also includes a follow-up version for repeated administration, which can serve as an outcome measure for the assessment of treatment effects. The follow-up versions generate scores for comparison with baseline outcomes, which the authors refer to as 'added values'. The mean value is the difference between the expected and observed outcome at follow-up (formula = 2.3 + 0.8 (× baseline total difficulties score) + 0.2 (× 1 baseline impact score) − 0.3 × baseline emotional problems subscale score − follow-up total difficulties score). The scores are normally distributed (with a mean of 0 and standard deviation of 5 SDQ points); therefore, higher than 0 scores mean better than predicted adjustment whereas scores lower than 0 indicate worse than predicted adjustment (Ford et al., 2003).

A substantive body of research exists on the psychometric properties of this tool. Several studies show a sound internal consistency on the original five factor structure (with a mean Cronbach alpha of 0.73) (Goodman, 1999; Goodman, 2001); and a satisfactory test-retest stability based on a survey of 10,000 UK children and young people (4- to 6-month retest stability of 0.72) (Goodman, 1999). Correlations among parent, teacher and self-report SDQ scores are moderate (Goodman, 1997; Goodman, 2001; Goodman et al., 1998).

*Eyberg Child Behavior Inventory*

The ECBI is a rating scale used to assess disruptive behaviour for children between the ages of 2 and 16 years. It is an informant scale aimed at the children's parents. The scale consists of 36 disruptive behaviour items (for example refusing to obey until threatened with punishment, stealing, fighting, short attention span, over activity and restlessness). It measures two dimensions: first, intensity, which is the frequency of the behaviour with responses measuring how often the behaviour occurs, with scores of 1 (never), 2 and 3 (seldom), 4 (sometimes), 5 and 6 (often), and 7 (always); and second, problem identification, which is measured by a 'yes' or 'no' answer (rated 1 if the answer is positive). The intensity score ranges from 36 to 252 and the problem score from 0 to 36.

Children are considered likely to have a disruptive behaviour if they score above the 90th percentile or with the established cut-offs of 127 for the intensity score and 11 for the problem score (Burns & Patterson, 2000). A recent study reported cut-offs of 132 for intensity and 15 for the problem score – the need for more research is also suggested by the authors (Colvin et al., 1999).

The ECBI has good psychometric properties (Axberg et al., 2008; Burns & Patterson, 1991; Burns & Patterson, 2000; Eyberg, 1992; McMahon & Estes, 1997). Scores are stable over time for both children (Robinson et al., 1980) and young people (Eyberg & Robinson, 1983). Regarding the structure of the scale, although the existence of three subscales has been supported by some authors (Burns & Patterson, 1991), the latest study examining re-standardisation of the scale did not find a structure in factor analysis (Colvin et al., 1999; Eyberg & Pincus, 1999) as stated by the original authors (Eyberg & Robinson, 1983; Robinson et al., 1980).

This scale has been developed in the US and standardised with US normative data; it is not freely available, with the copyright belonging to Psychological Assessment Resources, and permission to use it is required. The authors recommend that those scoring the instrument have at least a 4-year degree in psychology, counselling or a related field, including coursework in the administration of psychological tests.

*Sutter–Eyberg Student Behavior Inventory*

The SESBI-R is a teacher-rated scale of disruptive school behaviour for children between the ages of 2 and 16 years. This instrument was designed to identify children who are in need of treatment for behavioural problems. The SESBI-R is a revision of the original SESBI and was constructed as a complement to the ECBI. The scale consists of 38 items, 11 of which are identical to the ECBI. Twelve items were slightly modified to match the educational environment and 15 additional new items were selected from a list of problem behaviours often reported by teachers of children who have been referred for treatment for behavioural problems (Querido & Eyberg, 2003). For example, items such as 'teases or provokes other children' were replaced with 'teases or provokes other students' to match classroom language.

The SESBI-R consists of disruptive behaviour items and some examples of these are 'refuses to obey until threatened with punishment', 'steals', 'physically fights' and 'has difficulty staying on task is overactive and restless'. The instrument comprises two dimensions: the intensity score, which assesses the frequency of occurrence of a variety of child behaviour problems, and the problem score, which assesses the degree to which the child's behaviour is a problem to the teacher (Eyberg & Pincus, 1999). The intensity score is rated using a seven-point Likert-type scale ranging from 1 (never) to 7 (always).

The SESBI-R has demonstrated satisfactory psychometric properties. The intensity and problem scores have shown high internal consistency coefficients (between 0.96 and 0.98) (Burns & Owen, 1990; Funderburk & Eyberg, 1989), high test-retest correlations (0.87 to 0.90 and 0.89 to 0.93, respectively) (Funderburk & Eyberg, 1989; Funderburk et al., 1989; Rayfield et al., 1998; Schaughency et al., 1989) and also high inter-rates reliability (Dumas, 1992; Funderburk & Eyberg, 1989).

### 6.2.5    Studies considered[45]

The literature search was conducted to identify studies that considered the case identification, diagnosis and assessment of conduct disorders. The outcome of this search for RCTs, observational studies and systematic reviews resulted in 22,434 papers (22,328 came from database searches and 106 were hand searched). Scanning the titles and abstracts of these papers resulted in 20,794 studies being excluded from the review because they did not meet eligibility criteria. Of these, a number of studies were not relevant to this guideline (20,794) because either they were outside the scope or were duplicates. This resulted in a total of 1,628 potential studies that reported instruments used in the assessment of conduct disorder in children or young people.

Upon further inspection of these 1,628 potential studies, 1,534 assessed instruments that were not specific to case identification or were longer than 5 minutes to administer. This resulted in 93 articles (see Appendix 16b for a list of instruments that were not included in the review and the reasons why, and a list of excluded studies and the reasons why). Of those, 11 were excluded because the instrument did not specifically screen for conduct disorders, 53 did not report sensitivity or specificity data and 29 reported instruments that had been translated into other languages other than English. (Note that it was decided to exclude these studies in the first instance because the translation of the scale might have compromised the validity of the scale. Further information about the included studies can be found in Appendix 16b).

Of the seven studies (N = 11,257) included in the review, five assessed the sensitivity and specificity of the SDQ and two assessed the ECBI. For the SDQ, two of the studies included the same sample drawn from a survey of mental health in British children between the ages of 5 and 15 years that was carried out in 1999 by the Office for National Statistics (so those 7,984 have not been added to the total number): GOODMAN2000A (Goodman et al., 2000a) and GOODMAN2001 (Goodman, 2001). Another study included a sample drawn from a survey of mental

---

[45]Here and elsewhere in the guideline, each study considered for review is referred to by a study ID in capital letters (primary author and date of study publication, except where a study is in press or only submitted for publication, then a date is not used).

health of British looked-after children which was carried out by the same organisation in 2001–2002, GOODMAN2004 (Goodman et al., 2004), while the other two studies included a sample taken from new referrals to mental health clinics: GOODMAN2000B (Goodman et al., 2000b) and MATHAI2004 (Mathai et al., 2004). Regarding the assessment of discriminate validity of the ECBI, two studies were included and both had samples from archival data, one from studies of stress, affect and parenting in families with young children, WEIS2005 (Weis et al., 2005), and the other from mothers of preschool-age children: RICH2001 (Rich & Eyberg, 2001).

### 6.2.6 Clinical evidence for case identification instruments

Review Manager 5 (The Cochrane Collaboration, 2011) was used to summarise the test accuracy data reported in each study using forest plots and summary ROC plots. Where more than two studies reported appropriate data, a bivariate test accuracy meta-analysis was conducted in order to obtain pooled estimates of sensitivity, specificity and likelihood ratios. These were calculated with the statistical package Meta-DiSc (Zamora et al., 2006) (see Chapter 3 for further details on test accuracy terms).

*Case identification of conduct disorder and oppositional defiant disorder*
The SDQ, ECBI and SESBI-R were the only instruments that met the inclusion criteria for suitable screening instruments because they were designed to identify children with possible conduct disorder and could be completed within 5 minutes. However, only sensitivity and specificity data were reported in the literature for two of those instruments (SDQ and ECBI). The SDQ assesses conduct behaviour and the ECBI assesses identified behavioural disorders including conduct disorder and oppositional defiant disorder. Although the ECBI was created as a one-dimensional scale, some authors have also demonstrated the multidimensional structure and identified conduct disorder and oppositional defiant disorder subscales (Burns & Patterson, 1991).

*Strengths and Difficulties Questionnaire*
Five studies that reported sensitivity and specificity data were identified in the searched studies. Two of them included children from new referrals to CAMHS (GOODMAN2000B, MATHAI2004) and three of them were large samples of British children drawn from national mental health surveys (GOODMAN2000A, GOODMAN2001, GOODMAN2004).

The SDQ includes three different versions that can be completed by parents or carers, teachers and the children themselves. The analysis showed that the sensitivity and specificity for the SDQ ranged from 'excellent' to 'poor', depending on who the informant was and how many of them completed the scales.

The best values in terms of sensitivity were found in studies were the SDQ was completed by multi-informants. That is, when the three versions were completed and an overall score was calculated with algorithms developed by the authors, the values were considered 'excellent' to 'good', ranging from 0.93 to 0.76. The next best values were when two informants (parent or carer and teacher) assessed the child's behaviour. Those values were considered 'good' to 'moderate' and ranged from 0.82 to 0.55 (see Figure 4). However, when the SDQ was completed by just one informant (either parent/carer or teacher), the values were considered 'moderate' and ranged from 0.68 to 0.55 except for the self-report form, which was rated as 'poor' with values between 0.16 and 0.29 (see Figure 4).

Specificity was reported in only a few studies and ranged from 'excellent' for single informants (0.96 to 0.91) to 'low' when completed by multi-informants (0.47). A summary ROC plot is provided in Figure 5.

## Figure 4: Forest plot of sensitivity and specificity for the SDQ

Forest plot SDQ one informant: parent form (children 4 to 17 years).

| Study | TP | FP | FN | TN | Sensitivity | Specificity | Sensitivity | Specificity |
|---|---|---|---|---|---|---|---|---|
| GOODMAN2001 | 317 | 858 | 149 | 8674 | 0.68 [0.64, 0.72] | 0.91 [0.90, 0.92] | | |

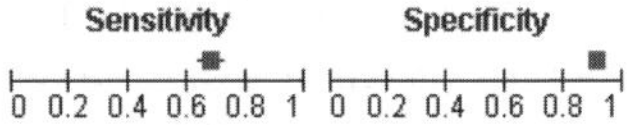

Forest plot SDQ one informant: teacher form (children 4 to 17 years).

| Study | TP | FP | FN | TN | Sensitivity | Specificity | Sensitivity | Specificity |
|---|---|---|---|---|---|---|---|---|
| GOODMAN2001 | 199 | 350 | 122 | 6642 | 0.62 [0.56, 0.67] | 0.95 [0.94, 0.95] | | |

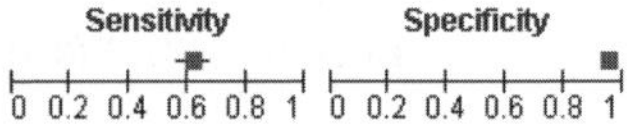

Forest plot of SDQ one informant: self-reported form (children 4 to 17 years)

| Study | TP | FP | FN | TN | Sensitivity | Specificity | Sensitivity | Specificity |
|---|---|---|---|---|---|---|---|---|
| GOODMAN2001 | 57 | 151 | 141 | 3634 | 0.29 [0.23, 0.36] | 0.96 [0.95, 0.97] | | |

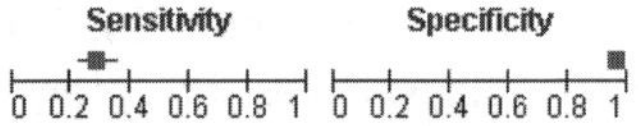

Forest plot of SDQ one informant: carer form (looked-after children 5 to 10 years).

| Study | TP | FP | FN | TN | Sensitivity | Specificity | Sensitivity | Specificity |
|---|---|---|---|---|---|---|---|---|
| GOOODMAN2004 | 51 | 0 | 42 | 0 | 0.55 [0.44, 0.65] | Not estimable | | |

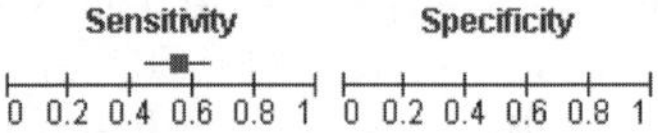

Forest plot of SDQ one informant: carer form (looked-after children 11 to 17 years).

| Study | TP | FP | FN | TN | Sensitivity | Specificity | Sensitivity | Specificity |
|---|---|---|---|---|---|---|---|---|
| GOOODMAN2004 | 58 | 0 | 38 | 0 | 0.60 [0.50, 0.70] | Not estimable | | |

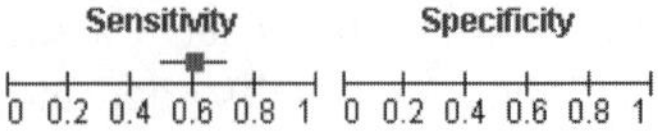

Forest plot of SDQ one informant: teacher form (looked-after children 5 to 10 years).

| Study | TP | FP | FN | TN | Sensitivity | Specificity | Sensitivity | Specificity |
|---|---|---|---|---|---|---|---|---|
| GOOODMAN2004 | 61 | 0 | 32 | 0 | 0.66 [0.55, 0.75] | Not estimable | | |

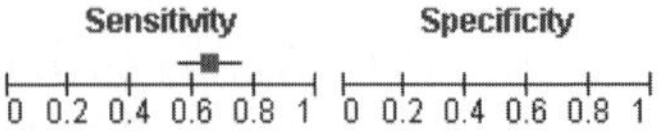

Forest plot of SDQ one informant: teacher form (looked-after children 11 to 17 years).

| Study | TP | FP | FN | TN | Sensitivity | Specificity | Sensitivity | Specificity |
|---|---|---|---|---|---|---|---|---|
| GOOODMAN2004 | 62 | 0 | 34 | 0 | 0.65 [0.54, 0.74] | Not estimable | | |

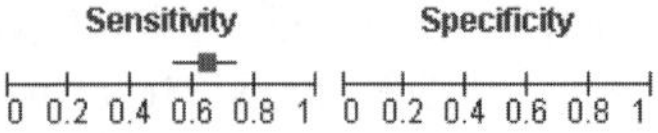

Forest plot of SDQ one informant: self-reported form (looked-after children 11 to 17 years).

| Study | TP | FP | FN | TN | Sensitivity | Specificity | Sensitivity | Specificity |
|---|---|---|---|---|---|---|---|---|
| GOOODMAN2004 | 15 | 0 | 81 | 0 | 0.16 [0.09, 0.24] | Not estimable | | |

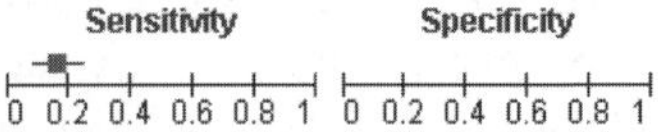

Forest plot of SDQ two informants: carer and teacher forms together (looked-after children 5 to 10 years).

| Study | TP | FP | FN | TN | Sensitivity | Specificity | Sensitivity | Specificity |
|---|---|---|---|---|---|---|---|---|
| GOOODMAN2004 | 79 | 0 | 14 | 0 | 0.85 [0.76, 0.92] | Not estimable | | |

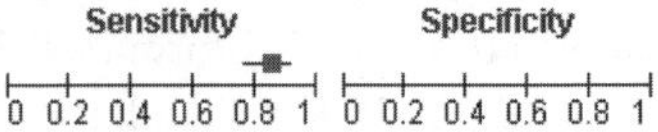

**Figure 4: (*Continued*)**

Forest plot of SDQ two informants: carer and teacher forms together (looked-after children 11 to 17 years).

| Study | TP | FP | FN | TN | Sensitivity | Specificity | Sensitivity | Specificity |
|---|---|---|---|---|---|---|---|---|
| GOOODMAN2004 | 86 | 0 | 10 | 0 | 0.90 [0.82, 0.95] | Not estimable | | |

0 0.2 0.4 0.6 0.8 1     0 0.2 0.4 0.6 0.8 1

Forest plot of SDQ two informants: carer and self-report forms together (looked-after children 11 to 17 years).

| Study | TP | FP | FN | TN | Sensitivity | Specificity | Sensitivity | Specificity |
|---|---|---|---|---|---|---|---|---|
| GOOODMAN2004 | 63 | 0 | 33 | 0 | 0.66 [0.55, 0.75] | Not estimable | | |

0 0.2 0.4 0.6 0.8 1     0 0.2 0.4 0.6 0.8 1

Forest plot of SDQ two informants: teacher and self-reported forms together (looked-after children 11 to 17 years)

| Study | TP | FP | FN | TN | Sensitivity | Specificity | Sensitivity | Specificity |
|---|---|---|---|---|---|---|---|---|
| GOOODMAN2004 | 66 | 0 | 30 | 0 | 0.69 [0.58, 0.78] | Not estimable | | |

0 0.2 0.4 0.6 0.8 1     0 0.2 0.4 0.6 0.8 1

Forest plot of SDQ three informants: carer, teacher and self-report forms (looked-after children 11 to 17 years).

| Study | TP | FP | FN | TN | Sensitivity | Specificity | Sensitivity | Specificity |
|---|---|---|---|---|---|---|---|---|
| GOOODMAN2004 | 87 | 0 | 9 | 0 | 0.91 [0.83, 0.96] | Not estimable | | |

0 0.2 0.4 0.6 0.8 1     0 0.2 0.4 0.6 0.8 1

Forest plot of SDQ three informants: multi-informant (parent, teacher and self-reported forms together) calculated with algorithms (children 4 to 17 years).

| Study | TP | FP | FN | TN | Sensitivity | Specificity | Sensitivity | Specificity |
|---|---|---|---|---|---|---|---|---|
| GOODMAN2000A | 292 | 0 | 91 | 0 | 0.76 [0.72, 0.80] | Not estimable | | |
| GOODMAN2000B | 43 | 28 | 5 | 25 | 0.90 [0.77, 0.97] | 0.47 [0.33, 0.61] | | |
| GOOODMAN2004 | 166 | 0 | 23 | 0 | 0.88 [0.82, 0.92] | Not estimable | | |
| MATHAI2004 | 111 | 0 | 8 | 0 | 0.93 [0.87, 0.97] | Not estimable | | |

0 0.2 0.4 0.6 0.8 1     0 0.2 0.4 0.6 0.8 1

*Note*: FN, false negative; FP, false positive; TN, true negative; TP, true positive.

### *Eyberg Child Behavior Inventory*

Two studies were identified that assessed discriminant validity of the ECBI (RICH2001, WEIS2005). Both studies included samples of mothers of children younger than 7 years old. The analysis showed excellent to good sensitivity for both sensitivity and specificity values in the two studies (sensitivity ranged from 0.75 to 0.96; specificity ranged from 0.87 to 0.94) (see Figures 6 and 7).

The pooled analysis for both sensitivity and specificity was rated as 'excellent', with values of 0.93 (95% CI, 0.24 to 0.91) for sensitivity and 0.91 (95% CI, 0.86 to 0.94) for specificity (see Figures 8 and 9 for forest plots, and see Figure 10 for ROC pane).

### 6.2.7 Clinical evidence summary

The initial review identified three instruments (the SDQ, ECBI and SESBI-R) that met the inclusion criteria as they screened for conduct disorders and took no longer than 5 minutes to complete. A total of seven studies were included in the review, five of them evaluated the test accuracy of the SDQ while two assessed the ECBI. No studies were identified that reviewed the sensitivity and specificity of the SESBI-R.

A summary of both scales' sensitivity and specificity data is presented in Table 37.

**Figure 5: Summary ROC plot for SDQ (note that only studies with both sensitivity and specificity values reported are charted here)**

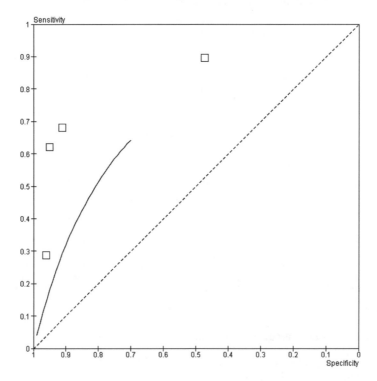

*Strengths and Difficulties Questionnaire*

The SDQ is a brief tool that, when parent and teacher versions are completed (to a lesser extent if only one version is completed), has the ability to identify children and young people with a conduct disorder. However, the self-report version does not appear to be a reliable method when used on its own and the detection values are not much improved when this form is combined with either the parent or teacher version.

It is important to note that although the evidence for the high sensitivity of the SDQ has been extracted from five studies, each of those studies assessed the discriminant validity of different forms and for different age groups. It is also important to mention that two of the five studies have the same sample. Because of this, it was not possible to carry out pooled analyses because the existing data could not be

**Figure 6: Forest plot of sensitivity and specificity for the ECBI**

| Study | TP | FP | FN | TN | Sensitivity | Specificity | Sensitivity | Specificity |
|-------|----|----|----|----|-------------|-------------|-------------|-------------|
| RICH2001 | 94 | 13 | 4 | 85 | 0.96 [0.90, 0.99] | 0.87 [0.78, 0.93] | | |
| WEIS2005 | 39 | 4 | 13 | 59 | 0.75 [0.61, 0.86] | 0.94 [0.85, 0.98] | | |

0 0.2 0.4 0.6 0.8 1  0 0.2 0.4 0.6 0.8 1

**Figure 7: Summary of ROC plot for ECBI**

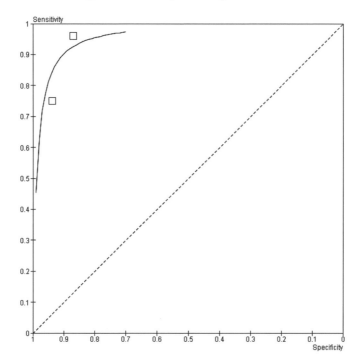

**Figure 8: Pooled data for sensitivity of the ECBI**

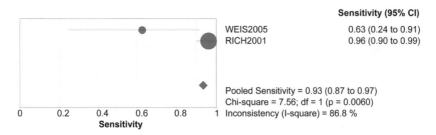

Sensitivity (95% CI)

WEIS2005    0.63 (0.24 to 0.91)
RICH2001    0.96 (0.90 to 0.99)

Pooled Sensitivity = 0.93 (0.87 to 0.97)
Chi-square = 7.56; df = 1 (p = 0.0060)
Inconsistency (I-square) = 86.8 %

**Figure 9: Pooled data for specificity of the ECBI**

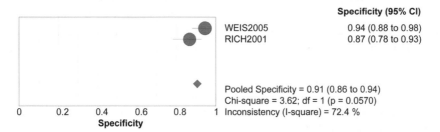

Specificity (95% CI)

WEIS2005    0.94 (0.88 to 0.98)
RICH2001    0.87 (0.78 to 0.93)

Pooled Specificity = 0.91 (0.86 to 0.94)
Chi-square = 3.62; df = 1 (p = 0.0570)
Inconsistency (I-square) = 72.4 %

**Figure 10: ROC pane for ECBI**

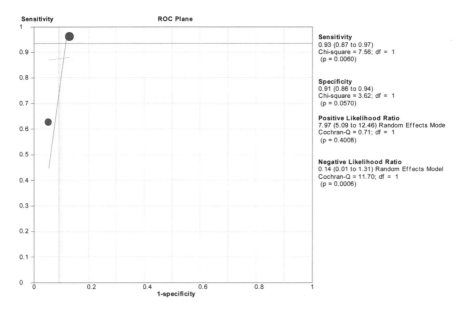

compared. In addition, some studies only reported sensitivity with no specificity, and ROC curves could not be generated for all studies. Therefore, the evidence comes from a small number of studies and should be treated with some caution.

The SDQ is a measure that allows for multi-informant reports and includes a supplement that assesses the impact of the disorder. In terms of scoring, it provides algorithms that calculate the probabilities of having the condition based on multi-informant reports and provides with 'added values' formulas to enable the scale to be used as a routinely outcome measure. The SDQ is freely available from the author's website (www.sdqinfo.org). The scale has been thoroughly validated and provides UK normative data.

*Eyberg Child Behavior Inventory*
The ECBI is a brief measure that assesses disruptive behaviour in children. This review identified two studies that assessed its discriminant validity (RICH2001, WEIS2005) and both included samples of children aged younger than 7 years.

The analysis showed excellent to good accuracy for both sensitivity and specificity values in both studies, and the analysis performed to pool the data was rated as excellent. However, it should be noted that the samples in both studies were relatively small and the prevalence of conduct disorders in each sample was also very low.

The ECBI is a parent-only scale and although there is a companion teacher scale available, no accuracy data were identified in the review. The scale is not freely available and can only be used with permission from the developers. The measure has been validated in a US population only.

**Table 37: Evidence summary table for all case identification instruments included in the review**[46]

| Instrument | Target condition | Number of informants/scale version | Cut-off | Participant age | Included studies | Sensitivity: specificity |
|---|---|---|---|---|---|---|
| SDQ | Conduct problems | 3 multi-informants (parent, teacher and self-reported) | 3 to 4 (conduct disorder subscale)/90th percentile | 4 to 17 years | 4 | 0.76 to 0.93: 0.47 |
| | Conduct problems | 3 multi-informants (parent, teacher and self-reported) | 3 to 4 (conduct disorder subscale)/90th percentile | 11 to 17 years* | 1 | 0.91: not estimable |
| | Conduct problems | 2 informants: (parent/carer and teacher) | 3 to 4 (conduct disorder subscale)/90th percentile | 5 to 10 years* | 1 | 0.85: not estimable |
| | Conduct problems | 2 informants: (parent/carer and teacher) | 3 to 4 (conduct disorder subscale)/90th percentile | 11 to 17 years* | 1 | 0.90: not estimable |
| | Conduct problems | 2 informants: (parent/carer and self-report) | 3 to 4 (conduct disorder subscale)/90th percentile | 11 to 17 years* | 1 | 0.66: not estimable |
| | Conduct problems | 2 informants: (teacher and self-report) | 3 to 4 (conduct disorder subscale)/90th percentile | 11 to 17 years* | 1 | 0.69: not estimable |
| | Conduct problems | 1 informant: (parent/carer) | 3 to 4 (conduct disorder subscale)/90th percentile | 4 to 17 years | 1 | 0.68: 0.91 |

*Continued*

[46]When data for an instrument is available from more than one study, a range of test data across the included studies is provided. See forest plots for individual data by study.

193

**Table 37:** (*Continued*)

| Instrument | Target condition | Number of informants/scale version | Cut-off | Participant age | Included studies | Sensitivity: specificity |
|---|---|---|---|---|---|---|
| | Conduct problems | 1 informant: (teacher) | 3 to 4 (conduct disorder subscale)/90th percentile | 4 to 17 years | 1 | 0.62: 0.95 |
| | Conduct problems | 1 informant (self-reported) | 3 to 4 (conduct disorder subscale)/90th percentile | 4 to 17 years | 1 | 0.29: not estimable |
| | Conduct problems | 1 informant (carer) | 3 to 4 (conduct disorder subscale)/90th percentile | 5 to 10 years* | 1 | 0.55: not estimable |
| | Conduct problems | 1 informant (carer) | 3 to 4 (conduct disorder subscale)/90th percentile | 11 to 17 years* | 1 | 0.60: not estimable |
| | Conduct problems | 1 informant (teacher) | 3 to 4 (conduct disorder subscale)/90th percentile | 5 to 10 years* | 1 | 0.66: not estimable |
| | Conduct problems | 1 informant (teacher) | 3 to 4 (conduct disorder subscale)/90th percentile | 11 to 17 years* | 1 | 0.65: not estimable |
| | Conduct problems | 1 informant (self-report) | 3 to 4 (conduct disorder subscale)/90th percentile | 11 to 17 years* | 1 | 0.16: not estimable |
| ECBI | Conduct disorder and oppositional defiant disorder | 1 informant: (parent) | 90th percentile | 2 to 6 years | 2 | 0.75 to 0.96: 0.87 to 0.94 |

*Looked-after children.

### 6.2.8    Assessment of conduct disorders

*The structure and content of the assessment process*
In the review of the literature, the GDG was unable to identify any formal evaluations of the structure and content of the overall clinical assessment process for children and young people with a suspected conduct disorder other than the data on the various case identification and assessment instruments described above. In light of this, the GDG drew on their expert knowledge and experience regarding the structure and content of a clinical assessment for children and young people and their parents and carers, and used informal consensus methods as set out in Chapter 3. When considering the assessment process, the GDG assumed that any child or young person referred for such an assessment would already have been identified as possibly having a conduct disorder or that there were concerns that they did.

*Assessment of conduct disorders.*  Given the variety of presentations of conduct disorders covered by this guideline, the need to be able to assess parental functioning and the family environment, and the high prevalence of comorbid conditions, the GDG was of the view that any assessment process should be undertaken by professionals who are trained and competent and have specific knowledge of conduct disorders and its assessment. The GDG were aware that many children with a conduct disorder may simply be regarded as being 'naughty or unpleasant'; in response to this, the GDG felt it was necessary to set out the criteria for a possible diagnosis and to alert those who are in contact with children and young people of these criteria and to have a proper index of suspicion. Equally importantly, the presence of comorbid conditions such as ADHD should not preclude a consideration of a diagnosis of conduct disorder.

The GDG was also of the view that the comprehensive assessment of children and young people and their parents or carers requires a broad range of skills and knowledge. The GDG considered it important that any professional undertaking an assessment should have access to support from a range of professionals with the requisite skills to contribute to a comprehensive assessment (for example the ability to undertake a full cognitive assessment). Given the variety of presentations of conduct disorder across different settings and situations, such as home, school and in peer groups, the GDG took the view that a family member or other carer with knowledge of the child or young person's personal history and a teacher or another person with knowledge of their school performance should be involved in the assessment. Although parental involvement was identified as key, it was also agreed by the GDG that the child or young person should be offered an interview on his or her own at some point in the assessment. This would provide an opportunity to explore issues such as potential abuse that may not always be possible to broach in the presence of a parent or carer. The GDG was also aware of the different context in which assessments may take place, for example at home, school or residential settings, and felt it was important that the structure and process of the assessment should be adapted to be compatible with the setting in which it was undertaken.

In considering the structure and content of an assessment for children and young people with a conduct disorder, the GDG was mindful of the mistrust that they might exhibit and potential difficulties in building a positive relationship with professionals, as described in Chapter 4. Clear explanations of the purpose of the assessment, prompt feedback and clarity about the communication of the outcome, along with a consistent person responsible for the assessment, would, in the view of the GDG, help to address these concerns and improve engagement with the assessment process. Being aware of a child's capacity to consent to be involved in the assessment process is also a crucial consideration.

The GDG took the view that the assessment of the family, and particularly parent functioning, was an important part of any comprehensive assessment. The key elements of such an assessment encompass positive and negative aspects of parenting including the use of coercion, the relationship with the wider family, the presence of domestic violence, the parent–child relationship, the physical and mental health of the parents and other family members and the involvement of any family members with the criminal justice system.

The GDG acknowledged that formal assessment tools might play a useful role in a comprehensive assessment of conduct disorder. The GDG agreed that the use of a measure such as the SDQ (Goodman, 1997), to help provide an overview of a child's difficulties, and the Child Behavior Checklist (CBCL) (Achenbach, 1991), to provide a more detailed quantitative assessment of a child or young person's behavioural problems, could be helpful when carrying out an assessment.

*Assessment of coexisting conditions.* The GDG recognised that comorbid conditions are very common in children and young people with a conduct disorder and can make the assessment of such disorders difficult. A number of commonly coexisting disorders should be considered as part of a comprehensive assessment, such as (a) learning disabilities or difficulties; (b) neurodevelopmental disorders, in particular, ADHD and autism; (c) mental disorders such as depression and bipolar disorder; (d) drug and alcohol misuse; (e) neurological disorders such as epilepsy; and (f) communication disorders such as speech and language problems. The GDG drew on their expert knowledge in a number of key areas. First, those comorbidities which, in their opinion, presented the most significant challenges in arriving at a diagnosis of conduct disorder, in that their presence may 'mask' the presence of conduct disorder and which may also have a significant bearing on the choice or likely success of the possible interventions available for the treatment of conduct disorder. The identified areas were cognitive ability, reading ability, ADHD, autism and comorbid mental health problems. Second, the GDG drew on its expert knowledge of well-validated measures of the areas identified above that are in use or are available for use in routine practice and therefore could readily be adopted (and, in a number of services, already are) for use as part of a comprehensive assessment. Based on this criteria, the GDG identified the following assessment instruments: the SDQ (Goodman, 1997) and the CBCL (Achenbach & Rescorla, 2001) for the identification of comorbid mental disorders; the Conners' Rating Scales – Revised (Conners et al., 1997) for ADHD; the Wechsler

Abbreviated Scale of Intelligence (Psychological Corporation, 1999; Wechsler, 2005) for the assessment of cognitive function, and the Wechsler Individual Achievement Test – Second UK Edition (Wechsler, 2005) for the assessment of reading difficulties. The GDG were unable to identify a single measure for the assessment of autism that, in their opinion, could be readily adopted into a comprehensive assessment for conduct disorder and therefore referred to the NICE guideline on the assessment and diagnosis of childhood autism (NICE, 2011a).

The CBCL has been well validated[47] and was frequently used as an outcome measure in the trials included in the review of treatment and prevention (see Chapter 5, Chapter 7 and Chapter 8). It also has the added advantage of having a number of syndrome and DSM-based scales. The empirically-based syndrome scales cover the following areas: anxious/depressed, withdrawn/depressed, somatic complaints, social problem, thought problems, attention problems, rule-breaking behaviour and aggressive behaviour. The six DSM-oriented scales are: affective problems, anxiety problems, somatic problems, attention deficit/hyperactivity problems, oppositional defiant problems and conduct problems. The SDQ[48] and Conners' Rating Scales – Revised[49] have been well validated and are recommended for use in the NICE clinical guideline for ADHD (NICE, 2009b).

*Risk assessment and management*
Children and young people with a conduct disorder are often vulnerable and at risk, because of their behaviour and the behaviour of others in their family or the surrounding environment; drug and alcohol misuse may further increase that risk. The GDG considered risk assessment and management to be an important area and, in developing their recommendations, drew on the advice developed for risk assessment in other relevant NICE guidelines – for example NICE (2009b). The GDG judged that any risk assessment of children and young people with conduct disorder should consider the risk of self-harm, in particular the risk of suicide in young people who are also depressed. Risk of harm to others also needs to be considered including harm to family members including siblings. Children and young people with a conduct disorder are perhaps most at risk of harm, including physical and sexual abuse from others, and the GDG was of the view that inquiry about this should form part of any comprehensive assessment.

*Assessing the needs of families and carers*
The GDG recognised the challenges faced by a family with a child or young person with a conduct disorder, and that consideration should be given to the assessment of parents' and carers' needs.

*Feedback following assessment*
The GDG considered how the outcome of a comprehensive assessment should be fed back to children and young people and their parents or carers. The view of the

---

[47]www.cebc4cw.org/assessment-tool/child-behavior-checklist-for-ages-6-18/
[48] www.cebc4cw.org/assessment-tool/strengths-and-difficulties-questionnaire/
[49] vinst.umdnj.edu/VAID/TestReport.asp?Code = CBRST

GDG was that there was a need for a comprehensive care plan, which should include specification of:

● the nature and extent of the conduct problems
● the nature and extent of any coexisting mental or physical disorders
● the level of personal, social, occupational, housing and educational needs
● the problems faced and their impact on families'/carers' needs
● the strengths and the needs of the young person and their family/carer
● which individuals and agencies may be involved in providing care
● how and to whom any information from the assessment will be communicated.

The GDG took the view that these should be fed back in a manner either that could be understood by a young person or in the presence of a family member or carer for a child.

The GDG also considered how the assessment might influence the choice and nature of the intervention offered to the child, young person and the family or carer. This topic was covered in the *Common Mental Health Disorders* (NICE, 2011b) guideline and was judged to be relevant to the current guideline. The GDG followed the methods outlined in Chapter 3 and adapted three recommendations relating to identifying the correct treatment options. Table 38 contains the original recommendations from *Common Mental Health Disorders* in column one, the original evidence base in column two and the adapted recommendations in column three. Where recommendations required adaptation, the rationale is provided in column four. In column one the numbers refer to the recommendations in the *Common Mental Health Disorders* NICE guideline (NICE, 2011b). In column three the numbers in brackets following the recommendation refer to Section 6.4 in this guideline.

*Common Mental Health Disorders* is an adult guideline; however, the GDG took the view that, as far as possible, the child or young person should be active participants in any decisions about the choice of intervention and that their preferences should be taken into account.

## 6.3    FROM EVIDENCE TO RECOMMENDATIONS

In drawing up recommendations on case identification and assessment, the GDG drew on the evidence review of case identification instruments in Sections 6.2.4 to 6.2.7 and the structured GDG discussion of the assessment process summarised in Section 6.2.8

### 6.3.1    Relative value placed on the outcomes considered

In considering case identification instruments, the primary outcome was the accurate detection of conduct disorders. A secondary concern was the clinical utility of the instrument and the possible generation of false positives with potentially negative consequences for a child or young person and their family or carers.

**Table 38: Recommendations from *Common Mental Health Disorders* (NICE, 2011b) for inclusion**

| Original recommendation from *Common Mental Health Disorders* | Evidence base of existing recommendation | Recommendation following adaptation for this guideline | Reasons for adaptation |
|---|---|---|---|
| 1.4.1.1  When discussing treatment options with a person with a common mental health disorder, consider:<br>• their past experience of the disorder<br>• their experience of, and response to, previous treatment<br>• the trajectory of symptoms<br>• the diagnosis or problem specification, severity and duration of the problem<br>• the extent of any associated functional impairment arising from the disorder itself or any chronic physical health problem<br>• the presence of any social or personal factors that may have a role in the development or maintenance of the disorder<br>• the presence of any comorbid disorders. | Review of five existing NICE guidelines covering common mental health disorders and six systematic reviews, and GDG expert opinon. See Chapter 6 (NCCMH, 2011). | When discussing treatment or care interventions with a child or young person with a conduct disorder and, if appropriate, their parents or carers, take account of:<br>• their past and current experience of the disorder<br>• their experience of, and response to, previous interventions and services<br>• the nature, severity and duration of the problem(s)<br>• the impact of the disorder on educational performance<br>• any chronic physical health problem<br>• any social or family factors that may have a role in the development or maintenance of the identified problem(s)<br>• any coexisting conditions. [6.4.1.18] | This recommendation was adapted to make it relevant to the specific needs of children and young people with a conduct disorder, such as the impact of the disorder on educational attainment. The impact of education was a recurrent theme identified in Chapter 4. |

*Continued*

199

**Table 38:** *(Continued)*

| Original recommendation from *Common Mental Health Disorders* | Evidence base of existing recommendation | Recommendation following adaptation for this guideline | Reasons for adaptation |
|---|---|---|---|
| 1.4.1.2   When discussing treatment options with a person with a common mental health disorder, provide information about:<br>• the nature, content and duration of any proposed intervention<br>• the acceptability and tolerability of any proposed intervention<br>• possible interactions with any current interventions<br>• the implications for the continuing provision of any current interventions. | Review of five existing NICE guidelines covering common mental health disorders and six systematic reviews, and GDG expert opion. See Chapter 6 (NCCMH, 2011). | When discussing treatment or care interventions with a child or young person and, if appropriate, their parents or carers, provide information about:<br>• the nature, content and duration of any proposed intervention<br>• the acceptability and tolerability of any proposed intervention<br>• the possible impact on interventions for any other behavioural or mental health problem | No significant adaptation required, except to clarify 'current interventions' in the original recommendation. |

| | | |
|---|---|---|
| • the implications for the continuing provision of any current interventions. [6.4.1.19] | | The original recommendation was adapted to refer to children and young people; no further adaptation was required. |
| 1.4.1.3   When making a referral for the treatment of a common mental health disorder, take account of patient preference when choosing from a range of evidence-based treatments. | Review of five existing NICE guidelines covering common mental health disorders and six systematic reviews, and GDG expert opion. See Chapter 6 (NCCMH, 2011). | When making a referral for treatment or care interventions for a conduct disorder, take account of the preferences of the child or young person and, if appropriate, their parents or carers when choosing from a range of evidence-based interventions. [6.4.1.20] |

### 6.3.2    Trade-off between clinical benefits and harms

Data were only available for two instruments for use as case identification instruments, the SDQ and the ECBI. For observer-administered forms, both had reasonable sensitivity and specificity, but the dataset for the SDQ was considerably larger and was based on UK samples. In addition, although the two instruments took the same time for administration, the SDQ provided important information about other aspects of a child or young person's mental health and is suitable for a wider age range. The SDQ can also be used as a routine outcome measure. For these reasons, the GDG decided to recommend the SDQ as an initial assessment instrument. However, it should be noted while the evidence suggests that the sensitivity of the SDQ is improved from moderate to excellent when multi-informants are used, the GDG recognised that for use in an initial assessment, for example in a primary care setting, it would not normally be feasible to use multiple informants.

No formal evaluation of systems for the assessment of children and young people with conduct disorder was identified. The GDG was therefore required to use its expert knowledge and experience in drawing up recommendations for the structure and content of the assessment process. The content of these discussions is described in Section 6.2.8. Given the limited formal evidence, for the process and content of the assessment as opposed to that for individual components of the assessment, the GDG was cautious in developing recommendations but was concerned to emphasise a number elements which it felt were essential to include in a comprehensive assessment for the child or young person with a conduct disorder. These included:

- responding to the concerns of parents, carers and professionals about the child or young person's behaviour
- being aware of comorbid disorders and their impact on both functioning and the assessment process itself
- ensuring competence in assessment skills
- actively involving the child or young person (with the opportunity to be interviewed alone) and the parents or carers
- fully assessing the child or young person's needs
- assessing parenting quality and the family environment
- using formal assessment scales to support the assessment process
- assessing risk
- developing a care plan that takes account of child or young person's and the parents' or carers' preferences and pays attention to the impact of previous interventions.

In developing the recommendations, the GDG sought to develop a structure for the assessment that: (a) took account of the different needs of children and young people and their parents or carers; (b) would facilitate the identification of effective interventions for the problems identified; (c) used well-validated instruments which were available for or were already in routine use; and (d) would best integrate with existing systems for the care and treatment of children and young people with a conduct disorder.

With regard to the assessment of coexisting conditions, the GDG recognised the importance of a comprehensive assessment, given the high rate of comorbidity. As part of this assessment, the GDG agreed that formal assessment instruments should be used to aid the diagnosis of coexisting conditions. Examples of validated instruments were given where appropriate.

With regard to developing recommendations for identifying effective treatment and care options, the technical team reviewed existing NICE mental health guidelines and found that the *Common Mental Health Disorders* guideline had covered this topic. After the technical team checked that the scope and review questions were appropriate, the GDG agreed that various degrees of adaptation were necessary (see Section 6.2.8). Regarding the evidence base that underpinned the existing guideline, as can be seen in Table 38, a relatively large number of existing NICE guidelines and published reviews were utilised, as well as considerable expert opinion. Because of the nature of the evidence utilised, and the fact the guideline was published relatively recently, it was agreed by the GDG that any new evidence was unlikely to change the existing recommendations and, therefore, adaptation was appropriate.

### 6.3.3 Quality of the evidence

The methodological quality of the evidence included in the review of case identification instruments was generally adequate. However, some important aspects covered by the checklist (for example whether the reference standard results were blinded) were rated as unclear. In addition, only two studies of the ECBI provided appropriate data and there were no studies of the SESBI-R.

## 6.4 RECOMMENDATIONS

### 6.4.1 Clinical practice recommendations

*Working safely and effectively with children and young people*
6.4.1.1 Health and social care professionals working with children and young people who present with behaviour suggestive of a conduct disorder, or who have a conduct disorder, should be trained and competent to work with children and young people of all levels of learning ability, cognitive capacity, emotional maturity and development.

*Initial assessment of children and young people with a possible conduct disorder*
6.4.1.2 Adjust delivery of initial assessment methods to:
● the needs of children and young people with a suspected conduct disorder **and**
● the setting in which they are delivered (for example, health and social care, educational settings or the criminal justice system).

6.4.1.3    Undertake an initial assessment for a suspected conduct disorder if a child or young person's parents or carers, health or social care professionals, school or college, or peer group raise concerns about persistent antisocial behaviour.

6.4.1.4    Do not regard a history of a neurodevelopmental condition (for example, attention deficit hyperactivity disorder [ADHD]) as a barrier to assessment.

6.4.1.5    For the initial assessment of a child or young person with a suspected conduct disorder, consider using the Strengths and Difficulties Questionnaire (completed by a parent, carer or teacher).

6.4.1.6    Assess for the presence of the following significant complicating factors:
● a coexisting mental health problem (for example, depression, post-traumatic stress disorder)
● a neurodevelopmental condition (in particular ADHD and autism)
● a learning disability or difficulty
● substance misuse in young people.

6.4.1.7    If any significant complicating factors are present refer the child or young person to a specialist CAMHS for a comprehensive assessment.

6.4.1.8    If no significant complicating factors are present consider direct referral for an intervention.

*Comprehensive assessment*

6.4.1.9    A comprehensive assessment of a child or young person with a suspected conduct disorder should be undertaken by a health or social care professional who is competent to undertake the assessment and should:
● offer the child or young person the opportunity to meet the professional on their own
● involve a parent, carer or other third party known to the child or young person who can provide information about current and past behaviour
● if necessary involve more than one health or social care professional to ensure a comprehensive assessment is undertaken.

6.4.1.10    Before starting a comprehensive assessment, explain to the child or young person how the outcome of the assessment will be communicated to them. Involve a parent, carer or advocate to help explain the outcome.

6.4.1.11    The standard components of a comprehensive assessment of conduct disorders should include asking about and assessing the following:
● core conduct disorders symptoms including:
  – patterns of negativistic, hostile, or defiant behaviour in children aged under 11 years
  – aggression to people and animals, destruction of property, deceitfulness or theft and serious violations of rules in children aged over 11 years
● current functioning at home, at school or college and with peers
● parenting quality
● history of any past or current mental or physical health problems.

6.4.1.12    Take into account and address possible coexisting conditions such as:
● learning difficulties or disabilities
● neurodevelopmental conditions such as ADHD and autism

- neurological disorders including epilepsy and motor impairments
- other mental health problems (for example, depression, post-traumatic stress disorder and bipolar disorder)
- substance misuse
- communication disorders (for example, speech and language problems).

6.4.1.13    Consider using formal assessment instruments to aid the diagnosis of coexisting conditions such as:

- the Child Behavior Checklist for all children and young people
- the Strengths and Difficulties Questionnaire for all children or young people
- the Conners Rating Scales – Revised for a child or young person with suspected ADHD
- a validated measure of autistic behaviour for a child or young person with a suspected autism spectrum disorder (see *Autism: Recognition, Referral and Diagnosis of Children and Young People on the Autistic Spectrum* [NICE clinical guideline 128])
- a validated measure of cognitive ability for a child or young person with a suspected learning disability
- a validated reading test for a child or young person with a suspected reading difficulty.

6.4.1.14    Assess the risks faced by the child or young person and if needed develop a risk management plan for self-neglect, exploitation by others, self-harm or harm to others.

6.4.1.15    Assess for the presence or risk of physical, sexual and emotional abuse in line with local protocols for the assessment and management of these problems.

6.4.1.16    Conduct a comprehensive assessment of the child or young person's parents or carers, which should cover:

- positive and negative aspects of parenting, in particular any use of coercive discipline
- the parent–child relationship
- positive and negative adult relationships within the child or young person's family, including domestic violence
- parental wellbeing, encompassing mental health, substance misuse (including whether alcohol or drugs were used during pregnancy) and criminal behaviour.

6.4.1.17    Develop a care plan with the child or young person and their parents or carers that includes a profile of their needs, risks to self or others, and any further assessments that may be needed. This should encompass the development and maintenance of the conduct disorder and any associated behavioural problems, any coexisting mental or physical health problems and speech, language and communication difficulties, in the context of:

- any personal, social, occupational, housing or educational needs
- the needs of parents or carers
- the strengths of the child or young person and their parents or carers.

*Case identification and assessment*

*Identifying effective treatment and care options*

6.4.1.18  When discussing treatment or care interventions with a child or young person with a conduct disorder and, if appropriate, their parents or carers, take account of:
- their past and current experience of the disorder
- their experience of, and response to, previous interventions and services
- the nature, severity and duration of the problem(s)
- the impact of the disorder on educational performance
- any chronic physical health problem
- any social or family factors that may have a role in the development or maintenance of the identified problem(s)
- any coexisting conditions[50].

6.4.1.19  When discussing treatment or care interventions with a child or young person and, if appropriate, their parents or carers, provide information about:
- the nature, content and duration of any proposed intervention
- the acceptability and tolerability of any proposed intervention
- the possible impact on interventions for any other behavioural or mental health problem
- the implications for the continuing provision of any current interventions[51].

6.4.1.20  When making a referral for treatment or care interventions for a conduct disorder, take account of the preferences of the child or young person and, if appropriate, their parents or carers when choosing from a range of evidence-based interventions[52].

---

[50]Adapted from *Common Mental Health Disorders* (NICE Clinical Guideline 123).
[51]Adapted from *Common Mental Health Disorders* (NICE Clinical Guideline 123).
[52]Adapted from *Common Mental Health Disorders* (NICE Clinical Guideline 123).

# 7 PSYCHOLOGICAL/PSYCHOSOCIAL INDICATED PREVENTION AND TREATMENT INTERVENTIONS

## 7.1 INTRODUCTION

Multifactorial causal factors have been identified in relation to conduct disorder (for example social deprivation issues, family interactions, individual developmental factors and peer relationships), and a wide potential spectrum of challenges are associated with a diagnosis of conduct disorder (for example problems at home, in school and in the community). For these reasons, psychological interventions for conduct disorders have been developed across a wide spectrum from those focused on the psychological wellbeing of the individual child to those which incorporate familial and social domains. The interventions currently available have also been developed from a range of theoretical frameworks, from those based on social learning theory to more individually conceptualised cognitive behavioural therapy (CBT) approaches, systemic approaches and psychodynamic approaches. This chapter reviews evidence of the clinical effectiveness (and, where possible, the cost effectiveness) for the range of interventions which can be described broadly as coming within the 'psychosocial' sphere. For the purposes of the review, the interventions have been grouped around their key focus of delivery (see Section 7.2.1). It should be noted that any system of categorisation has elements of arbitrariness and is subject to boundary disputes.

### 7.1.1 Indicated prevention and treatment interventions

As discussed in Chapter 5, a distinction can be made between prevention and treatment interventions, and within prevention interventions a further distinction can be made between universal, selective and indicated interventions. Separate review questions were initially developed for selective, indicated and treatment interventions (universal interventions were excluded from the scope; further information about each category can be found in the full review protocols presented in Appendix 15).

After the evidence had been synthesised, it became evident that there was considerable overlap between trials of indicated prevention and treatment interventions, both in terms of (a) the sample of participants recruited, as shown by recruitment methods and baseline symptom scores, and (b) the interventions offered. Although selective prevention interventions show some similarity with treatment interventions, the sample is by definition very different, as recruitment of children and young people is based on individual risk factors (for example low school achievement), family risk factors (for example antisocial parents) or socioeconomic risk factors (for example low family income).

Because of the overlap between indicated prevention and treatment intervention trials, a decision was made to combine these in the review presented in this chapter. The GDG suggested that doing this not only makes sense clinically but also allows for statistical methods to be used to examine whether there is any difference in intervention effectiveness.

## 7.2    CLINICAL EVIDENCE REVIEW

### 7.2.1    Categorisation of interventions

For the purposes of the guideline, interventions were categorised as:
● child-focused (delivered to child only)
● parent-focused (delivered to parent only)
● foster carer-focused (delivered to foster carer only)
● parent–child-based (separate interventions delivered to parent and child)
● parent–teacher-based (separate interventions delivered to parent and teacher)
● family-focused (delivered to the family)
● multimodal (integrated approach involving the family and community)
● multi-component (separate interventions delivered to parents, child, and family or school)
● classroom-based – teacher involved (programmes delivered in classrooms and involving a teacher[53])
● classroom-based – other, non-teacher, involved (programmes delivered in classrooms, but involving someone other than a teacher).

The guideline scope also included social care, vocational, educational and community interventions, and work with peer groups. However, no trials were identified that could be included in these categories and, therefore, these interventions are not reviewed further.

*Child-focused interventions*
Most carefully-evaluated methods of intervention for conduct disordered children are based on behavioural or cognitive behavioural principles. There are also treatments utilising humanistic or psychodynamic methods, including those based on attachment theory, but on the whole these have not been evaluated rigorously and are less supported by the existing evidence. The evidence base is more extensive for cognitive behavioural approaches, a broad term referring to a variety of methods that help a young person learn to identify the connections between their thoughts, feelings and behaviour, so that they can learn to change one by adjusting another

---

[53]The intervention could be delivered to a group of teachers who were trained to use the intervention in the classroom.

(for example learning to change their automatic thoughts about another person's hostile intentions in order to change their own standard behavioural response of being aggressive, or changing their behaviour starting to do an activity that gives them a sense of achievement in order to change their mood). Cognitive behavioural approaches typically involve three stages: first, psychoeducation (to help the young person understand more about their own thoughts, behaviour and mood and the links between these); second, identification with the young person of areas to try to work on; and third, a program of learning and practicing those new patterns and seeing what effect they have. Cognitive behavioural approaches for children or young people might be delivered individually or in the context of group sessions. Duration of treatment will vary with the severity of the problems, but could involve up to 25 or 30 weekly sessions. Programmes that intervene with individual children and young people include those that seek to improve social skills, often referred to as social skills training, helping them to utilise social behaviours that instigate and maintain positive responses from others. Other approaches focus on the control of negative mood, such as anger coping or management training, where techniques are learned to self-monitor changes of emotion, identify triggers of feelings of anger or aggression, and techniques developed to diffuse them. Problem-solving skills-training helps the individual to understand links between their own behaviour and its consequences, and generate responses that are more likely to produce prosocial outcomes. In all these methods, structured tasks may be introduced, based on real-life situations that are meaningful to the young person, and various treatment components are utilised such as in vivo practice, role play and homework. Finally, child-focused psychosocial interventions may be offered to individual children in the school setting rather than the clinic setting.

*Parent-focused interventions*
The main goals of parenting interventions are to enable parents to improve their child's behaviour and to improve their relationship with their child. In the majority of programmes, this is undertaken through helping parents learn behaviour-management principles grounded in social-learning theory. There are many different types of parent-focused interventions (often described as parent-training or education programmes). Many are conducted primarily with the parents and involve no direct intervention with the child. However, in some individual programmes both parent and child will be present in sessions and the therapist will coach the parent directly, in play with their child, to help them strengthen the relationship with their child and learn more effective parenting skills. There are two main types of programme, behavioural and relationship, but most parenting programmes combine elements of both (Gould & Richardson, 2006). Behavioural programmes focus on helping parents learn skills needed to address the causes of problem behaviours. Relationship programmes aim to help parents understand both their own and their child's emotions and behaviour, and to improve their communication with their child.

Parent-focused interventions tend to be intensive and short term, usually 1.5 to 2 hours every week for 8 to 12 weeks. They can be held in a variety of settings, including the hospital, clinic, community or home, and they can be conducted either in groups, typically of six to 12 participants, or individually. Ideally programmes are provided in a congenial setting, accessible by parents and with crèche facilities for children and siblings. Programmes can be run by a range of helping professionals including psychologists, therapists, nurses, counsellors, social workers or community workers, and, in some, parents who have been through programmes can themselves can be involved. Some parent-training/education programmes can also be self-administered in the home, using printed training materials or audiovisual training tools such as videos.

Some parent-training programmes contain specific additional elements to help address factors interfering with effective parenting, such as marital problems, depression and lack of adult social skills, as well as their children's behaviour problems. Programmes may also combine parent training with other interventions such as child programmes based on social learning theory.

*Parent-focused interventions (which include the child in at least some sessions)*
Parent–child interaction therapy was developed originally by Hanf and is based on a two-staged intervention model (Querido & Eyberg, 2005). The overall objective is to help parents learn the skills necessary to establish a nurturing and secure relationship with the child whose behaviour is disruptive, while shifting the balance of the child's behaviour from the negative to prosocial. The first phase focuses on building the parent–child bond through play, through which child social skills and parenting skills are supported, and the second phase is similar to CBT in helping the parent to set realistic expectations, improve consistency and fairness, and reducing reinforcement of negative behaviour. This mode of therapy draws at the theoretical level on Baumrind's developmental studies which identified associations between parenting styles, as well as attachment and social learning theories (Foote et al., 1998).

*Family-focused interventions*
Family therapy is a generic term for a range of approaches to engaging with the whole family, together with the child or young person, to address problematic behaviours including communication patterns, discipline or supervision. The assumption underpinning most forms of family therapy where conduct disorders are being addressed is that family interactions can maintain or worsen conduct problems; consequently, the family needs to be included as a critical agent of change. Various approaches to family therapy have been developed; those most prominent in the treatment of conduct disorders are described below.

Strategic family therapy takes as its therapeutic focus the internal organisation of the family, its cohesion and role structure. Conduct problems are viewed as resulting from malfunctioning of family systems, as a response to which the family seeks to regain or maintain equilibrium and any threats whether external or internal are met by attempts to attain self-stabilisation. Family therapists adopting a strategic approach attempt to influence family interactions or shared family assumptions and to reorganise or re-establish family hierarchies and patterns of emotional engagement that are adaptive and productive.

Functional family therapy is a manualised form of systemic family therapy for adolescent conduct disorders that is designed to intervene in ways that closely match the family relationships and culture. Conduct problems are conceptualised as communications that may serve some function in the family environment and which are maintained by family interactions. Functional family therapy is a phased and developmental model. In the initial phases, the focus is on engaging and motivating family members who are characteristically caught up in negative interaction cycles of negativity and blame. Family sessions typically take place in the family home and the emphasis is on breaking down barriers that could prevent the family members engaging in treatment. In the behaviour change phase, the focus is on facilitating competent family problem-solving, and using a range of parenting and CBT interventions to reduce child conduct problems and improve the parent–child relationship. In the generalisation phase, families learn to apply new skills in a range of situations and to deal with setbacks, and are assisted to engage more fully with community resources (Alexander & Robbins, 2010). Whole family sessions are conducted according to family need, often two or three times a week initially but reducing in intensity over the course of treatment, which spans between eight and 30 sessions over 3 to 6 months. Thus, functional family therapy attempts to influence and alter family interactions and beliefs, improve communication patterns to support more appropriate functioning, and help the child and parent develop specific skills.

## Multimodal interventions

Ecological or 'milieu' interventions aim to impact on the entire ecosystem or 'milieu' in which the child or young person operates – the focus is on changing the environment around the young person, in order to change the young person's behaviour. Multisystemic therapy was specifically developed for working with conduct-disordered adolescents (Henggeler et al., 1998) and takes antisocial behaviour to be caused and sustained by multiple factors, any of which may be intervened with during multisystemic therapy, using a range of evidence-based intervention methods. In keeping with parent-based approaches, the primary caregiver is seen as the primary agent of change, but rather than focusing primarily on the parent–child relationship as is done in parent training, which is aimed at younger children, the primary caregiver is instead encouraged to take part in developing and delivering interventions across home, school, the local community and so on. The aim of multisystemic therapy is to enable the 'systems' around the young person to effectively manage the young person in a way that reduces their antisocial behaviour. The particular foci of treatment vary between families, in keeping with the varied causes of conduct disorder between young people, so that in one family there may be a strong focus on helping the parent to manage peer relationships and school issues, whereas in another the focus may be on reducing conflict in the parental couple relationship to reduce the modelling of aggression in the home (Littell et al., 2005). A package of intervention is negotiated with the family and other key stakeholders that is complex, multifaceted and time limited but, crucially, is highly individualised to meet the needs of the young person and the family. Crucially, multisystemic therapy interventions are designed to be delivered in a way that engages hard-to-reach families, and so include a number of key differences from standard practice such as delivery via one multi-skilled therapist rather than several different agencies, delivery of interventions entirely in the community rather than a clinic at locations and times that suit the family (including evenings and weekends), and provision of a 24-hour duty cover system to ensure that families receive support from the multisystemic therapy team when crises are actually occurring. Finally, there is a significant focus from the outset on sustainability and generalisation of skills, so that the therapist will always be looking at how to develop the ability of the immediate network (that is, the primary caregiver, their social supports and the school) to create change, rather than expediting change by creating it themselves. For example, if it seems appropriate that a young person is encouraged to become involved in some new prosocial evening activities, a multisystemic therapy therapist would not simply arrange these and escort the young person to them, but would rather help the primary caregiver to think about whether such activities might make a difference to the young person's behaviour and, if they would, to learn how to find out about local activities and make a plan for how to get the young person there.

An alternative way of providing an ecological intervention is to temporarily move a young person out of their existing family system and into a network that is better equipped and supported to address their needs, in order to start to create change for them, and at the same time work with their original family system, with a view to rehabilitation at home. These are the key elements of MTFC, which could be considered as a fostering equivalent to multisystemic therapy because it also targets multiple settings and determinants of antisocial behaviour. Based on social learning theory and the work of the Oregon Social Learning Centre, MTFC uses the foster home as the primary site of intervention. The 'treatment team' is comprised of the foster carers and a multidisciplinary clinical team working together under the leadership of an experienced clinician. Treatment plans for the young person are highly individualised, and designed and co-ordinated across the treatment team including within the foster care home. MTFC works across family, school and peer settings but with specially trained and selected foster carers as key agents of change (Liabø & Richardson, 2007). The clinical team provides a range of CBT interventions that are specific to the child's problems. The young person also becomes involved in a range of activities that are selected to maximise exposure to positive influences. Foster carers have access to resources and support services on a 24-hour basis, which are provided by the clinical team. One key difference between MTFC and multisystemic therapy (apart from the difference in setting) is that in MTFC a number of clinical staff will be involved in delivering interventions related to a particular child, whereas in multisystemic therapy usually only one therapist would work directly with a family (although the whole team would be involved in treatment planning).

*Classroom-based interventions*
The school is one of the targets that may be the subject of interventions in multi-modal approaches such as multisystemic therapy and MTFC, but some approaches

to addressing conduct disorders take the school as the primary focus of intervention. The rationale for classroom-based approaches include the preponderance of time children spend in school, the variability of levels of conduct disturbance in schools that are matched on other relevant variables, the finding that children with conduct problems improve or deteriorate in their behaviour in the direction of the school milieu to which they move, and the finding that the level of behavioural disturbance in a school correlates with organisational characteristics (Fonagy et al., 2002). Classroom-based interventions targeted at children and young people with conduct disorders include interventions aimed at different system levels, from the behaviour of the teacher, to classroom-based contingency programmes, to so-called 'ecosystemic' approaches which seek to influence the culture of a whole school. Interventions tend to be broadly based on social learning theory, for example interventions aimed at teacher behaviour generally seek to encourage increased responsiveness in attending to and rewarding the prosocial behaviour of disruptive children, and refraining from responses that reward antisocial behaviour. Contingency management programmes have also been developed that seek to engage the class, using token economy methods or social learning approaches to decrease disruptive behaviour and reduce aggression. Ecosystemic approaches include school-wide methods such as that developed by Olweus (1994) to reduce bullying in schools. A number of other programmes designed to improve conflict resolution and reduce aggressive behaviour are relevant to the management of conduct disordered children, although evaluations of such programmes tend not to include clinical diagnosis of conduct disorder or oppositional defiant disorder as a variable.

*Multi-component interventions*
For the purposes of the guideline, multi-component interventions were defined as those that used any combination of the interventions described above. In practice, trials often tested the combination of child-focused, parent-focused and classroom-based interventions. Multi-component interventions are distinct from multimodal interventions, as there is no attempt to change the environment around the child.

### 7.2.2   Clinical review protocol

A summary of the review protocol, including the review questions, information about the databases searched, and the eligibility criteria used for this section of the guideline, can be found in Table 39 (a complete list of review questions can be found in Appendix 5; further information about the search strategy can be found in Appendix 7; the full review protocols can be found in Appendix 15).

The review strategy was to evaluate the clinical effectiveness of the interventions using meta-analysis. However, in the absence of adequate data, the available evidence was synthesised using narrative methods. Consideration was given as to whether any amendments due to common mental health disorders are needed. Studies of children with subaverage IQ (where mean of sample was above 60) will be analysed separately. Studies with a mean IQ of below 60 were excluded.

**Table 39:  Clinical review protocol for the review of indicated prevention and psychological/psychosocial treatment interventions**

| Component | Description |
|---|---|
| Review questions* | • What indicated prevention interventions for at risk individuals (including children/young people or their parents/families/carers) reduce the likelihood of children and young people developing a conduct disorder? (RQ-A1b)<br>• For children and young people with conduct disorders, what are the benefits and potential harms associated with individual and group psychosocial interventions? (RQ-E1)<br>• For children and young people with conduct disorders, what are the benefits and potential harms associated with parenting and family interventions? (RQ-E2)<br>• For children and young people with conduct disorders, what are the benefits and potential harms associated with multimodal interventions? (RQ-E3)<br>• For children and young people with conduct disorders, what are the benefits and potential harms associated with school behaviour management? (RQ-E6)<br>• For children and young people with conduct disorders, should interventions found to be safe and effective be modified in any way in light of coexisting conditions (such as ADHD, depression, anxiety disorders, attachment insecurity) or demographics (such as age, particular black and minority ethnic groups, or gender)? (RQ-E7) |
| Objectives | • To evaluate the clinical effectiveness and safety of indicated prevention and treatment interventions for conduct disorders<br>• To evaluate if any modifications should be made to interventions to take into account co-existing conditions or demographic variation. |
| Population | Children and young people (aged 18 years and younger), including looked-after children and those in contact with the criminal justice system, diagnosed with a conduct disorder, including oppositional defiant disorder, or with persistent offending behaviour, or high risk with minimal but detectable signs or symptoms foreshadowing a diagnosis (conduct disorder and ODD are characterised by repetitive and persistent patterns of antisocial, aggressive or defiant behaviour that amounts to significant and persistent violations of age-appropriate social expectations). |

*Continued*

**Table 39:** (***Continued***)

| Component | Description |
|---|---|
| Intervention(s) | • **Child-focused** (for example social skills training).<br>• **Parent-focused** (for example Incredible Years Parent Training; Triple P).<br>• **Foster carer focused** (for example Keeping Foster Parents Trained and Supported).<br>• **Parent–child-based** (for example Incredible Years Parent Training + Incredible Years Dina Dinosaur Child Training).<br>• **Parent–teacher-based** (for example the early impact intervention for parents and for teachers).<br>• **Family-focused** (for example functional family therapy).<br>• **Multimodal** (for example multisystemic therapy).<br>• **Multi-component** (for example Incredible Years – Teacher Classroom Management Program + Incredible Years Parent Training + Incredible Years Dina Dinosaur Child Training).<br>• **Classroom-based** (for example Incredible Years – Teacher Classroom Management Program). |
| Comparison | Treatment as usual, no treatment, waitlist control, active control, other active interventions. |
| Critical outcomes | Child outcomes:<br>• agency contact (for example residential care, criminal justice system)<br>• antisocial behaviour (at home, at school, in the community)<br>• drug/alcohol use<br>• educational attainment (that is, the highest level of education completed)<br>• offending behaviour<br>• school exclusion due to antisocial behaviour. |
| Electronic databases** | Mainstream databases:<br>• Embase, MEDLINE, PreMEDLINE, PsycINFO.<br><br>Topic specific databases and grey literature databases (see search strategy in Appendix 7). |
| Date searched | Inception to June 2012. |
| Study design | RCT |

*Under 'Review questions', the review question reference (for example RQ-A1) can be used to cross-reference against the full review protocol in Appendix 15.
**In addition to electronic databases, the following guidance documents were hand-reference searched: the NICE technology appraisal guidance 102 (NICE, 2006) and the NICE Clinical Practice Guideline Number 77 on antisocial personality disorder (NCCMH, 2010); four Cochrane reviews were also hand-reference searched (Furlong et al., 2012; Littell et al., 2005; Montgomery et al., 2006; Woolfenden et al., 1999).

### 7.2.3 Studies considered[54]

202 RCTs (N = 26,422) met the eligibility criteria for this review: AUGUST2001 (August et al., 2001), AUGUST2003 (August et al., 2003), AUGUST2006 (August et al., 2006), ADAMS2001 (Adams, 2001), ALEXANDER1973 (Alexander, 1973), ARBUTHNOT1986 (Arbuthnot & Gordon, 1986), AUGIMERI2007 (Augimeri et al., 2007), AZRIN2001 (Azrin et al., 2001), BAKER-HENNINGHAM2009 (Baker-Henningham et al., 2009), BAKER-HENNINGHAM2012 (Baker-Henningham et al., 2012), BANK1991 (Bank et al., 1991), BARRETT2000 (Barrett et al., 2000), BAUER2000 (Bauer et al., 2000), BEHAN2001 (Behan et al., 2001), BERNAL1980 (Bernal et al., 1980), BODENMANN2008 (Bodenmann, 2008), BORDUIN1995 (Borduin et al., 1995), BORDUIN2002 (Borduin & Schaeffer, 2002), BRADLEY2003 (Bradley et al., 2003), BRAET2009 (Braet et al., 2009), BRASWELL1997 (Braswell et al., 1997), BUSHMAN2010 (Bushman & Peacock, 2010), BUTLER2011 (Butler et al., 2011), BYWATER2011 (Bywater et al., 2011), CARNES-HOLT2010 (Carnes-Holt, 2010), CAVELL2000 (Cavell & Hughes, 2000), CEBALLOS2010 (Ceballos & Bratton, 2010), CHAMBERLAIN1998 (Chamberlain & Reid, 1998), CHAMBERLAIN2007 (Chamberlain et al., 2007), CHAMBERLAIN2008 (Chamberlain et al., 2008), CHAO2006 (Chao et al., 2006), CHENEY2009 (Cheney et al., 2009), CHOI2010 (Choi et al., 2010), CLARK1994 (Clark et al., 1994), COATSWORTH2001 (Coatsworth et al., 2001), CONNELL1997 (Connell et al., 1997), CPPRG1999 (Conduct Problems Prevention Research Group, 1999), CUMMINGS2008 (Cummings & Wittenberg, 2008), CUNNINGHAM1995 (Cunningham et al., 1995), DADDS1992 (Dadds & McHugh, 1992), DEFFENBACHER1996 (Deffenbacher et al., 1996), DEMBO1997 (Dembo et al., 1997), DEMBO2001 (Dembo et al., 2001), DESBIENS2003 (Desbiens & Royer, 2003), DIRKS-LINHORST2003 (Dirks-Linhorst, 2003), DISHION1995 (Dishion & Andrews, 1995), DISHION2008 (Dishion et al., 2008), DODGEN1995 (Dodgen, 1995), DOZIER2006 (Dozier et al., 2006), DRUGLI2006 (Drugli & Larsson, 2006), DUPPER1993 (Dupper & Krishef, 1993), ELIAS2003 (Elias et al., 2003), ELROD1992 (Elrod & Minor, 1992), EMSHOFF1983 (Emshoff & Blakely, 1983), FARMER2010 (Farmer et al., 2010), FEINDLER1984 (Feindler et al., 1984), FEINFIELD2004 (Feinfield & Baker, 2004), FISHER2007 (Fisher & Kim, 2007), FOREHAND2010 (Forehand et al., 2010), FOREHAND2011 (Forehand et al., 2011), FOWLES2009 (Fowles, 2009), FRASER2004 (Fraser et al., 2004), FRIEDEN2006 (Freiden, 2006), GALLART2005 (Gallart & Matthey, 2005), GARDNER2006 (Gardner et al., 2006), GARDNER2007 (Gardner et al., 2007), GARRISON1983 (Garrison & Stolberg, 1983), GARZA2004 (Garza, 2004), GLISSON2010 (Glisson et al., 2010), GREENE2004 (Greene et al., 2004), HANISCH2010 (Hanisch et al., 2010), HARWOOD2006 (Harwood, 2006), HENGGELER1992 (Henggeler et al., 1992), HENGGELER1997 (Henggeler et al., 1997), HENGGELER1999 (Henggeler et al., 1999), HENGGELER2006 (Henggeler et al., 2006), HERRMAN2003 (Herrmann &

---

[54] Here and elsewhere in the guideline, each study considered for review is referred to by a study ID in capital letters (primary author and date of study publication, except where a study is in press or only submitted for publication, then a date is not used).

McWhirter, 2003), HILYER1982 (Hilyer et al., 1982), HUTCHINGS2002 (Hutchings et al., 2002), HUTCHINGS2007 (Hutchings et al., 2007), IRELAND2003 (Ireland et al., 2003), ISON2001 (Ison, 2001), JOURILES2001 (Jouriles et al., 2001), JOURILES2009 (Jouriles et al., 2009), KACIR1999 (Kacir & Gordon, 1999), KANNAPPAN2008 (Kannappan & Bai, 2008), KAZDIN1987 (Kazdin et al., 1987), KAZDIN1989 (Kazdin et al., 1989), KAZDIN1992 (Kazdin et al., 1992), KENDALL1990 (Kendall et al., 1990), KETTLEWELL1983 (Kettlewell & Kausch, 1983), KING1990 (King & Kirschenbaum, 1990), KLING2010 (Kling et al., 2010), KOLKO2009 (Kolko et al., 2009), KOLKO2010 (Kolko et al., 2010), KRATOCHWILL2003 (Kratochwill et al., 2003), LANE1999 (Lane, 1999), LANGBERG2006 (Langberg, 2006), LARKIN1999 (Larkin & Thyer, 1999), LARMAR2006 (Larmar et al., 2006), LARSSON2009 (Larsson et al., 2009), LAU2011 (Lau et al., 2011), LAVIGNE2008 (Lavigne et al., 2008), LESCHIED2002 (Leschied & Cunningham, 2002), LETOURNEAU2009 (Letourneau et al., 2009), LEUNG2003 (Leung et al., 2003), LEWIS1983 (Lewis, 1983), LINARES2006 (Linares et al., 2006), LIPMAN2006 (Lipman et al., 2006), LOCHMAN1984 (Lochman et al., 1984), LOCHMAN2002 (Lochman & Wells, 2002), LOCHMAN2004 (Lochman & Wells, 2004), LOPATA2003 (Lopata, 2003), MACDONALD2005 (Macdonald & Turner, 2005), MACSRG2002 (Metropolitan Area Child Study Research Group, 2002), MAGEN1994 (Magen, 1994), MARKIE-DADDS2006 (Markie-Dadds & Sanders, 2006b), MARKIE-DADDS2006A (Markie-Dadds & Sanders, 2006a), MARTIN2003 (Martin & Sanders, 2003), MARTSCH2005 (Martsch, 2000), MCARDLE2002 (McArdle et al., 2002), MCCABE2009 (McCabe & Yeh, 2009), MCCABE2009B (McCabe, 2009), MCCART2006 (McCart, 2006), MCCONAUGHY1999 (McConaughy et al., 1999), MCGILLOWAY2012 (McGilloway et al., 2012), MCMAHON1981 (McMahon et al., 1981), MCPHERSON1983 (McPherson et al., 1983), MICHELSON1983 (Michelson et al., 1983), MORAWSKA2011 (Morawska et al., 2011), NESTLER2011 (Nestler & Goldbeck, 2011), NICHOLSON1999 (Nicholson & Sanders, 1999), NICKEL2005 (Nickel et al., 2005), NICKEL2006 (Nickel et al., 2006b), NICKEL2006A (Nickel et al., 2006a), NINNESS1985 (Ninness et al., 1985), NIXON2003 (Nixon et al., 2003), OGDEN2004 (Ogden & Halliday-Boykins, 2004), OGDEN2008 (Ogden & Hagen, 2008), OMIZO1988 (Omizo et al., 1988), PANTIN2009 (Pantin et al., 2009), PATTERSON2002 (Patterson et al., 2002), PEPLER1995 (Pepler et al., 1995), PETIT1998 (Petit, 1998), PETRA2001 (Petra, 2001), PIETRUCHA1998 (Pietrucha, 1998), PITTS2001 (Pitts, 2001), REID2007 (Reid et al., 2007), ROHDE2004 (Rohde et al., 2004), ROWLAND2005 (Rowland et al., 2005), SALMON2009 (Salmon et al., 2009), SANDERS1985 (Sanders & Christensen, 1985), SANDERS2000 (Sanders et al., 2000b), SANDERS2000A (Sanders et al., 2000a), SANDERS2000B (Sanders & McFarland, 2000), SANTISTEBAN2003 (Santisteban et al., 2003), SAYGER1988 (Sayger et al., 1988), SCHUHMANN1998 (Schuhmann et al., 1998), SCHUMANN2004 (Schumann, 2004), SCOTT2010:PALS (Scott et al., 2010a), SCOTT2010:SPOKES (Scott et al., 2010b), SEDA1992 (Seda, 1992), SEXTON2010 (Sexton & Turner, 2010), SHECHTMAN2000 (Shechtman, 2000), SHECHTMAN2006A (Shechtman & Birani-Nasaraladin, 2006), SHECHTMAN2006B (Shechtman, 2006), SHECHTMAN2009 (Shechtman & Ifargan, 2009), SHIN2009 (Shin, 2009), SIMONSEN2011 (Simonsen et al., 2011), SMITH2011 (Smith et al., 2011), SNYDER1999 (Snyder et al., 1999),

STALLMAN2007 (Stallman & Ralph, 2007), STOLK2008:MP (Stolk et al., 2008), STOLK2008:PP (Stolk et al., 2008), STRAYHORN1989 (Strayhorn & Weidman, 1989), SUKHODOLSKY2000 (Sukhodolsky et al., 2000), SUNDELL2008 (Sundell et al., 2008), SWIFT2009 (Swift et al., 2009), SZAPOCZNIK1989 (Szapocznik et al., 1989), TAYLOR1998 (Taylor et al., 1998), TIMMER2010 (Timmer et al., 2010), TIMMONS-M2006 (Timmons-Mitchell et al., 2006), TREMBLAY1992 (McCord & Tremblay, 1992), TURNER2006 (Turner & Sanders, 2006), TURNER2007 (Turner et al., 2007), VANDEWIEL2007 (Van De Wiel et al., 2007), VANMANEN2004 (van Manen et al., 2004), VERDUYN1990 (Verduyn et al., 1990), WALKER1998 (Walker et al., 1998), WALTON2010 (Walton et al., 2010), WANDERS2008 (Wanders et al., 2008), WEBSTER-S1984 (Webster-Stratton, 1984), WEBSTER-S1988 (Webster-Stratton et al., 1988), WEBSTER-S1990 (Webster-Stratton, 1990), WEBSTER-S1992 (Webster-Stratton, 1992), WEBSTER-S1994 (Webster-Stratton, 1994), WEBSTER-S1997 (Webster-Stratton & Hammond, 1997), WEBSTER-S2004 (Webster-Stratton et al., 2004), WESTERMARK2011 (Westermark et al., 2011), WIGGINS2009 (Wiggins et al., 2009), WILMSHURST2002 (Wilmshurst, 2002). Of these, 16 were unpublished doctoral theses and 186 were published in peer-reviewed journals between 1973 and 2011.

An additional trial, WEINBLATT2008 (Weinblatt & Omer, 2008), was highlighted by a stakeholder during consultation. Due to the nature of the intervention, this study did not fit into any of the existing categories and, therefore, is reviewed narratively in Section 7.2.5.

In addition, 311 studies were excluded from the review. Further information about both included and excluded studies can be found in Appendix 16a.

Of the 203 eligible trials, 135 (N = 18,144) included sufficient data to be included in statistical analysis. For the trials that reported critical outcomes but could not be included in the meta-analyses due to the way the data had been reported, a brief narrative synthesis is given to assess whether these support or refute the meta-analyses. All other eligible trials did not report any critical outcomes and, therefore, are not described further.

For the purposes of the guideline, interventions were categorised as:
- child-focused (delivered to child only)
- parent-focused (delivered to parent only)
- foster carer focused (delivered to foster carer only)
- parent–child-based (separate interventions delivered to parent and child)
- parent–teacher-based (separate interventions delivered to parent and teacher)
- family-focused (delivered to the family)
- multimodal (integrated approach involving the family and community)
- multi-component (separate interventions delivered to parents, child, and family or school)
- classroom-based – teacher involved (programmes delivered in classrooms involving a teacher, focusing on improving behaviour problems)
- classroom-based – other, non-teacher, involved (programmes delivered in classrooms involving someone other than a teacher, focusing on improving behaviour problems).

Table 40, Table 41, Table 42, Table 43 and Table 44 provide an overview of the trials included in each category.

Psychological/psychosocial indicated prevention and treatment interventions

**Table 40: Study information table for trials included in the meta-analysis of indicated prevention and treatment interventions (child-focused, parent-focused and foster carer-focused) versus any control**

| | Child-focused versus any control | Parent-focused versus any control | Foster carer-focused versus any control |
|---|---|---|---|
| Total no. of trials (N) | 27 RCTs (1,666) | 54 RCTs (4,150) | 3 RCTs (879) |
| Study ID | ARBUTHNOT1986<br>DODGEN1995<br>FEINDLER1984<br>FOWLES2009<br>FREIDEN2006<br>GARZA2004<br>ISON2001<br>KENDALL1990<br>KETTLEWELL1983<br>LANGBERG2006<br>LOCHMAN1984<br>LOCHMAN2004<br>MCARDLE2002<br>MICHELSON1983<br>NESTLER2011<br>OMIZO1988<br>PEPLER1995<br>SHECHTMAN2000<br>SHECHTMAN2006A | BEHAN2001<br>BODENMANN2008<br>BRADLEY2003<br>BRAET2009<br>CARNES-HOLT2010<br>CEBALLOS2010<br>CHAO2006<br>CONNELL1997<br>CUNNINGHAM1995<br>DRUGLI2006<br>FOREHAND2011<br>GALLART2005<br>GARDNER2006<br>HUTCHINGS2002<br>HUTCHINGS2007<br>JOURILES2001<br>JOURILES2009<br>KACIR1999<br>KLING2010 | BYWATER2011<br>CHAMBERLAIN2008<br>CLARK1994 |

219

**Table 40:** *(Continued)*

| Child-focused versus any control | Parent-focused versus any control | Foster carer-focused versus any control |
| --- | --- | --- |
| SHECHTMAN2006B | LARSSON2009 | |
| SHECHTMAN2009 | LAU2011 | |
| SNYDER1999 | LEUNG2003 | |
| SUKHODOLSKY2000 | LINARES2006 | |
| SZAPOCZNIK1989 | MAGEN1994 | |
| VANMANEN2004 | MARKIE-DADDS2006A | |
| WEBSTER-S1997 | MARKIE-DADDS2006 | |
| WEBSTER-S2004 | MARTIN2003 | |
| | MCCABE2009 | |
| | MCGILLOWAY2012 | |
| | MORAWSKA2011 | |
| | NICHOLSON1999 | |
| | NIXON2003 | |
| | OGDEN2008 | |
| | PATTERSON2002 | |
| | PITTS2001 | |
| | SANDERS2000 | |
| | SANDERS2000A | |
| | SCHUHMANN1998 | |
| | SCOTT2010:PALS | |
| | SCOTT2010:SPOKES | |
| | STALLMAN2007 | |
| | STOLK2008:MP | |
| | STOLK2008:PP | |
| | SWIFT2009 | |
| | TAYLOR1998 | |

|  |  |  |  |
|---|---|---|---|
|  |  |  | TURNER2006<br>TURNER2007<br>WEBSTER-S1984<br>WEBSTER-S1988<br>WEBSTER-S1990<br>WEBSTER-S1992<br>WEBSTER-S1997<br>WEBSTER-S2004<br>WIGGINS2009 |
| Country | Argentina (k = 1)<br>Canada (k = 1)<br>Germany (k = 1)<br>Israel (k = 4)<br>Netherlands (k = 1)<br>UK (k = 1)<br>US (k = 18) | Australia (k = 14)<br>Belgium (k = 1)<br>Canada (k = 2)<br>China (k = 1)<br>Ireland (k = 2)<br>Netherlands (k = 2)<br>Norway (k = 3)<br>Sweden (k = 1)<br>Switzerland (k = 1)<br>UK (k = 6)<br>US (k = 21) | UK (k = 1)<br>US (k = 2) |
| Year of publication | 1983 to 2011 (k = 27) | 1984 to 2012 (k = 54) | 1994 to 2011 (k = 3) |
| Age of children/ young people | 11+ (k = 10)<br><11 (k = 5)<br>Both (k = 12) | 11 + (k = 2)<br><11 (k = 52)<br>Both (k = 0) | 11+ (k = 0)<br><11 (k = 1)<br>Both (k = 2) |

*Continued*

*Psychological/psychosocial indicated prevention and treatment interventions*

Table 40: *(Continued)*

| | Child-focused versus any control | Parent-focused versus any control | Foster carer-focused versus any control |
|---|---|---|---|
| Gender of children/young people (% female) | 0 to 25% (k = 17)<br>26 to 50% (k = 7)<br>51 to 75% (k = 0)<br>76 to 100% (k = 0)<br>Not reported (k = 3) | 0 to 25% (k = 11)<br>26 to 50% (k = 36)<br>51 to 75% (k = 2)<br>76 to 100% (k = 1)<br>Not reported (k = 4) | 0 to 25% (k = 0)<br>26 to 50% (k = 2)<br>51 to 75% (k = 1)<br>76 to 100% (k = 0) |
| Ethnicity of children/young people (% white) | 0 to 25% (k = 9)<br>26 to 50%(k = 4)<br>51 to 75% (k = 1)<br>76 to 100% (k = 3)<br>Not reported (k = 10) | 0 to 25% (k = 3)<br>26 to 50% (k = 1)<br>51 to 75% (k = 0)<br>76 to 100% (k = 6)<br>Not reported (k = 44) | 0 to 25% (k = 1)<br>26 to 50% (k = 0)<br>51 to 75% (k = 1)<br>76 to 100% (k = 0)<br>Not reported (k = 1) |
| Timepoint (weeks) | Post-treatment: 4 to 117 (k = 27)<br>Follow-up: 12 to 117 (k = 8) | Post-treatment: 2 to 73 (k = 54)<br>Follow-up: 12 to 87 (k = 12) | Post-treatment: 12 to 78 (k = 3)<br>Follow-up: 182 (k = 1) |
| Intervention type | Indicated prevention (k = 9)<br>Treatment (k = 18) | Indicated prevention (k = 13)<br>Treatment (k = 41) | Indicated prevention (k = 0)<br>Treatment (k = 3) |
| Comparisons | Child-focused versus attention control (k = 7)<br>Child-focused versus no treatment (k = 10)<br>Child-focused versus treatment as usual (k = 4)<br>Child-focused versus waitlist control (k = 6) | Parent-focused versus no treatment (k = 9)<br>Parent-focused versus treatment as usual (k = 11)<br>Parent-focused versus waitlist control (k = 34) | Foster carer-focused versus attention control (k = 0)<br>Foster carer-focused versus no treatment (k = 1)<br>Foster carer-focused versus treatment as usual (k = 1)<br>Foster carer-focused versus waitlist control (k = 1) |

**Table 41: Study information table for trials included in the meta-analysis of indicated prevention and treatment interventions (parent–child-based, parent–teacher-based and family-focused) versus any control**

| | Parent–child-based versus any control | Parent–teacher-based versus any control | Family-focused versus any control |
|---|---|---|---|
| Total no. of trials (N) | 12 RCTs (1,138) | 7 RCTs (797) | 8 RCTs (1,685) |
| Study ID | DRUGLI2006<br>FRASER2004<br>KANNAPPAN2008<br>KAZDIN1987<br>LARSSON2009<br>LOCHMAN2002<br>LOCHMAN2004<br>MCCART2006<br>MCPHERSON1983<br>STRAYHORN1989<br>TREMBLAY1992<br>WEBSTER-S1997 | HANISCH2010<br>KING1990<br>KRATOCHWILL2003<br>LARMAR2006<br>WEBSTER-S2004 | ALEXANDER1973<br>COATSWORTH2001<br>DEMBO2001<br>NICKEL2006A<br>SANTISTEBAN2003<br>SAYGER1988<br>SEXTON2010<br>SZAPOCZNIK1989 |
| Country | Canada (k = 1)<br>India (k = 1)<br>Norway (k = 2)<br>US (k = 8) | Australia (k = 1)<br>Germany (k = 1)<br>US (k = 3) | Germany (k = 1)<br>US (k = 7) |
| Year of publication | 1983 to 2009 (k = 12) | 1990 to 2010 | 1973 to 2006 |
| Age of children/young people | 11+ (k = 3)<br><11 (k = 6)<br>Both (k = 3) | 11+ (k = 0)<br><11 (k = 5)<br>Both (k = 0) | 11+ (k = 5)<br><11 (k = 2)<br>Both (k = 1) |

*Continued*

**Table 41:** *(Continued)*

| | Parent–child-based versus any control | Parent–teacher-based versus any control | Family-focused versus any control |
|---|---|---|---|
| Gender of children/ young people (% female) | 0 to 25% (k = 6) <br> 26 to 50% (k = 3) <br> 51 to 75% (k = 1) <br> 76 to 100% (k = 1) <br> Not reported (k = 1) | 0 to 25% (k = 1) <br> 26 to 50% (k = 4) <br> 51 to 75% (k = 0) <br> 76 to 100% (k = 0) | 0 to 25% (k = 5) <br> 26 to 50% (k = 1) <br> 51 to 75% (k = 1) <br> 76 to 100% (k = 1) |
| Ethnicity of children/ young people (% white) | 0 to 25% (k = 1) <br> 26 to 50% (k = 1) <br> 51 to 75% (k = 1) <br> 76 to 100% (k = 3) <br> Not reported (k = 6) | Not reported (k = 5) | 0 to 25% (k = 3) <br> 26 to 50% (k = 1) <br> 51 to 75% (k = 1) <br> 76 to 100% (k = 0) <br> Not reported (k = 3) |
| Timepoint (weeks) | Post-treatment: 10 to 117 (k = 11) <br> Follow-up: 30 to 624 (k = 6) | Post-treatment: 10 to 39 (k = 4) <br> Follow-up: 26 (k = 1) | Post-treatment: 5 to 52 (k = 8) <br> Follow-up: 52 (k = 1) |
| Intervention type | Indicated prevention (k = 5) <br> Treatment (k = 7) | Indicated prevention (k = 3) <br> Treatment (k = 2) | Indicated prevention (k = 0) <br> Treatment (k = 8) |
| Comparisons | Parent–child-based versus attention control (k = 1) <br> Parent–child-based versus no treatment (k = 5) <br> Parent–child-based versus treatment as usual (k = 3) <br> Parent–child-based versus waitlist control (k = 3) | Parent–teacher-based versus no treatment (k = 3) <br> Parent–teacher-based versus treatment as usual (k = 1) <br> Parent–child-based versus waitlist control (k = 1) | Family-focused versus attention control (k = 2) <br> Family-focused versus no treatment/ treatment as usual (k = 1) <br> Family-focused versus placebo (k = 1) <br> Family-focused versus treatment as usual (k = 3) <br> Family-focused versus waitlist control (k = 1) |

**Table 42: Study information table for trials included in the meta-analysis of indicated prevention and treatment interventions (multimodal and multi-component interventions) versus any control**

|  | **Multimodal versus any control** | **Multi-component versus any control** |
|---|---|---|
| Total no. of trials (N) | 14 RCTs (1,874) | 16 RCTs (5,211) |
| Study ID | BORDUIN1995<br>BORDUIN2002<br>BUTLER2011<br>DIRKS-LINHORST2003<br>HENGGELER1992<br>HENGGELER1997<br>HENGGELER1999<br>HENGGELER2006<br>LESCHIED2002<br>LETOURNEAU2009<br>OGDEN2004<br>ROWLAND2005<br>SUNDELL2008<br>TIMMONS-M2006 | AUGUST2001<br>AUGUST2003<br>AUGUST2006<br>BARRETT2000<br>BRASWELL1997<br>CAVELL2000<br>CPPRG1999<br>FEINFIELD2004<br>HENGGELER2006<br>KING1990<br>KOLKO2010<br>LIPMAN2006<br>LOCHMAN2002<br>MACSRG2002<br>REID2007<br>WEBSTER-S2004 |
| Country | Canada (k = 1)<br>Norway (k = 1)<br>Sweden (k = 1)<br>UK (k = 1)<br>US (k = 10) | Australia (k = 1)<br>Canada (k = 1)<br>US (k = 14) |
| Year of publication | 1992 to 2011 (k = 14) | 1990 to 2010 (k = 16) |
| Age of children/young people | 11+ (k = 14)<br><11 (k = 0)<br>Both (k = 0) | 11+ (k = 1)<br><11 (k = 13)<br>Both (k = 2) |
| Gender of children/young people | 0 to 25% (k = 7)<br>26 to 50% (k = 6)<br>51 to 75% (k = 0)<br>76 to 100% (k = 0)<br>Not reported (k = 1) | 0 to 25% (k = 7)<br>26 to 50% (k = 8)<br>51 to 75% (k = 1)<br>76 to 100% (k = 0) |

*Continued*

**Table 42: (*Continued*)**

| | Multimodal versus any control | Multi-component versus any control |
|---|---|---|
| Ethnicity of children/ young people | 0 to 25% (k = 3)<br>26 to 50% (k = 5)<br>51 to 75% (k = 2)<br>76 to 100% (k = 0)<br>Not reported (k = 4) | 0 to 25% (k = 3)<br>26 to 50% (k = 4)<br>51 to 75% (k = 0)<br>76 to 100% (k = 2)<br>Not reported (k = 7) |
| Timepoint (weeks) | Post-treatment: 17 to 156 (k = 14)<br>Follow-up: 48 to 467 (k = 7) | Post-treatment: 10 to 104 (k = 16)<br>Follow-up: 52 to 156 (k = 3) |
| Intervention type | Indicated prevention (k = 0)<br>Treatment (k = 14) | Indicated prevention (k = 9)<br>Treatment (k = 7) |
| Comparisons | Multimodal versus treatment as usual (k = 14) | Multi-component versus attention control (k = 2)<br>Multi-component versus no treatment (k = 7)<br>Multi-component versus treatment as usual (k = 5)<br>Multi-component versus waitlist control (k = 2) |

**Table 43: Study information table for trials included in the meta-analysis of indicated prevention and treatment interventions (classroom-based interventions) versus any control**

| | Classroom-based (teacher involved) versus any control | Classroom-based (other, non-teacher involved) versus any control |
|---|---|---|
| Total no. of trials (N) | 5 RCTs (2,753) | 5 RCTs (576) |
| Study ID | BAKER-HENNINGHAM2009<br>BAKER-HENNINGHAM2012<br>MACSRG2002<br>REID2007<br>WEBSTER-S2004 | CHENEY2009<br>DESBIENS2003<br>SHECHTMAN2009<br>SIMONSEN2011<br>WALKER1998 |

*Continued*

**Table 43:** (*Continued*)

| | Classroom-based (teacher involved) versus any control | Classroom-based (other, non-teacher involved) versus any control |
|---|---|---|
| Country | Jamaica (k = 2)<br>US (k = 3) | Canada (k = 1)<br>Israel (k = 1)<br>US (k = 3) |
| Year of publication | 2002 to 2012 (k = 5) | 1998 to 2011 (k = 5) |
| Age of children/ young people | <11 (k = 4)<br>Both (k = 1) | <11 (k = 3)<br>Both (k = 2) |
| Gender of children/ young people | 0 to 25% (k = 1)<br>26 to 50% (k = 4)<br>51 to 75% (k = 0)<br>76 to 100% (k = 0) | 0 to 25% (k = 3)<br>26 to 50% (k = 2)<br>51 to 75% (k = 0)<br>76 to 100% (k = 0) |
| Ethnicity of children/young people | 0 to 25% (k = 2)<br>26 to 50% (k = 1)<br>51 to 75% (k = 0)<br>76 to 100% (k = 1)<br>Not reported (k = 1) | 0 to 25% (k = 2)<br>26 to 50% (k = 1)<br>51 to 75% (k = 0)<br>76 to 100% (k = 0)<br>Not reported (k = 2) |
| Timepoint (weeks) | Post-treatment: 22 to 104 (k = 5) | Post-treatment: 6 to 78 (k = 5) |
| Intervention type | Indicated prevention (k = 4)<br>Treatment (k = 1) | Indicated prevention (k = 4)<br>Treatment (k = 1) |
| Comparisons | Classroom-based (teacher involved) versus attention control (k = 2)<br>Classroom-based (teacher involved) versus no treatment (k = 1)<br>Classroom-based (teacher involved) versus treatment as usual (k = 1)<br>Classroom-based (teacher involved) versus waitlist control (k = 1) | Classroom-based (other, non-teacher involved) versus attention control (k = 0)<br>Classroom-based (other, non-teacher involved) versus no treatment (k = 3)<br>Classroom-based (other, non-teacher involved) versus treatment as usual (k = 1)<br>Classroom-based (other, non-teacher involved) versus waitlist control (k = 1) |

**Table 44: Study information table for trials included in the
meta-analysis of head-to-head indicated prevention and treatment
intervention trials (parent-focused versus parent–child-based and
family-focused versus child-based)**

| | Parent-focused versus parent–child-based | Family-focused versus child-based |
|---|---|---|
| Total no. of trials (N) | 5 RCTs (615) | 2 RCTs (140) |
| Study ID | DISHION1995<br>DRUGLI2006<br>KAZDIN1992<br>LARSSON2009<br>WEBSTER-S1997 | AZRIN2001<br>SZAPOCZNIK1989 |
| Country | Norway (k = 2)<br>US (k = 3) | US (k = 2) |
| Year of publication | 1992 to 2009 (k = 5) | 1989 to 2001 (k = 2) |
| Age of children/young people | 11+ (k = 0)<br><11 (k = 3)<br>Both (k = 2) | 11+ (k = 1)<br><11 (k = 1) |
| Gender of children/ young people (% female) | 0 to 25% (k = 3)<br>26 to 50% (k = 2)<br>51 to 75% (k = 0)<br>76 to 100% (k = 0) | 0 to 25% (k = 2)<br>26 to 50% (k = 0)<br>51 to 75% (k = 0)<br>76 to 100% (k = 0) |
| Ethnicity of children/ young people (% white) | 0 to 25% (k = 0)<br>26 to 50% (k = 0)<br>51 to 75% (k = 1)<br>76 to 100% (k = 1)<br>Not reported (k = 3) | 0 to 25% (k = 1)<br>26 to 50% (k = 0)<br>51 to 75% (k = 0)<br>76 to 100% (k = 1)<br>Not reported (k = 0) |
| Timepoint (weeks) | Post-treatment: 12 to 35 (k = 5)<br>Follow-up: 52 to 87 (k = 5) | Post-treatment: 26 (k = 2)<br>Follow-up: 52 to 78 (k = 2) |
| Intervention type | Indicated prevention (k = 1)<br>Treatment (k = 4) | Indicated prevention (k = 0)<br>Treatment (k = 2) |

**7.2.4    Clinical evidence for the review of an intervention versus any control**

The critical outcomes of antisocial behaviour, offending behaviour and drug and/or alcohol use were sub-categorised according to the person who rated the outcome: (a) observer rated, (b) researcher/clinician rated, (c) peer rated, (d) teacher rated and (e) parent rated. The GDG recognised that blinding of outcome raters who received the intervention was not possible; therefore, congruence of the effect between outcome raters was considered to be stronger evidence. Because few trials reported offending behaviour as a continuous outcome, data from this outcome were combined in the meta-analyses with antisocial behaviour measured by rating scale. Because few trials reported composite outcomes, these were combined in the meta-analyses with researcher-/clinician-rated outcomes. No other critical outcomes were reported in adequate numbers to be included in meta-analyses. It should be noted that harms associated with treatment are possible (for example problems associated with stigmatisation), but the GDG felt the risk was small. Furthermore, the included trials do not measure harm. Therefore, this issue is not examined further within this section.

In the included trials, the interventions were compared with a variety of control groups that were categorised as: treatment as usual, attention control, waitlist control and no treatment. Further information about the control group used in each trial can be found in the forest plots presented in Appendix 17.

Summary of findings tables are used below to summarise the evidence. The full GRADE evidence profiles can be found in Appendix 18.

*Child-focused interventions*
From the 27 trials with appropriate data for meta-analysis (see Table 40 for study characteristics), moderate quality evidence from up to 25 comparisons with 1,335 participants showed that child-focused interventions reduced antisocial behaviour when rated by researchers/clinicians, teachers and parents at post-treatment (Table 45). The direction of effect was consistent for observer and peer-rated antisocial behaviour, although not conclusive. Effect sizes were small across all raters and there was moderate to substantial heterogeneity between comparisons reporting teacher- and parent-rated outcomes. At follow-up, six to seven comparisons with 246 to 300 participants presented low quality evidence in favour of child-focused interventions when rated by teachers and by parents (Table 46).

To explore the heterogeneity between study effect sizes (for parent-rated outcomes), a series of meta-regressions were conducted (see Section 7.2.6).

With regard to trials not included in the meta-analyses, eight reported the intervention to be effective on the outcomes of interest (CHOI2010, DEFFENBACHER1996, DUPPER1993, GARRISON1983, HILYER1982, LOPATA2003, SHECHTMAN2006A, SHIN2009). A further six trials found no treatment group effects (LEWIS1983, MCCABE2009B, PETIT1998, PIETRUCHA1998, ROHDE2004, SEDA1992).

**Table 45: Summary of findings table for child-focused interventions compared with a control group (post-treatment)**

**Patient or population:** children and young people with, or at high risk of, conduct disorders (follow-up)

**Intervention:** child-focused

**Comparison:** any control group

| Outcomes | Illustrative comparative risks (95% CI) | | No. of participants (studies) | Quality of the evidence (GRADE) |
|---|---|---|---|---|
| | Assumed risk | Corresponding risk | | |
| | Any control group | Child-focused | | |
| **Observer-rated antisocial behaviour** Any valid method | – | The mean observer-rated antisocial behaviour in the intervention groups was **0.20 standard deviations lower** (0.61 lower to 0.21 higher) | 90 (2) | ⊕⊕⊕⊝ **moderate**[1] |
| **Researcher-/clinician-rated antisocial/ offending behaviour** Any valid rating scale/any measure of offending behaviour | – | The mean researcher-/clinician-rated antisocial/ offending behaviour in the intervention groups was **0.42 standard deviations lower** (0.69 to 0.16 lower) | 221 (4) | ⊕⊕⊕⊝ **moderate**[1] |
| **Peer-rated antisocial behaviour** Any valid rating scale | – | The mean peer-rated antisocial behaviour in the intervention groups was **0.25 standard deviations lower** (0.72 lower to 0.23 higher) | 79 (2) | ⊕⊕⊕⊝ **moderate**[1] |
| **Teacher-rated antisocial behaviour** Any valid rating scale | – | The mean teacher-rated antisocial behaviour in the intervention groups was **0.37 standard deviations lower** (0.55 to 0.19 lower) | 1335 (25) | ⊕⊕⊕⊝ **moderate**[2] |
| **Parent-rated antisocial behaviour** Any valid rating scale | – | The mean parent-rated antisocial behaviour in the intervention groups was **0.34 standard deviations lower** (0.67 to 0.01 lower) | 469 (11) | ⊕⊕⊕⊝ **moderate**[3] |

[1]OIS (for dichotomous outcomes, OIS = 300 events; for continuous outcomes, OIS = 400 participants) not met.
[2]There is evidence of moderate heterogeneity of study effect sizes.
[3]There is evidence of substantial heterogeneity of study effect sizes.

**Table 46: Summary of findings table for child-focused interventions compared with a control group (follow-up)**

**Patient or population:** children and young people with, or at high risk of, conduct disorders (follow-up)

**Intervention:** child-focused

**Comparison:** any control group

| Outcomes | Illustrative comparative risks (95% CI) | | No. of participants (studies) | Quality of the evidence (GRADE) |
|---|---|---|---|---|
| | Assumed risk | Corresponding risk | | |
| | Any control group | Child-focused | | |
| **Teacher-rated antisocial behaviour** Any valid rating scale Follow-up: 12 to 52 weeks | – | The mean teacher-rated antisocial behaviour in the intervention groups was **0.45 standard deviations lower** (0.88 to 0.03 lower) | 246 (6) | ⊕⊕⊕⊝ **low**[1,2] |
| **Parent-rated antisocial behaviour** Any valid rating scale Follow-up: 52 to 117 weeks | – | The mean parent-rated antisocial behaviour in the intervention groups was **0.26 standard deviations lower** (0.66 lower to 0.14 higher) | 300 (7) | ⊕⊕⊕⊝ **low**[1,2] |

[1]There is evidence of substantial heterogeneity of study effect sizes.
[2]OIS (for dichotomous outcomes, OIS = 300 events; for continuous outcomes, OIS = 400 participants) not met.

*Psychological/psychosocial indicated prevention and treatment interventions*

*Parent-focused interventions*
From the 54 trials with appropriate data for meta-analysis (see Table 40 for study characteristics), moderate quality evidence from up to 63 comparisons with 3,550 participants showed that parent-focused interventions reduced antisocial behaviour when rated by observers, researchers/clinicians and parents at post-treatment (Table 47). Effect sizes were small to medium and there was moderate heterogeneity between studies reporting observer- and parent-rated outcomes. For teacher-rated outcomes, there was high quality evidence from ten comparisons with 671 participants suggesting no benefit. At follow-up, high quality evidence from 12 comparisons with 762 participants demonstrated a favourable effect in terms of parent-rated outcomes (Table 48). However, moderate quality evidence from one to three comparisons with 154 to 245 participants did not find benefit when antisocial behaviour was rated by observers, researchers/clinicians and teachers.

To examine the effect of excluding attenuated parent-focused interventions (that is, those that were self-directed or of very few sessions), a sensitivity analysis was conducted excluding 24 comparisons (Table 49 and Table 50). The evidence was not qualitatively different from the analysis of all comparisons.

To explore the heterogeneity between study effect sizes (for observer- and parent-rated outcomes), a series of meta-regressions were conducted (see Section 7.2.6).

With regard to trials not included in the meta-analyses, two demonstrated effects on antisocial behaviour outcomes favouring the intervention group (GARDNER2007, PETRA2001), while one found mixed findings on official crime outcomes (BANK1991) and two found no intervention effects (LAVIGNE2008, STRAYHORN1989).

*Foster carer-focused interventions*
From the three trials with appropriate data for meta-analysis (see Table 40 for study characteristics), high quality evidence from all three comparisons (855 participants) showed that foster carer-focused interventions reduced antisocial behaviour when rated by parents at post-treatment (Table 51). No data were available for other raters or at follow-up.

With regard to trials not included in the meta-analyses, two reported results favouring the intervention (FARMER2010, SMITH2011) and two others reported no significant effects favouring intervention for the outcomes of interest (DOZIER2006, MACDONALD2005).

*Parent–child-based interventions*
From the 12 trials with appropriate data for meta-analysis (see Table 41 for study characteristics), low quality evidence from up to eight comparisons with up to 588 participants showed that parent–child-based interventions reduced antisocial behaviour when rated by teachers and parents at post-treatment (Table 52). Effect sizes were small to medium, although there was substantial heterogeneity between studies. In addition, one small study of 44 participants showed moderate quality evidence of a small effect in favour of the parent–child-based intervention, but wide confidence intervals make this inconclusive. At follow-up, two to three comparisons with 84 to 169 participants demonstrated large effects in favour of the intervention (Table 53).

**Table 47: Summary of findings table for parent-focused interventions compared with a control group (post-treatment)**

**Patient or population:** children and young people with, or at high risk of, conduct disorders (post-treatment)

**Intervention:** any parent-focused

**Comparison:** any control group

| Outcomes | Illustrative comparative risks (95% CI) | | No. of participants (studies) | Quality of the evidence (GRADE) |
|---|---|---|---|---|
| | **Assumed risk** Any control group | **Corresponding risk** Any parent-focused | | |
| **Observer-rated antisocial behaviour** Any valid method | — | The mean observer-rated antisocial behaviour in the intervention groups was **0.40 standard deviations lower** (0.58 to 0.21 lower) | 1,026 (19) | ⊕⊕⊕⊕ moderate[1] |
| **Researcher-/clinician-rated antisocial behaviour** Any valid rating scale | — | The mean researcher-/clinician-rated antisocial behaviour in the intervention groups was **0.69 standard deviations lower** (1.22 to 0.16 lower) | 56 (1) | ⊕⊕⊕⊕ moderate[2] |
| **Teacher-rated antisocial behaviour** Any valid rating scale | — | The mean teacher-rated antisocial behaviour in the intervention groups was **0.04 standard deviations lower** (0.22 lower to 0.13 higher) | 671 (10) | ⊕⊕⊕⊕ high |
| **Parent-rated antisocial behaviour** Any valid rating scale | — | The mean parent-rated antisocial behaviour in the intervention groups was **0.54 standard deviations lower** (0.65 to 0.44 lower) | 3,550 (63) | ⊕⊕⊕⊕ moderate[1] |

[1] There is evidence of moderate heterogeneity of study effect sizes.
[2] OIS (for dichotomous outcomes, OIS = 300 events; for continuous outcomes, OIS = 400 participants) not met.

**Table 48: Summary of findings table for parent-focused interventions compared with a control group (follow-up)**

**Patient or population:** children and young people with, or at high risk of, conduct disorders (follow-up)

**Intervention:** any parent-focused

**Comparison:** any control group

| Outcomes | Illustrative comparative risks (95% CI) | | No. of participants (studies) | Quality of the evidence (GRADE) |
| --- | --- | --- | --- | --- |
| | Assumed risk | Corresponding risk | | |
| | Any control group | Any parent-focused | | |
| **Observer-rated antisocial behaviour**<br>Any valid method<br>Follow-up: 38 to 52 weeks | – | The mean observer-rated antisocial behaviour in the intervention groups was **0.18 standard deviations higher** (0.07 lower to 0.43 higher) | 245 (3) | ⊕⊕⊕⊕<br>**moderate**[1] |
| **Researcher-/clinician-rated antisocial behaviour**<br>Any valid rating scale<br>Follow-up: 52 weeks | – | The mean researcher-/clinician-rated antisocial behaviour in the intervention groups was **0.28 standard deviations higher** (0.04 lower to 0.59 higher) | 154 (1) | ⊕⊕⊕⊕<br>**moderate**[1] |
| **Teacher-rated antisocial behaviour**<br>Any valid rating scale<br>Follow-up: 25 to 52 weeks | – | The mean teacher-rated antisocial behaviour in the intervention groups was **0.16 standard deviations higher** (0.09 lower to 0.42 higher) | 240 (2) | ⊕⊕⊕⊕<br>**moderate**[1] |
| **Parent-rated antisocial behaviour**<br>Any valid rating scale<br>Follow-up: 13 to 87 weeks | – | The mean parent-rated antisocial behaviour in the intervention groups was **0.28 standard deviations lower** (0.48 to 0.08 lower) | 762 (12) | ⊕⊕⊕⊕<br>**high** |

OIS (for dichotomous outcomes, OIS = 300 events; for continuous outcomes, OIS = 400 participants) not met.

**Table 49: Summary of findings table for standard parent-focused interventions (excluding attenuated interventions) compared with a control group (post-treatment)**

**Patient or population:** children and young people with, or at high risk of, conduct disorders (post-treatment)

**Intervention:** standard parent-focused (excluding attenuated interventions)

**Comparison:** any control group

| Outcomes | Illustrative comparative risks (95% CI) | | No. of participants (studies) | Quality of the evidence (GRADE) |
|---|---|---|---|---|
| | **Assumed risk**<br>Any control group | **Corresponding risk**<br>Any parent-focused | | |
| **Observer-rated antisocial behaviour**<br>Any valid method | – | The mean observer-rated antisocial behaviour in the intervention groups was **0.40 standard deviations lower** (0.6 to 0.2 lower) | 714 (10) | ⊕⊕⊕⊕<br>**high** |
| **Researcher-/clinician-rated antisocial behaviour**<br>Any valid rating scale | – | The mean researcher-/clinician-rated antisocial behaviour in the intervention groups was **0.69 standard deviations lower** (1.22 to 0.16 lower) | 56 (1) | ⊕⊕⊕⊝<br>**moderate**[1] |
| **Teacher-rated antisocial behaviour**<br>Any valid rating scale | – | The mean teacher-rated antisocial behaviour in the intervention groups was **0.03 standard deviations higher** (0.16 lower to 0.21 higher) | 520 (7) | ⊕⊕⊕⊕<br>**high** |
| **Parent-rated antisocial behaviour**<br>Any valid rating scale | – | The mean parent-rated antisocial behaviour in the intervention groups was **0.50 standard deviations lower** (0.63 to 0.38 lower) | 2413 (39) | ⊕⊕⊕⊝<br>**moderate**[2] |

[1]OIS (for dichotomous outcomes, OIS = 300 events; for continuous outcomes, OIS = 400 participants) not met.
[2]There is evidence of moderate heterogeneity of study effect sizes.

235

**Table 50: Summary of findings table for standard parent-focused interventions (excluding attenuated interventions) compared with a control group (follow-up)**

**Patient or population:** children and young people with, or at high risk of, conduct disorders (follow-up)

**Intervention:** standard parent-focused (excluding attenuated interventions)

**Comparison:** any control group

| Outcomes | Illustrative comparative risks (95% CI) | | No. of participants (studies) | Quality of the evidence (GRADE) |
|---|---|---|---|---|
| | **Assumed risk** | **Corresponding risk** | | |
| | **Any control group** | **Standard parent-focused (excluding attenuated interventions)** | | |
| **Observer-rated antisocial behaviour**<br>Any valid method<br>Follow-up: 38 to 52 weeks | – | The mean observer-rated antisocial behaviour in the intervention groups was **0.18 standard deviations higher** (0.07 lower to 0.43 higher) | 245 (3) | ⊕⊕⊕⊕ **moderate**[1] |
| **Researcher-/clinician-rated antisocial behaviour**<br>Any valid rating scale<br>Follow-up: 52 weeks | – | The mean researcher-/clinician-rated antisocial behaviour in the intervention groups was **0.28 standard deviations higher** (0.04 lower to 0.59 higher) | 154 (1) | ⊕⊕⊕⊕ **moderate**[1] |
| **Teacher-rated antisocial behaviour**<br>Any valid rating scale<br>Follow-up: 25 to 52 weeks | – | The mean teacher-rated antisocial behaviour in the intervention groups was **0.16 standard deviations higher** (0.09 lower to 0.42 higher) | 240 (2) | ⊕⊕⊕⊕ **moderate**[1] |
| **Parent-rated antisocial behaviour**<br>Any valid rating scale<br>Follow-up: 13 to 87 weeks | – | The mean parent-rated antisocial behaviour in the intervention groups was **0.26 standard deviations lower** (0.47 to 0.05 lower) | 724 (11) | ⊕⊕⊕⊕ **high** |

[1] OIS (for dichotomous outcomes, OIS = 300 events; for continuous outcomes, OIS = 400 participants) not met.

**Table 51: Summary of findings table for foster carer-focused interventions compared with a control group (post-treatment)**

| Patient or population: children and young people with, or at high risk of, conduct disorders (follow-up)<br>Intervention: foster carer-focused<br>Comparison: any control group | | | | |
|---|---|---|---|---|
| **Outcomes** | **Illustrative comparative risks (95% CI)** | | **No. of participants (studies)** | **Quality of the evidence (GRADE)** |
| | **Assumed risk** | **Corresponding risk** | | |
| | **Any control group** | **Foster carer-focused** | | |
| **Parent-rated antisocial behaviour**<br>Any valid rating scale | – | The mean parent-rated antisocial behaviour in the intervention groups was **0.19 standard deviations lower** (0.39 lower to 0.02 higher) | 855 (3) | ⊕⊕⊕⊕<br>**high** |

With regard to trials not included in the meta-analyses, one showed significant intervention effects on all reported antisocial behaviour measures (SHECHTMAN2006A). Another trial reported three parent-rated outcomes (parent daily report of overt aggression, parent daily report of oppositional behaviour, CBCL – Externalising Behaviour) and one teacher-rated outcome (Teacher Report Form – Externalising Behaviour). Of the four outcomes, only parent daily report of overt aggression showed a statistically significant effect in favour of the parent–child-based intervention (VANDEWIEL2007). A final study found no statistically significant differences between the intervention and control groups (ELROD1992).

*Parent–teacher-based interventions*
From the seven trials with appropriate data for meta-analysis (see Table 41 for study characteristics), low to moderate quality evidence from up to four comparisons with 304 participants showed that parent–teacher-based interventions did not reduce antisocial behaviour when rated by observers, researchers/clinicians, teachers and parents at post-treatment (Table 54). At follow-up, one comparison with 108 participants was inconclusive with regard to antisocial behaviour when rated by parents (Table 55).

*Family-focused interventions*
From the eight trials with appropriate data for meta-analysis (see Table 41 for study characteristics), low to moderate quality evidence from four comparisons with 209 participants showed that family-focused interventions reduced antisocial behaviour when rated by parents at post-treatment (Table 56). In addition, one small trial with 29 participants presented moderate quality evidence of a large effect favouring the intervention when rated by teachers. However, another larger comparison with 303 participants found no evidence of a reduction in offending

**Table 52: Summary of findings table for parent–child-based interventions compared with a control group (post-treatment)**

**Patient or population:** children and young people with, or at high risk of, conduct disorders (post-treatment)
**Intervention:** parent-child based
**Comparison:** any control group

| Outcomes | Illustrative comparative risks (95% CI) | | No. of participants (studies) | Quality of the evidence (GRADE) |
| --- | --- | --- | --- | --- |
| | Assumed risk | Corresponding risk | | |
| | Any control group | Parent–child-based | | |
| **Observer-rated antisocial behaviour** Any valid method | – | The mean observer-rated antisocial behaviour in the intervention groups was **0.20 standard deviations lower** (0.78 lower to 0.38 higher) | 44 (1) | ⊕⊕⊕⊝ moderate[1] |
| **Teacher-rated antisocial behaviour** Any valid rating scale | – | The mean teacher-rated antisocial behaviour in the intervention groups was **0.44 standard deviations lower** (0.86 to 0.01 lower) | 588 (7) | ⊕⊕⊝⊝ low[2,3] |
| **Parent-rated antisocial behaviour** Any valid rating scale | – | The mean parent-rated antisocial behaviour in the intervention groups was **0.52 standard deviations lower** (0.96 to 0.08 lower) | 524 (8) | ⊕⊕⊝⊝ low[2,3] |

[1] OIS (for dichotomous outcomes, OIS = 300 events; for continuous outcomes, OIS = 400 participants) not met.
[2] Risk of bias across domains was generally high or unclear.
[3] There is evidence of moderate heterogeneity of study effect sizes.

**Table 53: Summary of findings table for parent–child-based interventions compared with a control group (follow-up)**

**Patient or population:** children and young people with, or at high risk of, conduct disorders (follow-up)
**Intervention:** parent–child based
**Comparison:** any control group

| Outcomes | Illustrative comparative risks (95% CI) | | No. of participants (studies) | Quality of the evidence (GRADE) |
|---|---|---|---|---|
| | Assumed risk | Corresponding risk | | |
| | Any control group | Parent–child-based | | |
| **Teacher-rated antisocial behaviour** Any valid rating scale Follow-up: 76 to 156 weeks | – | The mean teacher-rated antisocial behaviour in the intervention groups was **1.29 standard deviations lower** (1.79 to 0.78 lower) | 84 (2) | ⊕⊕⊕⊖ **low**[1,2] |
| **Parent-rated antisocial behaviour** Any valid rating scale Follow-up: 76 to 156 weeks | – | The mean parent-rated antisocial behaviour in the intervention groups was **1.40 standard deviations lower** (2.35 to 0.45 lower) | 169 (3) | ⊕⊕⊕⊖ **low**[1,2] |

[1] Risk of bias across domains was generally high or unclear.
[2] OIS (for dichotomous outcomes, OIS = 300 events; for continuous outcomes, OIS = 400 participants) not met.

239

**Table 54: Summary of findings table for parent–teacher-based interventions compared with a control group (post-treatment)**

**Patient or population:** children and young people with, or at high risk of, conduct disorders (post-treatment)
**Intervention:** parent–teacher based
**Comparison:** any control group

| Outcomes | Illustrative comparative risks (95% CI) | | No. of participants (studies) | Quality of the evidence (GRADE) |
|---|---|---|---|---|
| | Assumed risk<br>Any control group | Corresponding risk<br>Parent–teacher-based | | |
| **Observer-rated antisocial behaviour**<br>Any valid method | – | The mean observer-rated antisocial behaviour in the intervention groups was **0.03 standard deviations lower** (0.34 lower to 0.29 higher) | 155 (1) | ⊕⊕⊕⊕<br>**moderate**[1] |
| **Researcher-/clinician-rated antisocial behaviour**<br>Any valid rating scale | – | The mean researcher-/clinician-rated antisocial behaviour in the intervention groups was **0.26 standard deviations lower** (0.81 lower to 0.3 higher) | 50 (1) | ⊕⊕⊕⊕<br>**moderate**[1] |
| **Teacher-rated antisocial behaviour**<br>Any valid rating scale | – | The mean teacher-rated antisocial behaviour in the intervention groups was **0.05 standard deviations lower** (0.29 lower to 0.19 higher) | 304 (4) | ⊕⊕⊕⊕<br>**low**[1,2] |
| **Parent-rated antisocial behaviour**<br>Any valid rating scale | – | The mean parent-rated antisocial behaviour in the intervention groups was **0.11 standard deviations lower** (0.40 lower to 0.17 higher) | 245 (4) | ⊕⊕⊕⊕<br>**low**[1,2] |

[1] OIS (for dichotomous outcomes, OIS = 300 events; for continuous outcomes, OIS = 400 participants) not met.
[2] Risk of bias across domains was generally high or unclear.

**Table 55:  Summary of findings table for parent–teacher-based interventions compared with a control group (follow-up)**

**Patient or population:** children and young people with, or at high risk of, conduct disorders (follow-up)
**Intervention:** parent–teacher based
**Comparison:** any control group

| Outcomes | Illustrative comparative risks (95% CI) | | No. of participants (studies) | Quality of the evidence (GRADE) |
|---|---|---|---|---|
| | **Assumed risk** | **Corresponding risk** | | |
| | Any control group | Parent–teacher-based | | |
| **Parent-rated antisocial behaviour** Any valid rating scale Follow-up: 26 to 82 weeks | – | The mean parent-rated antisocial behaviour in the intervention groups was **0.20 standard deviations lower** (0.58 lower to 0.17 higher) | 108 (1) | ⊕⊕⊕⊝ **low**[1,2] |

[1]OIS (for dichotomous outcomes, OIS = 300 events; for continuous outcomes, OIS = 400 participants) not met.
[2]Risk of bias across domains was generally high or unclear.

**Table 56: Summary of findings table for family-focused interventions compared with a control group (post-treatment)**

**Patient or population:** children and young people with, or at high risk of, conduct disorders (post-treatment)
**Intervention:** family focused
**Comparison:** any control group

| Outcomes | Illustrative comparative risks (95% CI) | | No. of participants (studies) | Quality of the evidence (GRADE) |
| --- | --- | --- | --- | --- |
| | **Assumed risk** | **Corresponding risk** | | |
| | **Any control group** | **Family-focused** | | |
| **Researcher-/clinician-rated offending behaviour** frequency of arrests/charges | – | The mean researcher-/clinician-rated offending behaviour in the intervention groups was **0.01 standard deviations lower** (0.24 lower to 0.21 higher) | 303 (1) | ⊕⊕⊕⊕ **moderate**[1] |
| **Teacher-rated antisocial behaviour** Any valid rating scale | – | The mean teacher-rated antisocial behaviour in the intervention groups was **0.95 standard deviations lower** (1.7 to 0.2 lower) | 29 (1) | ⊕⊕⊕⊕ **low**[1,2] |
| **Parent-rated antisocial behaviour** Any valid rating scale | – | The mean parent-rated antisocial behaviour in the intervention groups was **0.26 standard deviations lower** (0.55 lower to 0.02 higher) | 209 (4) | ⊕⊕⊕⊕ **low**[1,2] |

[1]OIS (for dichotomous outcomes, OIS = 300 events; for continuous outcomes, OIS = 400 participants) not met.
[2]Risk of bias across domains was generally high or unclear.

behaviour (recorded by researchers/clinicians). Two comparisons also reported dichotomous outcomes at post-treatment. Of these, one comparison with 86 participants reported moderate quality evidence suggesting reduced risk of offending behaviour. The other comparison with 40 participants found no evidence (moderate quality) of benefit with regard to drug and/or alcohol use (Table 57). At follow-up, one small comparison with 37 participants found no evidence in favour of family-focused interventions with regard to parent-rated antisocial behaviour (Table 58). In addition, one large comparison with 761 participants produced inconclusive moderate quality evidence with regard to researcher-/clinician-rated offending behaviour (Table 59).

With regard to trials not included in the meta-analyses, two reported statistically significant effects in favour of the family-focused intervention when behaviour was measured with the State-Trait Anger Expression Inventory (NICKEL2005, NICKEL2006). Another trial found that the family-focused intervention produced less recidivism on violent felony charges, but not any new offence (DEMBO1997). One trial found no treatment specific effects (EMSHOFF1983).

**Table 57: Summary of findings table for family-focused interventions compared with a control group (dichotomous outcomes) (post-treatment)**

**Patient or population:** children and young people with, or at high risk of, conduct disorders (dichotomous outcomes) (post-treatment)
**Intervention:** family focused
**Comparison:** any control group

| Outcomes | Relative effect (95% CI) | No. of participants (studies) | Quality of the evidence (GRADE) |
|---|---|---|---|
| **Researcher-/clinician-rated drug and/or alcohol use** <br> Drug screen – percentage positive for cannabis | **RR 1.0** (0.16 to 6.42) | 40 (1) | ⊕⊕⊕⊖ **moderate**[1] |
| **Researcher-/clinician-rated offending behaviour** <br> Recidivism | **RR 0.47** (0.27 to 0.83) | 86 (1) | ⊕⊕⊕⊖ **moderate**[1] |

[1]OIS (for dichotomous outcomes, OIS = 300 events; for continuous outcomes, OIS = 400 participants) not met.

**Table 58: Summary of findings table for family-focused interventions compared with a control group (follow-up)**

**Patient or population:** children and young people with, or at high risk of, conduct disorders (follow-up)
**Intervention:** family focused
**Comparison:** any control group

| Outcomes | Illustrative comparative risks (95% CI) | | No. of participants (studies) | Quality of the evidence (GRADE) |
|---|---|---|---|---|
| | Assumed risk | Corresponding risk | | |
| | Any control group | Family-focused | | |
| **Parent-rated antisocial behaviour** Any valid rating scale Follow-up: 78 weeks | – | The mean parent-rated antisocial behaviour in the intervention groups was **0.43 standard deviations higher** (0.22 lower to 1.09 higher) | 37 (1) | ⊕⊕⊝⊝ **low**[1,2] |

[1]Risk of bias across domains was generally high or unclear.
[2]OIS (for dichotomous outcomes, OIS = 300 events; for continuous outcomes, OIS = 400 participants) not met.

**Table 59: Summary of findings table for family-focused interventions compared with a control group (dichotomous outcomes) (follow-up)**

**Patient or population:** children and young people with, or at high risk of, conduct disorders (dichotomous outcomes) (follow-up)
**Intervention:** family focused
**Comparison:** any control group

| Outcomes | Relative effect (95% CI) | No. of participants (studies) | Quality of the evidence (GRADE) |
|---|---|---|---|
| **Researcher-/clinician-rated offending behaviour** Recidivism Follow-up: 52 weeks | **RR 1.00** (0.76 to 1.31) | 761 (1) | ⊕⊕⊕⊝ **moderate**[1] |

[1]OIS (for dichotomous outcomes, OIS = 300 events; for continuous outcomes, OIS = 400 participants) not met.

**Table 60: Summary of findings table for multimodal interventions compared with a control group (post-treatment)**

**Patient or population:** children and young people with, or at high risk of, conduct disorders (post-treatment)
**Intervention:** multimodal
**Comparison:** any control group

| Outcomes | Illustrative comparative risks (95% CI) | | No. of participants (studies) | Quality of the evidence (GRADE) |
| --- | --- | --- | --- | --- |
| | Assumed risk | Corresponding risk | | |
| | Any control group | Multimodal | | |
| **Researcher-/clinician-rated antisocial/offending behaviour** Any valid rating scale/any measure of offending behaviour | – | The mean researcher-/clinician-rated antisocial/offending behaviour in the intervention groups was **0.47 standard deviations lower** (0.74 to 0.21 lower) | 617 (7) | ⊕⊕⊕⊕ **high** |
| **Researcher-/clinician-rated drug and/or alcohol use** urine screen-cocaine/ marijuana; drug screen percentage positive-cannabis | – | The mean researcher-/clinician-rated drug and/or alcohol use in the intervention groups was **0.62 standard deviations lower** (2.07 lower to 0.83 higher) | 187 (2) | ⊕⊕⊕⊖ **low**[1,2] |
| **Parent-rated antisocial behaviour** Any valid rating scale | – | The mean parent-rated antisocial behaviour in the intervention groups was **0.25 standard deviations lower** (0.52 lower to 0.02 higher) | 786 (8) | ⊕⊕⊖⊖ **low**[1,3] |

[1]There is evidence of substantial heterogeneity of study effect sizes.
[2]OIS (for dichotomous outcomes, OIS = 300 events; for continuous outcomes, OIS = 400 participants) not met.
[3]CI includes both 1) no effect and 2) appreciable benefit or appreciable harm.

*Multimodal interventions*

From the 14 trials with appropriate data for meta-analysis (see Table 42 for study characteristics), high quality evidence from seven to eight comparisons with 617 to 786 participants showed that multimodal interventions reduced antisocial/offending behaviour when rated by researchers/clinicians and parents at post-treatment (Table 60). Effect sizes were small, and there was moderate to substantial heterogeneity between studies. In addition, two comparisons with 187 participants reported low quality evidence that was inconclusive with regard to drug and/or alcohol use. Also at post-treatment, three comparisons with 657 participants reported offending behaviour as a dichotomous outcome (researcher/clinician recorded) and provided moderate quality evidence in favour of the intervention, although this was not conclusive (Table 61). At follow-up, low quality evidence from five comparisons with 872 participants showed that multimodal interventions reduced antisocial/offending behaviour, and two comparisons with 136 participants reduced drug and/or alcohol use (Table 62). For both outcomes, there was substantial heterogeneity between comparisons, and the evidence was not conclusive due to wide confidence intervals. Dichotomous outcomes (of moderate quality) were also reported at follow-up, which supported the finding of benefit with regard to antisocial/offending behaviour (six comparisons with 943 participants), but not drug and/or alcohol use (one comparison with 80 participants) (Table 63).

With regard to trials not included in the meta-analyses, two trials of MTFC reported intervention effects on all reported antisocial behaviour outcome measures (CHAMBERLAIN1998, CHAMBERLAIN2007). However, two other trials of MTFC did not find treatment group specific effects on antisocial behaviour (FISHER2007, WESTERMARK2011). One trial of a programme called 'SNAP (Stop Now and Plan) under 12 outreach project' found results favouring the intervention for some antisocial behaviour measures, but not others (AUGIMERI2007). Finally, two trials did not find treatment group specific effects on antisocial behaviour (EMSHOFF1983 [Adolescent Diversion Project], GLISSON2010 [multisystemic therapy]).

**Table 61: Summary of findings table for multimodal interventions compared with a control group (dichotomous outcomes) (post-treatment)**

| Patient or population: children and young people with, or at high risk of, conduct disorders (dichotomous outcomes) (post-treatment) Intervention: multimodal Comparison: any control group | | | |
|---|---|---|---|
| **Outcomes** | **Relative effect (95% CI)** | **No. of participants (studies)** | **Quality of the evidence (GRADE)** |
| **Researcher-/clinician-rated offending behaviour** Any measure of offending behaviour | **RR 0.77** (0.53 to 1.11) | 657 (3) | ⊕⊕⊕⊖ **moderate** |

**Table 62: Summary of findings table for multimodal interventions compared with a control group (follow-up)**

**Patient or population:** children and young people with, or at high risk of, conduct disorders (follow-up)
**Intervention:** multimodal
**Comparison:** any control group

| Outcomes | Illustrative comparative risks (95% CI) | | No. of participants (studies) | Quality of the evidence (GRADE) |
| --- | --- | --- | --- | --- |
| | Assumed risk | Corresponding risk | | |
| | Any control group | Multimodal | | |
| **Researcher-/clinician-rated antisocial/offending behaviour** Any valid rating scale/any measure of offending behaviour Follow-up: 52 to 208 weeks | – | The mean researcher-/clinician-rated antisocial/offending behaviour in the intervention groups was **0.41 standard deviations lower** (0.93 lower to 0.1 higher) | 872 (5) | ⊕⊕⊕⊕ **low**[1,2] |
| **Researcher-/clinician-rated drug and/or alcohol use** Urine screen – cocaine/ marijuana; drug screen percentage positive for cocaine Follow-up: 52 to 226 weeks | – | The mean researcher-/clinician-rated drug and/or alcohol use in the intervention groups was **0.58 standard deviations lower** (1.91 lower to 0.75 higher) | 136 (2) | ⊕⊕⊕⊕ **low**[1,3] |

[1]There is evidence of substantial heterogeneity of study effect sizes.
[2]CI includes both 1) no effect and 2) appreciable benefit or appreciable harm.
[3]OIS (for dichotomous outcomes, OIS = 300 events; for continuous outcomes, OIS = 400 participants) not met.

**Table 63: Summary of findings table for multimodal interventions compared with a control group (dichotomous outcomes at follow-up)**

**Patient or population:** children and young people with, or at high risk of, conduct disorders (dichotomous outcomes) (follow-up)
**Intervention:** multimodal
**Comparison:** any control group

| Outcomes | Relative effect (95% CI) | No. of participants (studies) | Quality of the evidence (GRADE) |
|---|---|---|---|
| **Researcher-/clinician-rated antisocial/offending behaviour** Any valid rating scale/any measure of offending behaviour Follow-up: 48 to 1143 weeks | **RR 0.72** (0.52 to 1.02) | 943 (6) | ⊕⊕⊖⊖ **low**[1,2] |
| **Researcher-/clinician-rated drug and/or alcohol use** Drug screen percentage positive for cocaine Follow-up: 226 weeks | **RR 1.61** (0.94 to 2.76) | 80 (1) | ⊕⊕⊕⊖ **moderate**[3] |

[1]There is evidence of substantial heterogeneity of study effect sizes.
[2]CI includes both 1) no effect and 2) appreciable benefit or appreciable harm.
[3]OIS (for dichotomous outcomes, OIS = 300 events; for continuous outcomes, OIS = 400 participants) not met.

*Multi-component interventions*
From the 16 trials with appropriate data for meta-analysis (see Table 42 for study characteristics), moderate to high quality evidence from up to ten comparisons with 1,939 participants showed little evidence that multi-component interventions reduced antisocial behaviour when rated by observers, researchers/clinicians, peers and teachers at post-treatment (Table 64). In addition, 12 comparisons with 2,222 participants presented moderate quality evidence of a small effect in favour of the intervention when antisocial behaviour was rated by parents. At follow-up, there was much less evidence (ranging from very low to high quality) that was inconclusive (Table 65).

*Classroom-based interventions*
The ten trials of classroom-based interventions with appropriate data for meta-analysis were sub-categorised by whether teachers or non-teachers were involved in the intervention (see Table 43 for study characteristics). For those interventions involving teachers, high quality evidence from three comparisons with 499 participants showed a small effect in favour of the intervention when antisocial behaviour was rated by teachers at post-treatment (Table 66). However, the evidence was inconclusive when

**Table 64: Summary of findings table for multi-component interventions compared with a control group (post-treatment)**

**Patient or population:** children and young people with, or at high risk of, conduct disorders (post-treatment)
**Intervention:** multi-component
**Comparison:** any control group

| Outcomes | Illustrative comparative risks (95% CI) | | No. of participants (studies) | Quality of the evidence (GRADE) |
| --- | --- | --- | --- | --- |
| | Assumed risk | Corresponding risk | | |
| | Any control group | Multi-component | | |
| **Observer-rated antisocial behaviour**<br>Any valid method | – | The mean observer-rated antisocial behaviour in the intervention groups was **0.07 standard deviations higher** (0.07 lower to 0.2 higher) | 879 (3) | ⊕⊕⊕⊕<br>**high** |
| **Researcher-/clinician-rated antisocial/offending behaviour**<br>Any valid rating scale/any measure of offending behaviour | – | The mean researcher-/clinician-rated antisocial/offending behaviour in the intervention groups was **0.06 standard deviations lower** (0.37 lower to 0.24 higher) | 467 (3) | ⊕⊕⊕⊕<br>**moderate**[1] |
| **Peer-rated antisocial behaviour**<br>Any valid rating scale | – | The mean peer-rated antisocial behaviour in the intervention groups was **0.10 standard deviations higher** (0.05 lower to 0.26 higher) | 632 (1) | ⊕⊕⊕⊕<br>**high** |
| **Teacher-rated antisocial behaviour**<br>Any valid rating scale | – | The mean teacher-rated antisocial behaviour in the intervention groups was **0.08 standard deviations lower** (0.2 lower to 0.03 higher) | 1939 (10) | ⊕⊕⊕⊕<br>**high** |
| **Parent-rated antisocial behaviour**<br>Any valid rating scale | – | The mean parent-rated antisocial behaviour in the intervention groups was **0.23 standard deviations lower** (0.37 to 0.09 lower) | 2222 (12) | ⊕⊕⊕⊕<br>**moderate**[1] |

There is evidence of moderate heterogeneity of study effect sizes.

249

**Table 65: Summary of findings table for multi-component interventions compared with a control group (follow-up)**

**Patient or population:** children and young people with, or at high risk of, conduct disorders (follow-up)
**Intervention:** multi-component
**Comparison:** any control group

| Outcomes | Illustrative comparative risks (95% CI) | | No. of participants (studies) | Quality of the evidence (GRADE) |
| --- | --- | --- | --- | --- |
| | Assumed risk | Corresponding risk | | |
| | Any control group | Multi-component | | |
| **Researcher-/clinician-rated offending behaviour** <br> Frequency of arrest <br> Follow-up: 52 weeks | – | The mean researcher-/clinician-rated offending behaviour in the intervention groups was **0.36 standard deviations lower** (0.79 lower to 0.08 higher) | 61 (1) | ⊕⊕⊕⊝ **moderate**[1] |
| **Peer-rated antisocial behaviour** <br> Any valid method <br> Follow-up: 156 weeks | – | The mean peer-rated antisocial behaviour in the intervention groups was **0.15 standard deviations lower** (0.32 lower to 0.03 higher) | 495 (1) | ⊕⊕⊕⊕ **high** |
| **Teacher-rated antisocial behaviour** <br> Any valid rating scale <br> Follow-up: 122 to 156 weeks | – | The mean teacher-rated antisocial behaviour in the intervention groups was **0.16 standard deviations lower** (0.31 to 0.01 lower) | 669 (2) | ⊕⊕⊕⊝ **moderate**[2] |
| **Parent-rated antisocial behaviour** <br> Any valid rating scale <br> Follow-up: 122 to 156 weeks | – | The mean parent-rated antisocial behaviour in the intervention groups was **0.01 standard deviations higher** (0.5 lower to 0.53 higher) | 644 (2) | ⊕⊕⊕⊝ **very low**[2,3,4] |

[1]OIS (for dichotomous outcomes, OIS = 300 events; for continuous outcomes, OIS = 400 participants) not met.
[2]Risk of bias across domains was generally high or unclear.
[3]There is evidence of substantial heterogeneity of study effect sizes.
[4]CI includes no effect, and appreciable benefit or appreciable harm.

**Table 66:  Summary of findings table for classroom-based (teacher involved) interventions compared with a control group (post-treatment)**

**Patient or population:** children and young people with, or at high risk of, conduct disorders (post-treatment)
**Intervention:** classroom-based (teacher involved)
**Comparison:** any control group

| Outcomes | Illustrative comparative risks (95% CI) | | No. of participants (studies) | Quality of the evidence (GRADE) |
| --- | --- | --- | --- | --- |
| | Assumed risk | Corresponding risk | | |
| | Any control group | Classroom-based (teacher involved) | | |
| **Observer-rated antisocial behaviour** Any valid method | – | The mean observer-rated antisocial behaviour in the intervention groups was **0.09 standard deviations lower** (0.58 lower to 0.4 higher) | 359(2) | ⊕⊕⊕⊕ **low**[1,2] |
| **Researcher-/clinician-rated antisocial behaviour** Any valid rating scale | – | The mean researcher-/clinician-rated antisocial behaviour in the intervention groups was **0.13 standard deviations lower** (0.79 lower to 0.53 higher) | 275(2) | ⊕⊕⊕⊕ **low**[1,2] |
| **Teacher-rated antisocial behaviour** Any valid rating scale | – | The mean teacher-rated antisocial behaviour in the intervention groups was **0.43 standard deviations lower** (0.63 to 0.24 lower) | 499(3) | ⊕⊕⊕⊕ **high** |
| **Parent-rated antisocial behaviour** Any valid rating scale | – | The mean parent-rated antisocial behaviour in the intervention groups was **0.19 standard deviations lower** (0.4 lower to 0.02 higher) | 383(2) | ⊕⊕⊕ **moderate**[2] |

[1]There is evidence of moderate heterogeneity of study effect sizes.
[2]OIS (for dichotomous outcomes, OIS = 300 events; for continuous outcomes, OIS = 400 participants) not met.

**Table 67: Summary of findings table for classroom-based (other, non-teacher, involved) interventions compared with a control group (post-treatment)**

**Patient or population:** children and young people with, or at high risk of, conduct disorders (post-treatment)
**Intervention:** classroom-based (other, non-teacher, involved)
**Comparison:** any control group

| Outcomes | Illustrative comparative risks (95% CI) | | No. of participants (studies) | Quality of the evidence (GRADE) |
|---|---|---|---|---|
| | Assumed risk | Corresponding risk | | |
| | Any control group | Classroom-based (other, non-teacher, involved) | | |
| **Observer-rated antisocial behaviour** Any valid method | – | The mean observer-rated antisocial behaviour in the intervention groups was **0.39 standard deviations lower** (1.02 lower to 0.23 higher) | 42 (1) | ⊕⊕⊕⊝ **moderate**[1] |
| **Researcher-/clinician-rated antisocial behaviour** Any valid rating scale | – | The mean researcher-/clinician-rated antisocial behaviour in the intervention groups was **0.17 standard deviations lower** (0.79 lower to 0.45 higher) | 42 (1) | ⊕⊕⊕⊝ **moderate**[1] |
| **Peer-rated antisocial behaviour** Any valid rating scale | – | The mean peer-rated antisocial behaviour in the intervention groups was **0.15 standard deviations lower** (0.75 lower to 0.46 higher) | 31 (1) | ⊕⊕⊕⊝ **moderate**[1] |
| **Teacher-rated antisocial behaviour** Any valid rating scale | – | The mean teacher-rated antisocial behaviour in the intervention groups was **0.45 standard deviations lower** (0.88 to 0.02 lower) | 367 (5) | ⊕⊕⊝⊝ **low**[1,2] |

[1]OIS (for dichotomous outcomes, OIS = 300 events; for continuous outcomes, OIS = 400 participants) not met.
[2]There is evidence of substantial heterogeneity of study effect sizes.

antisocial behaviour was rated by observers, researchers/clinicians, and parents. No comparisons reported follow-up data. The pattern of results was similar for classroom-based interventions delivered by non-teachers (Table 67). That is, five comparisons with 367 participants showed low quality evidence of benefit when antisocial behaviour was rated by teachers, but the evidence was inconclusive for other raters and no follow-up data were reported.

With regard to trials not included in the meta-analyses, one reported that all students in the intervention group decreased their acting-out behaviours whereas only half of the control group did (NINNESS1985).

*Other interventions*

One RCT (WEINBLATT2008) did not fit into any of the intervention categories, and is therefore described narratively here. The trial, conducted in Israel, randomised 41 families to either an intervention directed at parents but involving the child (called 'non-violent resistance') or a waitlist control. Children and young people (4 to 17 years old) were eligible if they displayed acute behavioural problems according to parent report. Of those included, the mean age was 12.57 (standard deviation [SD] 3.53) years and 32% were female. The non-violent resistance intervention included five weekly 1-hour sessions with the family and telephone support conversations (of 30 to 40 minutes) every week. During treatment, four intervention areas were addressed: resistance by presence, support and public opinion, prevention of escalation, and reconciliation gestures. At post-treatment, the results favoured the non-violent resistance intervention when assessed using parent-rated antisocial behaviour using the CBCL (SMD -0.81, 95% CI, −0.19 to −1.44).

### 7.2.5 Clinical evidence for the review of head-to-head comparisons of interventions

There were relatively few trials that made relevant direct (head-to-head) comparisons of one category of an intervention with another category; therefore, meta-analysis could only be used for two comparisons: (a) parent-focused interventions versus parent–child-based interventions (five trials) and (b) family-focused interventions versus child-focused interventions (two trials) (see Table 44 for study characteristics and see below for a summary of the evidence). In addition, there were a number of other comparisons where neither intervention was shown to be effective when compared with a control group (see Section 7.2.4) and so the GDG did not review the evidence further (LOCHMAN2002 compared a multi-component intervention with a parent–child-based intervention; KING1990 compared a multi-component intervention with a parent–teacher-based intervention; MACSRG2002 and REID2007 compared a multi-component intervention with a classroom-based intervention).

**Table 68: Summary of findings table for parent-focused interventions compared with parent–child-based interventions (post-treatment)**

**Patient or population:** children and young people with, or at high risk of, conduct disorders (post-treatment)
**Intervention:** parent focused
**Comparison:** parent–child based

| Outcomes | Illustrative comparative risks (95% CI) | | No. of participants (studies) | Quality of the evidence (GRADE) |
| --- | --- | --- | --- | --- |
| | Assumed risk<br>Parent–child-based | Corresponding risk<br>Parent-focused | | |
| **Observer-rated antisocial behaviour**<br>Any valid method | – | The mean observer-rated antisocial behaviour in the intervention groups was **0.15 standard deviations lower** (0.71 lower to 0.41 higher) | 48 (1) | ⊕⊕⊕⊝<br>**moderate**[1] |
| **Researcher-/clinician-rated antisocial behaviour**<br>Any valid rating scale | – | The mean researcher-/clinician-rated antisocial behaviour in the intervention groups was **0.68 standard deviations higher** (0.12 to 1.24 higher) | 51 (1) | ⊕⊕⊕⊝<br>**low**[1,2] |
| **Teacher-rated antisocial behaviour**<br>Any valid rating scale | – | The mean teacher-rated antisocial behaviour in the intervention groups was **0.25 standard deviations higher** (0.14 lower to 0.64 higher) | 198 (3) | ⊕⊕⊕⊝<br>**low**[1,2] |
| **Parent-rated antisocial behaviour**<br>Any valid rating scale | – | The mean parent-rated antisocial behaviour in the intervention groups was **0.19 standard deviations higher** (0.54 lower to 0.91 higher) | 248 (4) | ⊕⊕⊝⊝<br>**very low**[1,2,3] |

[1] OIS (for dichotomous outcomes, OIS = 300 events; for continuous outcomes, OIS = 400 participants) not met.
[2] Risk of bias across domains was generally high or unclear.
[3] There is evidence of substantial heterogeneity of study effect sizes.

*Parent-focused versus parent–child-based interventions*

Very low quality evidence from four comparisons with 248 participants favoured parent–child-based interventions when antisocial behaviour was rated by parents at post-treatment, although this was not conclusive (Table 68). There was also inconclusive low quality evidence from three comparisons (198 participants) that reported teacher-rated antisocial behaviour, and inconclusive low quality evidence from one comparison (48 participants) that reported observer-rated antisocial behaviour. In addition, one comparison with 51 participants reported low quality evidence that favoured parent–child-based interventions when antisocial behaviour was rated by researchers/ clinicians. At follow-up, low to moderate quality evidence from the two comparisons that reported observer–rated (48 participants) and researcher-/clinician-rated (51 participants) antisocial behaviour were clearly in favour of parent–child-based interventions (Table 69). Similarly to post-treatment, very low to low quality evidence from comparisons reporting teacher-rated and parent-rated outcomes was inconclusive.

*Family-focused versus child-based interventions*

Low quality evidence from two comparisons with 108 participants favoured family-focused interventions when antisocial behaviour was rated by parents at post-treatment, although baseline differences in the outcome raises doubt about this finding (Table 70). There was also inconclusive moderate quality evidence from one comparison (88 participants) that reported researcher-/clinician-rated offending behaviour. At follow-up, moderate quality evidence from one trial favoured child-based interventions when offending behaviour was rated by a researcher/clinician, and low quality evidence from the two comparisons that reported parent-rated antisocial behaviour was inconclusive (Table 71).

### 7.2.6 Moderators of intervention effectiveness

Where sufficient data were available, meta-regression was used to explore unexplained between-study variation in effect size. There were two categories of interventions where meta-regression was possible: child-focused interventions (but only for teacher-rated outcomes) and parent-focused interventions (for observer and parent-rated outcomes). In the latter case, there was also sufficient data to conduct a sensitivity analysis excluding attenuated parent-focused interventions (for parent-rated outcomes). Attenuated interventions were defined as very brief or self-directed with little or no healthcare, social care or other professional involvement.

Some variables that the GDG specified before data extraction as being important to examine (that is, coexisting conditions, ethnicity, gender, looked-after children and young people, contact with the criminal justice system) could not be included in the meta-regression due to insufficient data. With regard to the variables that could be included in the meta-regression, for the child-focused interventions one was specified after the initial meta-regression models had been run (dose). For parent-focused interventions, three variables were specified after running the initial model (attenuation of the intervention, inclusion of child in the intervention and severity of antisocial behaviour at baseline). However, given that by definition meta-regression is observational in nature, all findings need to be interpreted with caution.

**Table 69: Summary of findings table for parent-focused interventions compared with parent–child-based interventions (follow-up)**

**Patient or population:** children and young people with, or at high risk of, conduct disorders (follow-up)
**Intervention:** parent-focused
**Comparison:** parent–child-based

| Outcomes | Illustrative comparative risks (95% CI) | | No. of participants (studies) | Quality of the evidence (GRADE) |
|---|---|---|---|---|
| | Assumed risk<br>Parent–child-based | Corresponding risk<br>Parent-focused | | |
| **Observer-rated antisocial behaviour**<br>Any valid method | – | The mean observer-rated antisocial behaviour in the intervention groups was **0.65 standard deviations higher** (0.07 to 1.22 higher) | 48 (1) | ⊕⊕⊕⊕<br>moderate[1] |
| **Researcher-/clinician-rated antisocial behaviour**<br>Any valid rating scale | – | The mean researcher-/clinician-rated antisocial behaviour in the intervention groups was **0.92 standard deviations higher** (0.34 to 1.49 higher) | 51 (1) | ⊕⊕⊕⊕<br>low[1,2] |
| **Teacher-rated antisocial behaviour**<br>Any valid rating scale | – | The mean teacher-rated antisocial behaviour in the intervention groups was **0.08 standard deviations lower** (0.36 lower to 0.20 higher) | 190 (3) | ⊕⊕⊕⊕<br>low[1,2] |
| **Parent-rated antisocial behaviour**<br>Any valid rating scale | – | The mean parent-rated antisocial behaviour in the intervention groups was **0.34 standard deviations higher** (0.10 lower to 0.77 higher) | 248 (4) | ⊕⊕⊕⊕<br>very low[1,2,3] |

[1]OIS (for dichotomous outcomes, OIS = 300 events; for continuous outcomes, OIS = 400 participants) not met.
[2]Risk of bias across domains was generally high or unclear.
[3]There is evidence of substantial heterogeneity of study effect sizes.

**Table 70: Summary of findings table for family-focused interventions compared with child-based interventions (post-treatment)**

**Patient or population:** children and young people with, or at high risk of, conduct disorders (post-treatment)
**Intervention:** family focused
**Comparison:** child-based

| Outcomes | Illustrative comparative risks (95% CI) | | No. of participants (studies) | Quality of the evidence (GRADE) |
| --- | --- | --- | --- | --- |
| | Assumed risk | Corresponding risk | | |
| | Parent–child based | Family focused | | |
| **Researcher-/clinician-rated offending behaviour** Any valid rating scale | – | The mean researcher-/clinician-rated offending behaviour in the intervention groups was **0.21 standard deviations lower** (0.73 lower to 0.31 higher) | 56 (1) | ⊕⊕⊕⊝ **moderate**[1] |
| **Parent-rated antisocial behaviour** Any valid rating scale | – | The mean parent-rated antisocial behaviour in the intervention groups was **0.47 standard deviations lower** (0.77 to 0.16 lower) | 108 (2) | ⊕⊕⊝⊝ **low**[1,2] |

[1] OIS (for dichotomous outcomes, OIS = 300 events; for continuous outcomes, OIS = 400 participants) not met.
[2] Baseline differences were as large at endpoint; analysis of change scores suggested the effect favoured child-focused intervention for AZRIN2001.

**Table 71: Summary of findings table for family-focused interventions compared with child-based interventions (follow-up)**

**Patient or population:** children and young people with, or at high risk of, conduct disorders (follow-up)
**Intervention:** family focused
**Comparison:** child-based

| Outcomes | Illustrative comparative risks (95% CI) | | No. of participants (studies) | Quality of the evidence (GRADE) |
|---|---|---|---|---|
| | Assumed risk | Corresponding risk | | |
| | Parent–child-based | Family-focused | | |
| **Researcher-/clinician-rated offending behaviour**<br>Any valid rating scale | – | The mean researcher-/clinician-rated offending behaviour in the intervention groups was **0.57 standard deviations higher** (0.04 to 1.09 higher) | 56 (1) | ⊕⊕⊕⊖<br>**moderate**[1] |
| **Parent-rated antisocial behaviour**<br>Any valid rating scale | – | The mean parent-rated antisocial behaviour in the intervention groups was **0.47 standard deviations lower** (0.10 lower to 0.77 higher) | 108 (2) | ⊕⊕⊖⊖<br>**low**[1,2] |

[1] OIS (for dichotomous outcomes, OIS = 300 events; for continuous outcomes, OIS = 400 participants) not met.
[2] Baseline differences were at large at endpoint; analysis of change scores suggested the effect favoured child-focused intervention for AZRIN2001.

**Table 72: Meta-regression results for child-focused interventions versus any control for the outcome of antisocial behaviour, rated by teachers (post-treatment)**

| Covariate | Categories of covariate | β | 95% CI | p value | Adjusted $R^2$ |
|---|---|---|---|---|---|
| **Univariate model** | | | | | |
| Characteristics of the study methods | | | | | |
| Country | US (k = 14) versus other Western (k = 11) | 0.14 | −0.25 to 0.53 | 0.465 | 0% |
| Year | 1983 to 2011 (k = 25) | −0.02[1] | −0.04 to 0.005 | 0.122 | 8% |
| Time point | 4 to 35 weeks (k = 25) | 0.01 | −0.02 to 0.04 | 0.615 | 0% |
| Intervention type | Indicated prevention (k = 9) versus treatment (k = 16) | 0.04 | −0.37 to 0.45 | 0.845 | 0% |
| Intervention theory base | Behaviour only (k = 6) versus cognitive and behavioural (k = 18) | −0.31 | −0.77 to 0.15 | 0.183 | 0% |
| Treatment setting | Clinic (k = 7) versus school (k = 17) | −0.47[2] | −0.91 to −0.04 | 0.035 | 19% |
| Intervention format | Individual (k = 3) versus group (k = 22) | 0.31[3] | −0.32 to 0.95 | 0.317 | 0.5% |
| Control group category | Attention control/treatment as usual (k = 11) versus no treatment/waitlist control (k = 14) | −0.26[4] | −0.65 to 0.13 | 0.188 | 6% |
| Intervention dose | 3 to 139 hours (k = 25) | 0.001 | −0.01 to 0.01 | 0.698 | 0% |
| **Multivariate model** | | | | | |
| Step 1 | | | | | |
| Treatment setting | | −0.47[2] | −0.91 to −0.04 | 0.035 | 19% |
| Step 2 | | | | | |
| Treatment setting | | −0.42[2] | −0.86 to 0.03 | 0.066 | 20% |
| Year | | −0.01[1] | −0.04 to 0.01 | 0.234 | |

*Continued*

259

**Table 72:** *(Continued)*

| Covariate | Categories of covariate | β | 95% CI | p value | Adjusted $R^2$ |
|---|---|---|---|---|---|
| **Multivariate model** | | | | | |
| Step 3 | | | | | |
| | Treatment setting | −0.43[2] | −0.93 to 0.08 | 0.092 | 13% |
| | Control group category | −0.08[4] | −0.52 to 0.36 | 0.491 | |
| Step 4 | | | | | |
| | Treatment setting | −0.49[2] | −0.92 to −0.05 | 0.029 | 23% |
| | Intervention format | 0.36[3] | −0.24 to 0.96 | 0.219 | |
| Sensitivity analysis: intervention type | | | | | |
| | Treatment setting | −0.63[2] | −1.12 to −0.15 | 0.013 | 31% |
| | Intervention format | 0.47[3] | −0.15 to 1.08 | 0.127 | |
| | Intervention type | −0.28 | −0.70 to 0.15 | 0.193 | |
| Sensitivity analysis: dose | | | | | |
| | Treatment setting | −0.49[2] | −0.93 to −0.05 | 0.031 | 17% |
| | Intervention format | 0.35[3] | −0.26 to 0.97 | 0.245 | |
| | Intervention dose | 0.001 | −0.01 to 0.01 | 0.723 | |

[1]Negative (regression coefficient) β favours more recently published trials relative to older trials.
[2]Negative β favours school relative to clinic setting.
[3]Positive β favours individual relative to group format.
[4]Negative β favours no treatment/waitlist control relative to attention control/treatment as usual control.
[5]Negative β favours treatment intervention relative to indicated prevention.

For the meta-analysis of child-focused interventions, there were 25 comparisons included in the analysis of teacher-rated antisocial behaviour at post-treatment. A visual inspection of the forest plot indicated that most comparisons favour the intervention, with some large effects and some small or negative effects; with moderate between-study heterogeneity ($I^2 = 58\%$, $p = 0.001$). As can be seen in Table 72, the univariate meta-regression results suggest that four factors (year of publication, treatment setting, intervention format and control group category) explain between 0.5% and 19% of the between trial variability in effect sizes. Using a forward step-wise approach, a multivariate model that included two variables (treatment setting and intervention format – see Step 4 of the model) explained the most variance (23%). The model suggested that interventions administered in schools produced, on average, a larger effect than those in clinics when controlling for intervention format (individual or group). In addition, to check that the effect was not caused by differences in severity of conduct disorder or intervention dose, sensitivity analyses were conducted. To control for severity, type of intervention (indicated prevention or treatment) was used as a proxy for severity[55] and entered into the model. As can be seen in Table 72, controlling for intervention type increased the variance explained to 31% and strengthens the finding that interventions administered in schools are more effective than clinic-based interventions. With regard to intervention dose, adding this variable to the model accounted for no more variance than treatment setting and intervention format alone.

For the meta-analysis of all (standard and attenuated) parent-focused interventions, there were 19 comparisons included in the analysis of observer-rated antisocial behaviour at post-treatment. A visual inspection of the forest plot indicated that most comparisons favoured the intervention, with some large effects and some small or negative effects, and with moderate heterogeneity ($I^2 = 44\%$, $p = 0.02$). As can be seen in Table 73, the univariate meta-regression results suggest that three factors (severity of symptoms at baseline, intervention format and intervention supervision) explain between 11% and 24% of the between-trial variability in effect sizes. Using a forward step-wise approach, a multivariate model, which included three variables (severity of symptoms at baseline, intervention format and intervention supervision – see Step 3 of the model) explained the most variance (45%). The model suggested that group interventions produced, on average, a larger effect than individual interventions when controlling for intervention supervision (yes/no) and baseline severity.

In addition, there were 63 comparisons included in the analysis of parent-rated antisocial behaviour at post-treatment. A visual inspection of the forest plot indicated that most comparisons favour the intervention, with some large effects and some small or negative effects, and with moderate heterogeneity ($I^2 = 54\%$, $p < 0.001$). As can be seen in Table 74, the univariate meta-regression results suggest that five factors (intervention theory base, control group category, time point, method of analysis and attenuation of the intervention) explain between 1% and 17% of the between trial

---

[55]Baseline severity of conduct problems could not be included as a variable due to the wide range of scales reported, many of which do not have published norms allowing standardisation.

**Table 73: Meta-regression results for parent-focused interventions versus any control for the outcome of antisocial behaviour, rated by observers (post-treatment)**

| Covariate | Categories of covariate | β | 95% CI | p value | Adjusted $R^2$ |
|---|---|---|---|---|---|
| **Univariate model** | | | | | |
| Characteristics of the sample (children and young people) | | | | | |
| Severity of symptoms at baseline | T score: 59 to 71 | −0.05[1] | −0.11 to 0.01 | 0.078 | 24% |
| Characteristics of the study methods | | | | | |
| Country | US (k = 11) versus other Western (k = 8) | −0.22 | −0.63 to 0.19 | 0.273 | 0% |
| Year | 1984 to 2012 (k = 19) | 0.02 | −0.01 to 0.04 | 0.236 | 0% |
| Intervention supervision | No (k = 8) versus yes (k = 11) | 0.32[2] | −0.08 to 0.73 | 0.113 | 11% |
| Intervention format | Individual (k = 12) versus group (k = 7) | −0.29[3] | −0.70 to 0.13 | 0.162 | 20% |
| Attenuation of parent-focused | Attenuated (k = 7) versus standard (k = 12) | −0.19 | −0.63 to 0.26 | 0.390 | 0% |

| Multivariate model | | | | |
|---|---|---|---|---|
| **Step 1** | | | | |
| Severity at baseline | −0.05 | −0.11 to 0.01 | 0.078 | 24% |
| **Step 2** | | | | |
| Severity at baseline | −0.05 | −0.11 to 0.004 | 0.068 | 45% |
| Intervention format | −0.29 | −0.67 to 0.09 | 0.126 | |
| **Step 3** | | | | |
| Severity at baseline | −0.04 | −0.10 to 0.02 | 0.203 | 45% |
| Intervention format | −0.35 | −0.73 to 0.04 | 0.074 | |
| Intervention supervision | 0.29 | −0.11 to 0.70 | 0.192 | |

[1] Negative regression coefficient ($\beta$) favours more severe symptoms relative to less severe.
[2] Positive $\beta$ favours no supervision relative to supervision.
[3] Negative $\beta$ favours group relative to individual interventions.

**Table 74: Meta-regression results for parent-focused interventions versus any control for the outcome of antisocial behaviour, rated by parents (post-treatment)**

| Covariate | Categories of covariate | $\beta$ | 95% CI | p value | Adjusted $R^2$ |
|---|---|---|---|---|---|
| **Univariate model** | | | | | |
| Characteristics of the sample (children and young people) | | | | | |
| Mean age | 2 to 14 (k = 63) | 0.04 | −0.02 to 0.09 | 0.181 | 0% |
| Severity of symptoms at baseline | T score: 53 to 84 | 0.001 | −0.02 to 0.02 | 0.929 | 0% |
| Characteristics of the study methods | | | | | |
| Country | US (k = 26) versus other Western (k = 36) | 0.02 | −0.21 to 0.26 | 0.841 | 0% |
| Year | 1984 to 2012 (k = 63) | 0.01 | −0.01 to 0.02 | 0.518 | 0% |
| Time point | 2 to 73 weeks (k = 63) | 0.008[1] | −0.0002 to 0.01 | 0.058 | 13% |
| Intervention type | Indicated prevention (k = 14) versus treatment (k = 49) | −0.14 | −0.41 to 0.14 | 0.332 | 0% |
| Intervention theory base | Behavioural only (k = 17) versus cognitive and behavioural (k = 42) | −0.23[2] | −0.47 to 0.01 | 0.059 | 17% |
| Intervention supervision | No (k = 31) versus yes (k = 32) | 0.06 | −0.16 to 0.29 | 0.574 | 0% |
| Intervention fidelity | No (k = 17) versus yes (k = 46) | −0.01 | −0.28 to 0.26 | 0.923 | 0% |

| Variable | Comparison | Estimate | 95% CI | p | % |
|---|---|---|---|---|---|
| Intervention format | Individual (k = 21) versus group (k = 26) | 0.06 | −0.22 to 0.35 | 0.652 | 0% |
| Control group category | Attention control/treatment as usual (k = 9) versus no treatment/waitlist control (k = 54) | −0.30[3] | −0.59 to −0.02 | 0.035 | 15% |
| Attenuation of parent-focused intervention | Attenuated (k = 19) versus standard (k = 44) | 0.20[4] | −0.06 to 0.45 | 0.123 | 1% |
| Method of analysis | Available case (k = 42) versus imputation (k = 13) | 0.25[5] | −0.02 to 0.52 | 0.068 | 9% |
| **Multivariate model** | | | | | |
| Step 1 | | | | | |
| Intervention theory base | | −0.23 | −0.47 to 0.01 | 0.059 | 17% |
| Step 2 | | | | | |
| Intervention theory base | | −0.20 | −0.43 to 0.04 | 0.094 | 31% |
| Control group category | | −0.26 | −0.53 to 0.01 | 0.055 | |
| Step 3 | | | | | |
| Intervention theory base | | −0.18 | −0.42 to 0.07 | 0.153 | 28% |
| Control group category | | −0.21 | −0.54 to 0.11 | 0.198 | |
| Time point[3] | | 0.003 | −0.72 to 1.30 | 0.570 | |

*Continued*

**Table 74:** *(Continued)*

| Covariate | Categories of covariate | β | 95% CI | *p* value | Adjusted $R^2$ |
|---|---|---|---|---|---|
| **Multivariate model** | | | | | |
| Step 4 | | | | | |
| Control group category | | −0.23 | −0.53 to 0.06 | 0.122 | |
| Method of analysis | | 0.07 | −0.20 to 0.35 | 0.585 | |
| Step 5 | | | | | 27% |
| Intervention theory base | | −0.20 | −0.44 to 0.03 | 0.093 | |
| Control group category | | −0.22 | −0.51 to 0.06 | 0.121 | |
| Attenuation of intervention | | 0.13 | −0.13 to 0.38 | 0.323 | |
| Sensitivity analysis | | | | | 26% |
| Intervention theory base | | −0.20 | −0.45 to 0.04 | 0.099 | |
| Control group category | | −0.27 | −0.55 to 0.01 | 0.058 | |
| Severity of symptoms at baseline | | −0.002 | −0.02 to 0.02 | 0.841 | |

[1]Positive β favours shorter relative to longer interventions.
[2]Negative β favours cognitive and behavioural based interventions relative to behavioural only.
[3]Negative β favours no treatment/waitlist control relative to attention control/treatment as usual.
[4]Positive β favours attenuated relative to standard interventions.
[5]Positive β favours available case relative to imputation.

variability in effect sizes. Using a forward step-wise approach, a multivariate model that included two variables (intervention theory base and control group category – see Step 2 of the model) explained the most variance (31%). The model suggested that cognitive and behavioural interventions produced on average a larger effect than behavioural-only interventions when controlling for control group category. To check that the effect was not caused by differences in severity of conduct disorder, a sensitivity analysis was conducted controlling for baseline severity. The addition of severity did not materially change the findings (see Table 74).

For standard (non-attenuated) parent-focused interventions, there were 39 comparisons included in the meta-analysis of parent-rated antisocial behaviour at post-treatment, with moderate heterogeneity ($I^2 = 52\%, p < 0.001$). A visual inspection of the forest plot indicated that most comparisons favour the intervention, with some large effects and some small or negative effects. As can be seen in Table 75, the univariate meta-regression results suggest that five factors (programme type, control group category, intervention theory base, method of analysis and inclusion of child) explain between 1% and 16% of the between trial variability in effect sizes. Using a forward step-wise approach, a multivariate model, which included four variables (programme type, control group category, intervention theory base and inclusion of child – see Step 5 of the model), explained the most variance (39%). The model suggested that standard Triple P and Incredible Years programmes produced, on average, a larger effect than other standard programmes when controlling for control group category, theory base and inclusion of the child in the intervention. To check that the effect was not caused by differences in severity of conduct disorder, a sensitivity analysis was conducted controlling for baseline severity. The addition of severity did not materially change the findings (see Table 75).

### 7.2.7     Clinical evidence summary

Overall, the clinical evidence suggests that parent-focused interventions are effective for reducing antisocial behaviour in younger children (<11 years old) with a conduct disorder (or those at high risk based on symptoms). The meta-regression analyses provide no consistent evidence (across outcome raters) with regard to moderators of effectiveness. However, the limited evidence suggests that group parent-focused interventions, those based on cognitive and behavioural principles and those using the Triple P or Incredible Years programmes may be especially effective. There was no evidence suggesting that indicated prevention and treatment interventions differ in effectiveness. For children in foster care there is some evidence that foster carer-focused interventions are also effective.

Child-focused interventions appear to be effective for reducing antisocial behaviour in children and young people with a conduct disorder (or at high risk based on symptoms). Thirty-seven percent of the included trials were conducted in the 11+ age group, 19% in the <11 age group and 44% in both age groups. Further inspection of the trials indicated that the average age in the trials ranged from 7 to 14 years. The meta-regression provides limited evidence that child-focused interventions delivered in school settings may be more effective than those delivered in the clinical setting.

**Table 75: Meta-regression results for standard (non-attenuated) parent-focused interventions versus any control for the outcome of antisocial behaviour, rated by parents (post-treatment)**

| Covariate | Categories of covariate | β | 95% CI | p value | Adjusted $R^2$ |
|---|---|---|---|---|---|
| **Univariate model** | | | | | |
| Characteristics of the sample (children and young people) | | | | | |
| Mean age | 3 to 10 (k = 44) | 0.04 | −0.04 to 0.12 | 0.357 | 0% |
| Severity of symptoms at baseline | T score: 54 to 84 (k = 44) | 0.003 | −0.02 to 0.02 | 0.727 | 0% |
| Characteristics of the study methods | | | | | |
| Country | US (k = 21) versus other Western (k = 22) | −0.05 | −0.31 to 0.21 | 0.721 | 0% |
| Year | 1984 to 2012 (k = 44) | 0.007 | −0.01 to 0.03 | 0.489 | 0% |
| Time point | 6 to 73 weeks (k = 44) | 0.006 | −0.002 to 0.01 | 0.114 | 0% |
| Intervention type | Indicated prevention (k = 8) versus treatment (k = 36) | −0.16 | −0.49 to 0.17 | 0.325 | 0% |
| Intervention theory base | Behavioural only (k = 13) versus cognitive and behavioural (k = 28) | −0.22[1] | −0.48 to 0.04 | 0.089 | 11% |
| Intervention supervision | No (k = 15) versus yes (k = 29) | −0.04 | −0.32 to 0.24 | 0.785 | 0% |
| Intervention fidelity | No (k = 10) versus yes (k = 34) | −0.13 | −0.44 to 0.19 | 0.414 | 0% |
| Intervention format | Individual (k = 14) versus group (k = 30) | 0.01 | −0.27 to 0.28 | 0.967 | 0% |

| | | | | | |
|---|---|---|---|---|---|
| Control group category | Attention control/treatment as usual (k = 9) versus no treatment/waitlist control (k = 35) | −0.26[2] | −0.54 to 0.02 | 0.067 | 15% |
| Programme type | Triple P and Incredible Years (k = 18) versus other (k = 21) | 0.25[3] | 0.01 to 0.49 | 0.041 | 16% |
| Inclusion of child | Parent only (k = 35) versus parent with child (k = 9) | −0.17[4] | −0.49 to 0.15 | 0.301 | 1% |
| Method of analysis | Available case (k = 31) versus imputation (k = 13) | 0.17[5] | −0.10 to 0.43 | 0.205 | 5% |
| **Multivariate model** | | | | | |
| Step 1 | | | | | |
| Programme type | | 0.25 | 0.01 to 0.49 | 0.041 | 16% |
| Step 2 | | | | | |
| Programme type | | 0.22 | −0.02 to 0.46 | 0.069 | 25% |
| Control group category | | −0.22 | −0.50 to 0.05 | 0.111 | |
| Step 3 | | | | | |
| Programme type | | 0.25 | −0.08 to 0.58 | 0.135 | 29% |
| Control group category | | −0.20 | −0.47 to 0.06 | 0.132 | |
| Intervention theory base | | 0.002 | −0.35 to 0.36 | 0.993 | |
| Step 4 | | | | | |
| Programme type | | 0.25 | −0.09 to 0.59 | 0.142 | 24% |
| Control group category | | −0.19 | −0.47 to 0.09 | 0.185 | |
| Method of analysis | | 0.04 | −0.23 to 0.31 | 0.772 | |

*Continued*

**Table 75: (*Continued*)**

| Covariate | Categories of covariate | β | 95% CI | *p* value | Adjusted $R^2$ |
|---|---|---|---|---|---|
| **Multivariate model** | | | | | |
| Step 5 | | | | | |
| Programme type | | 0.30 | −0.04 to 0.63 | 0.079 | 39% |
| Control group category | | −0.25 | −0.52 to 0.02 | 0.064 | |
| Intervention theory base | | 0.03 | −0.32 to 0.38 | 0.867 | |
| Inclusion of child | | −0.23 | −0.55 to 0.10 | 0.166 | |
| Sensitivity analysis | | | | | |
| Programme type | | 0.30 | −0.04 to 0.64 | 0.084 | 32% |
| Control group category | | −0.25 | −0.53 to 0.03 | 0.075 | |
| Intervention theory base | | 0.03 | −0.34 to 0.40 | 0.872 | |
| Inclusion of child | | −0.23 | −0.56 to 0.11 | 0.177 | |
| Severity of symptoms at baseline | | 0.001 | −0.02 to 0.02 | 0.991 | |

[1]Negative β favours cognitive and behavioural based interventions relative to behavioural only.
[2]Negative β favours no treatment/waitlist control relative to attention control/treatment as usual.
[3]Positive β favours standard Triple P and Incredible Years programmes relative to other programmes.
[4]Negative β favours parent with child interventions relative to parent only.
[5]Positive β favours available case relative to imputation.

There was inconclusive evidence regarding whether indication prevention and treatment interventions differ in effectiveness.

For young people (11+ years old) with a conduct disorder (or at high risk based on symptoms), multimodal treatment interventions may be effective for reducing antisocial and offending behaviour. The evidence was consistent across outcome raters with small- to medium-sized effects at both post-treatment and follow-up, although wide confidence intervals and substantial heterogeneity for some outcomes means that a null effect cannot be ruled out. It should be noted that there were no indicated prevention trials available for inclusion in the meta-analysis.

Based on comparisons with a treatment-as-usual or no-treatment control group, interventions given separately to both the parents and the child are not clearly more effective than parent-focused interventions alone. An intervention given to families called 'non-violent resistance' may be effective, but at present only one trial involving 41 families has been conducted. In addition, it is not clear whether interventions given separately to the parents and to teachers, or classroom-based interventions, or multi-component interventions are effective.

Based on head-to-head trials, interventions given separately to both the parents and the child are not clearly more effective than parent-focused interventions alone. The evidence was inconclusive with regard to whether family-focused interventions differed in effectiveness when compared with child-focused interventions.

## 7.3 HEALTH ECONOMIC EVIDENCE

### 7.3.1 Child-focused interventions

*Systematic literature review*
No studies assessing the cost effectiveness of child-focused programmes for children and young people with conduct disorder were identified by the systematic search of the economic literature undertaken for this guideline. Details on the methods used for the systematic search of the economic literature are described in Chapter 3.

*Economic modelling*
**Introduction – objective of economic modelling**
The systematic review of clinical evidence (summarised in Section 7.2.7) demonstrated that child-focused programmes in addition to treatment as usual are more clinically effective than treatment as usual alone in improving the behaviour of children and young people with conduct disorder. Given the resource implications of conduct disorder, which could potentially be significant, the GDG considered a cost-effectiveness analysis of child-focused programmes to be of high priority. In the absence of any existing economic evidence on child-focused programmes, a de novo economic model was developed to assess whether the intervention cost would be off-set by potential cost savings resulting from improvement in the behaviour of children and young people with conduct disorder. The model population consisted of children and young people between the age of 7 and 14 years with conduct disorder.

The perspective adopted was that of the NHS and personal social services (PSS) in the main analysis, as recommended by NICE (2009d). A secondary analysis was also conducted adopting a wider perspective because the GDG considered other costs such as education and crime to be significant. These costs are expected to be reduced greatly following successful treatment of a person with conduct disorder.

Available evidence on health utilities for conduct disorder was poor. Literature searches identified only one study on health utilities for conduct disorder (Petrou et al., 2010). The study was based on small study population of 17 children with any conduct disorder problem who also had other psychiatric problems, including developmental disabilities. The health utility values for the three health states considered in the model were not provided in that study. Moreover, the GDG was concerned about the relevance of health utilities in conduct disorder because the benefits resulting from improving children's behaviour could be far greater than the health-related quality of life. As a result of the poor health-related quality of life data available, quality adjusted life years (QALYs) were not estimated.

## Economic modelling methods

*Interventions assessed*
Child-focused interventions were estimated by the GDG to comprise ten to 18 weekly sessions lasting 2 hours each, based on a cognitive-behavioural problem-solving model. The programme is delivered to 7- to 14-year-olds, mostly in a school setting and in groups of six, by a therapist of NHS Band 7c equivalent. The programme is often delivered in addition to usual management services for this population. More details about the child-focused programme are given in Section 7.2.1. The child-focused intervention plus treatment as usual is compared with treatment as usual only.

*Model structure*
The starting population consisted of a cohort of children aged 7 to 14 years with a clinical diagnosis of conduct disorder. The model structure below (Figure 11) depicts the initial outcome of conduct disorder after treatment for (a) conduct disorder, (b) conduct problems or (c) no conduct problems, depending on the extent of improvement

**Figure 11:  Model structure for conduct problems**

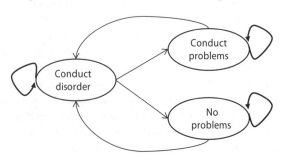

in the primary outcome of antisocial behaviour, and then the following possible progression through a Markov process where the absorbing state is conduct disorder. In the absence of sufficient data, the following assumptions were made to propagate the outcomes and costs over time:

● Children with an improved behaviour state (conduct problems or no conduct problems) were assumed to relapse to conduct disorder only, with none relapsing from no conduct problems to conduct problems.
● The relapse rate was assumed to be 50% (GDG consensus).
● For conduct disorder, children who were not offered the intervention were assumed to remain in the same state over time.

The model builds on the three possible health states of children and young people who have antisocial behavioural problems: conduct disorder, conduct problems and no conduct problems. The GDG was of the opinion that such categorisation could be based on the CBCL total T-score, a commonly reported antisocial behaviour primary outcome that is reflective of the impact of treatment on behaviour and the severity of the condition. To establish the categories of conduct problems from a continuous outcome measure, the CBCL T-score cut-off points used in *Parent-Training/Education Programmes in the Management of Children with Conduct Disorders*, NICE technology appraisal guidance 102 (NICE, 2006), were discussed and adopted for use by the GDG with definition of each state as follows:

● no conduct problems: <60
● conduct problems: 60 to 64
● conduct disorder: ≥ 65.

The mean baseline CBCL total T-score of 68.23 (SD 9.26) was derived by pooling the mean and variance of baseline CBCL total T-scores reported in the studies that were included in the systematic review of clinical evidence.

*Clinical input parameters*
From the meta-analysis of the clinical evidence, the effect size reported as a SMD was estimated to be 0.37 (95% CI, 0.19, 0.55) at post-treatment. This estimate was based on the teacher-rated antisocial behaviour outcome, demonstrating an overall low to moderate effect relative to treatment as usual.

Taking the CBLC score as the representative scale for the measurement of the antisocial behaviour treatment outcome, the magnitude of change in the CBCL score was estimated by re-expressing SMDs in the CBCL total T-score. This approach is one of the methods of interpreting the SMD as indicated in the *Cochrane Handbook for Systematic Reviews of Intervention* (Higgins & Green, 2011) and is described below.

The magnitude of change in score is equal to the standard deviation of a representative scale at baseline multiplied by the SMD. The variance of the absolute change in score is also estimated from the standard deviation of the representative score and 95% CI of the SMD. For example, if the SMD is 0.37 (95% CI, 0.19 to 0.55) and the standard deviation of the CBCL score at baseline is 9.26, then the magnitude of change in score is 0.37*9.26 (95% CI, 0.19*9.26, 0.55*9.26) = 3.34 (95% CI, 1.76 to 5.09).

The impact of child-focused programmes on behaviour is then deduced from the extent of reduction in the mean CBCL score using the absolute change in CBCL score derived from the formula above. Using the final CBCL score (post-intervention) and the cut-off points for conduct disorder, conduct problems and no conduct problems, on the CBCL score, it is possible to estimate the percentage of children with conduct disorder, conduct problems and no conduct problems post-intervention. For the control group, the treatment effect of the comparator was assumed to be zero given that the estimated effect size represents the relative effect between the intervention and comparator. As a result, the starting population of conduct disorder in the control group remained in the same state at the end of the programme.

*Time horizon*

Evidence on the natural history of conduct disorder as well as the sustained treatment effect of child-focused intervention is limited. None of the longitudinal studies have sufficient data to allow for modelling long-term transitions between the states of conduct disorder, conduct problems and no conduct problems (Cohen et al., 1993; Fergusson et al., 1995). Because of the lack of good quality data on the natural history, the model adopted an 8-year time horizon to represent children who received an intervention at 7 years of age and then were followed-up until 15 years of age. This time period covers the age range for which the intervention is expected to be offered.

*Cost data*

**Estimation of intervention cost**

The cost of child-focused intervention was based on the content of a child-focused programme that consisted of an average of 14 weekly 2-hour sessions delivered to a group of six children by a therapist of NHS Band 7 equivalent under the supervision of a senior therapist of NHS Band 8c. The cost was estimated to be £901.39 (see Table 76). Because both arms of the model included treatment as usual, the cost of treatment as usual was not estimated.

**Estimation of cost of states relating to conduct disorder**

The cost of states relating to conduct disorder considered in this analysis included NHS and PSS costs, education costs and crime costs for each health state considered in the model. NHS and PSS costs consisted of primary care services, psychiatric services, and hospital and social service costs, while education costs were mainly special education costs. The estimate of these service costs was based on those reported in Bonin and colleagues (2011) using conduct problem cost ratios as reported in Scott and colleagues (2001). Bonin and colleagues (2011) reported a comprehensive review of the mean annual cost of health, social and education service provisions to children with conduct disorder in the UK. The average annual costs associated with health states relating to conduct disorder are shown in Table 77.

The costs of crime associated with conduct disorder are usually found to be incurred by people aged 10 years and older. The crime cost estimates are based on those from the Home Office report by Dubourg and colleagues (2005). The total estimate of the cost of crime against individuals and households by young and adult offenders was £36.2 billion in 2003/04 prices. This includes the costs of violent crime

**Table 76: Cost of child-focused interventions**

| Resource use | Description | Unit cost | Total cost | Source |
|---|---|---|---|---|
| Staff cost | One therapist (Band 7 equivalent), one weekly 2-hour session for 14 weeks. Travel time: assumed 30 minutes each way. Total of 42 hours | £83 per hour | £3,486.00 | Resource use: expert opinion. Unit cost: (Curtis, 2011) |
| Supervision cost | One supervisor (Band 8c equivalent), assumed 7 hour's supervision for 14 weeks. Travel time: assumed 30 minutes each way for seven visits. Total of 14 hours | £135 per hour | £1,890.00 | Resource use: expert opinion. Unit cost: (Curtis, 2011) |
| Travel cost | 14 visits by a therapist and seven by a supervisor. Total of 21 visits | £1.54 per visit | £32.34 | Resource use: expert opinion. Unit cost: (Curtis, 2011) |
| Total | For six children | | £5,408.34 | |
| Total | Cost per child | | £901.39 | |

**Table 77: Mean annual cost of conduct disorder states**

| Public service | Cost for individual with no conduct problems | Cost for individual with conduct problems | Cost for individual with conduct disorder |
|---|---|---|---|
| NHS and social services | £144 | £459 | £1,312 |
| Education | £100 | £319 | £911 |
| Crime | £1,093 | £3,470 | £11,686 |

against individuals, of the criminal justice system and of the impact of violent crime on victims (including the emotional and physical impact, the healthcare costs of treating injuries and the longer-term health impact of violence).

To estimate the average cost of crime per person with conduct disorder, conduct problems or no conduct problem in the UK from the above total estimated cost, the following approach was taken:

- Estimation of the total population with conduct disorder, conduct problems and no conduct problems in the UK was achieved by weighting the total population of people aged 10 to 17 years (Office for National Statistics, 2011) with the relative proportion of children with conduct disorder, conduct problems and no conduct problems (Fergusson et al., 1995).
- Estimation of the total cost of crime attributable to conduct disorder, conduct problems and no conduct problems was achieved by weighting the total cost of crime attributable to those aged 10 to 17 years. This was estimated by multiplying the total crime cost of £36.2 billion by the percentage of offenders in a given year who were between 10 and 17 years old, as reported in the 2003 Home Office's Crime and Justice Survey (Budd et al., 2005); this cost figure was then attributed to conduct disorder, conduct problems and no conduct problem using estimated figures of the percentage of crime specifically attributed to each of these three conditions (Sainsbury Centre for Mental Health, 2009).
- Finally, estimation of the average cost of crime per person with conduct disorder, conduct problems or no conduct problem was achieved by dividing the total cost of crime attributable to individuals with conduct disorder, conduct problems and no conduct problem by the total number of children aged 10 to 17 years with conduct disorder, conduct problems and no conduct problem.

All prices were in 2011 UK pounds and the summary of the cost data is presented in Table 77.

**Discounting**
Discounting was applied at an annual rate of 3.5%, as recommended by NICE (2009); prices were expressed in 2011 UK pounds and uplifted, when necessary, using the Hospital and Community Health Service Pay and Price Index (Curtis, 2011).

*Data analysis and presentation of the results*
The difference in the mean costs over the time horizon of analysis between the treated and untreated groups was estimated, to determine the extent of potential cost savings due to improvement in the behaviour state of the target population. The results are presented in two parts: the main analysis, where only NHS and PSS costs were considered, and the secondary analysis, where wider costs to other sectors were considered. Sensitivity analysis was conducted for the secondary analysis to test the impact of potential uncertainty around the rate of relapse, cost of intervention and cost of crime by varying the base case value by 50%. In addition to deterministic analysis, a probabilistic analysis in which input parameters were assigned probabilistic distributions rather than being expressed as point estimates was undertaken. Probability distributions around the cost data and treatment effect as shown in Table 78 were generated

**Table 78: Summary of input parameters and their distributions**

| Parameter | Distribution | Point estimate | Probability distribution | Reference and comment |
|---|---|---|---|---|
| Effect size (child-focused + treatment as usual versus treatment as usual) | Normal | 0.37 | 95% CI, 0.19 to 0.55 | Meta-analysis |
| Baseline CBCL T-score | Normal | 68.23 | Standard error: 9.26 | Pooled baseline CBCL T-score from studies included in meta-analysis |
| Crime cost for conduct disorder | Gamma | £11,686 | Alpha = 2.04 Beta = 5,725.96 | See Table 77 |
| Crime cost for conduct problems | Gamma | £3,470 | Alpha = 2.04 Beta = 1,700.49 | See Table 77 |
| Crime cost for no conduct problems | Gamma | £1,093 | Alpha = 2.04 Beta = 535.65 | See Table 77 |
| NHS and PSS cost for conduct disorder | Gamma | £1,312 | Alpha = 2.04 Beta = 643.28 | See Table 77 |
| NHS and PSS cost for conduct problems | Gamma | £459 | Alpha = 2.04 Beta = 225.15 | See Table 77 |
| NHS and PSS cost for no conduct problems | Gamma | £144 | Alpha = 2.04 Beta = 70.76 | See Table 77 |
| Education cost for conduct disorder | Gamma | £911 | Alpha = 2.04 Beta = 446.75 | See Table 77 |
| Education cost for conduct problems | Gamma | £319 | Alpha = 2.04 Beta = 156.36 | See Table 77 |
| Education cost for no conduct problems | Gamma | £100 | Alpha = 2.04 Beta = 156.36 | See Table 77 |
| Cost of child-focused intervention | Gamma | £901 | Alpha = 2.04 Beta = 441.68 | See Table 76 |

using gamma distribution for cost parameters and normal distribution for effect sizes. Subsequently, 10,000 iterations of the economic model were run, each drawing random values out of the distributions fitted onto the model input parameters. Mean costs for the two treatment groups (intervention and control) were calculated by averaging across 10,000 iterations. Results of probabilistic analysis are also presented in the form of cost-effectiveness acceptability curves, which show the probability of the intervention being cost-effective at different levels of willingness-to-pay per extra person with conduct disorder improved to having no conduct problems following treatment.

**Economic modelling results**

*Results of analysis*
Treatment involving a child-focused programme plus treatment as usual compared with treatment as usual resulted in a reduction in the proportion of children with conduct disorder from 100% before treatment to 49% after treatment, because a proportion of children improved to an improved behaviour state of either conduct problems or no conduct problems (18% and 33%, respectively) (see Table 79). In the cost analysis, this improvement resulted in a net saving of £132 for the NHS and PSS (Table 80), and an overall net saving of up to £1,900 per child over an 8-year period when a wider perspective was considered (Table 81). For the three sectors considered, 26% of the savings were made in education while 37% were equally in health and social services and the criminal justice system.

**Table 79:  Estimated proportion of children with conduct disorder treated with child-focused intervention at post-treatment**

| Health state | Proportion at post-treatment |
|---|---|
| Conduct disorder | 0.49 |
| Conduct problems | 0.18 |
| No conduct problem | 0.33 |

**Table 80:  Results of main economic analysis of child-focused intervention for children and young people with conduct disorder**

| Cost component | Child focused + treatment as usual | Treatment as usual | Incremental cost |
|---|---|---|---|
| Intervention cost | £901 | – | £901 |
| NHS and PSS cost | £8,307 | £9,340 | –£1,033 |
| Total cost | **£9,208** | **£9,340** | **–£132** |

**Table 81: Results of secondary economic analysis of child-focused intervention for children and young people with conduct disorder**

| Cost component | Child-focused + treatment as usual | Treatment as usual | Incremental cost |
|---|---|---|---|
| Intervention cost | £901 | – | £901 |
| NHS and PSS cost | £8,307 | £9,340 | −£1,033 |
| Education cost | £5,769 | £6,486 | −£717 |
| Crime cost | £48,204 | £49,253 | −£1,049 |
| **Total cost (deterministic)** | **£63,181** | **£65,079** | **−£1,898** |
| **Total incremental cost (probabilistic)** | | | **−£1,881** |

**Table 82: Sensitivity analysis of child-focused programme**

| Variable | Value | Net cost |
|---|---|---|
| Relapse rate | 25% | −£7,607 |
| Relapse rate | 75% | −£386 |
| Intervention cost | 50% higher | −£1,450 |
| Intervention cost | 50% lower | −£2,350 |
| Crime cost | 50% lower | −£1,374 |

According to the sensitivity analysis shown in Table 82, the model results were robust under different scenarios. Results of the probabilistic analysis were essentially the same as with deterministic estimates. Further to the sensitivity analysis above, Figure 12 shows that the probability of child-focused programmes being cost-effective is 86% at zero willingness-to-pay per child with conduct disorder improved to having no conduct problems and consequently increases with increasing levels of willingness-to-pay.

**Discussion – limitations of the analysis**

*Discussion*
The analysis was based on evidence from the meta-analysis as well as from various assumptions on relapse rates and the persistence of the condition in children who were not offered treatment. It focused on estimating the savings that could be achieved by reducing the chance of conduct disorder persisting over time. Taking a narrow

**Figure 12: Probability of child-focused programmes being cost-effective at different levels of willingness-to-pay per child with conduct disorder improved to having no conduct problem**

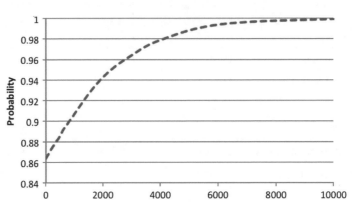

perspective of NHS and PSS only, adding a child-focused programme to treatment as usual was shown to result in a net saving of £132 over an 8-year period. This net saving increased to £1,898 when a wider perspective was considered. Overall, the results suggest that child-focused programme plus treatment as usual is potentially a cost-effective programme, compared with treatment as usual only.

The model considered the potential impact of relapse after treatment. Given that there is limited data available to model the relapse rate for those with improved states after the treatment of conduct problems, a 50% relapse rate was assumed. For those who had conduct problems after treatment, it was assumed that they could relapse to conduct disorder; similarly, those who had no conduct problems after treatment were also assumed to relapse to conduct disorder. That is, all children relapsing were assumed to move to the worst state. This is still conservative because there is the possibility that children with no conduct problems could relapse to having conduct problems and not conduct disorder. However, there is no data to determine such differential relapse, from no conduct problems to conduct problems or to conduct disorder. Recovery was not considered in the analysis due to lack of data on differential recovery from conduct disorder to conduct problems or no conduct problems, as well as from conduct problems to no conduct problems.

The model estimate of the cost of crime was based on the Home Office's crime-cost report of £36.2 billion (Dubourg et al., 2005), with the mean annual cost of crime for people with a severe form of conduct disorder estimated to be £11,686 and with an average cost of £5,416 per young offender across all three categories of the conduct disorder state. However, there is the possibility that this cost could be higher than estimated. A recent report on the cost of young offenders to the criminal justice system put the cost at £29,000 for those falling under 10% of potentially severe cases, and an average cost of £8,000 across all three conduct disorder states (National Audit Office, 2011). Elsewhere, the cost has been consistently reported to be higher (Sainsbury

Centre for Mental Health, 2009). As a result, it is possible that the model may have under-estimated the potential savings that may accrue from delivering a child-focused programme to children and young people with conduct disorder.

*Limitation of analysis*
The major limitation of this model, as indicated in *Parent-Training/Education Programmes in the Management of Children with Conduct Disorders* (NICE, 2006), is the arbitrary cut-off points of CBCL scores and the assumption of a normal distribution of children and young people's CBCL scores around this scale. There is a potential for the loss of information as a result of the cut-off points. However, the use of these points was essential in order to estimate the percentage of children in different health states and subsequently attach costs associated with different health states relating to conduct disorder.

*Overall conclusions from economic evidence*
Child-focused interventions delivered in addition to treatment as usual to children and young people with a conduct disorder were found to be cost-effective compared with treatment as usual alone.

## 7.3.2    Parent-focused interventions

*Systematic literature review*
The systematic literature review of economic evidence on parent-focused programmes for parents of children and young people with conduct disorder identified six existing studies (Bonin et al., 2011; Dretzke et al., 2005; Edwards et al., 2007; McCabe et al., 2005; Muntz et al., 2004; Sharac et al., 2011) that met the inclusion criteria (see Chapter 3 for details of the inclusion criteria). All studies were conducted in the UK; four adopted a short time horizon of 6 months to 1 year (Dretzke et al., 2005; Edwards et al., 2007; McCabe et al., 2005; Sharac et al., 2011) while the rest adopted a longer time horizon of about 4 to 25 years.

Edwards and colleagues (2007) compared a 6-month Webster-Stratton Incredible Years group parenting programme with a waitlist control for children aged 36 to 59 months in the UK who were 'at risk' of developing a conduct disorder. The 'at risk' group were defined as children with an ECBI score above a clinical cut-off point. Using a public perspective (NHS, education and social services) and costs in 2003/04 prices, they estimated the mean total cost for the intervention group at 6 months to be £2,881 while that of the control group was estimated to be £523. The incremental cost-effectiveness ratio (ICER) was £71 (95% CI, £42 to £140) per additional point scored in the ECBI Intensity scale. The programme had an 83.9% probability of being cost effective at the willingness-to-pay of £100 per additional point scored in the ECBI Intensity scale. In addition, the cost of bringing the child with the highest intensity score below the clinical cut-off point was estimated to be £5,486.

Sharac and colleagues (2011) evaluated the cost-effectiveness of home-based, manualised parenting programmes delivered to adoptive parents of children aged between

3 and 8 years who had been placed for non-relative adoption in the previous 3 to 18 months. The adopted children were identified as being at risk of conduct disorder from their high scores on the SDQ. The programmes were compared with routine care, and primary outcome measures were parent satisfaction and the SDQ. The time horizon for the analysis was 6 months, and the costs considered were the programme and service costs (NHS, social service and education costs). One of the home-based parenting programmes followed a cognitive approach, and the other educational; both lasted for 10 weeks with weekly sessions of 1 hour's duration. The mean (standard deviation) costs in 2006/07 over the 6-month period of intervention and follow-up were estimated to be £5,043 (£3,309) for the intervention group and £3,378 (£5,285) for the routine care group. Routine care was the dominant strategy when the SDQ outcome was considered.

Dretzke and colleagues (2005) assessed the cost-effectiveness of three types of parenting training/education programme (group community-based, group clinic-based and individual home-based) targeted at parents or carers of children or adolescents up to 18 years old where at least 50% have a behavioural disorder. Comparing the three types of programme with a control of no treatment, the treatment effect obtained through meta-analysis as the weighted mean difference of the CBCL score was estimated to be −4.36 (95% CI, −7.90 to −0.81), which was assumed to be the same across the various types of parenting programmes. The cost of the intervention was considered and no potential cost saving to the NHS or other sectors was reflected in the analysis. On average, the individual-based programme cost was about £3,000 more than the group programmes. No evidence on the impact of the programme on quality of life was identified but, based on the assumption of some level of improvement in the quality of life, ICERs for the three types of programmes were estimated to vary from £12,600 per QALY to £76,800 per QALY at 5% improvement in quality of life and £6,300 per QALY to £38,400 per QALY at 10% improvement in quality of life.

An additional study (McCabe et al., 2005) carried out for the technology appraisal (NICE, 2006) on parenting programmes assessed the incremental cost of each type of parenting programme compared with no treatment over a 1-year time horizon using an effect size derived from a meta-analysis, with the primary outcome measured by the CBCL scores. The estimated weighted mean difference of the CBCL was −5.96 (95% CI, −8.52 to −3.4), which was again assumed to be the same across the different types of parenting programme. The intervention costs ranged from £500 for the group clinic-based programme to £3,000 for the individual clinic-based programme, with the mean intervention cost reaching £1,279. Potential cost savings to the public sector were evaluated as the total cost savings due to a reduction in the proportion of individuals with conduct disorder or conduct problems following treatment. The analysis showed that the mean net cost of a parenting programme in conduct disorder alone was £99. The mean net cost of a parenting programme in conduct problems was £781. The mean net cost of a parenting programme for conduct problems and conduct disorder combined was £503. Probabilistic analysis showed that the probability of a parenting programme being cost-neutral or cost-saving was 35% in conduct disorder but only 15% in conduct problems.

Muntz and colleagues (2004) assessed the cost-effectiveness of an intensive practice-based parenting programme compared with standard treatment for children aged 2 to 10 years with conduct disorder. Using CBCL scores as the primary outcome measure, the intervention group showed a reduction in the baseline score of 12.8 compared with 4.2 in the control group after 4 years. The costs considered in the analysis were intervention costs and service costs (health, education and social services), which amounted to £1,005 per child in the intervention group and £4,400 per child in the control group. The intensive practice-based parenting programme was assessed as being a dominant strategy.

Out of all of the existing evidence on the economic analysis of parenting programmes, a study by Bonin and colleagues (2011) demonstrated the potential longer-term impact of a parenting programme over 20 years. They assessed a generic parenting programme versus no treatment delivered to a 5-year-old with conduct disorder. Costs considered included the intervention costs and potential downstream cost savings to the NHS, social services, education sector, voluntary sector and criminal justice system. The model made some assumptions around the natural course of conduct disorder in a 5-year-old child, based on the risk of persistence of the problem from age 3 to 8 years and from childhood to 18 years. Using an effect size from a published systematic review, the proportion of individuals with conduct disorder at 1-year post-treatment was derived to be 34%, and 50% of these individuals were assumed to remain problem free for the next 1 year after which the subsequent outcome is dependent on the natural course of conduct disorder. The results from this model showed that the potential cost savings to public services over 20 years were about 2.8 to 6.1 times the intervention costs. An explanation for this substantial cost saving could be due to the crime costs included in the analysis.

Overall, the results of these analyses indicate that parenting programmes are potentially cost-effective both in the short-term and in the long-term.

*Economic modelling*
**Introduction – objective of economic modelling**
Existing economic evidence on the parenting programme suggests it is a cost-effective option compared with no treatment for parents of children and young people with conduct disorder. Nonetheless, the GDG considered a cost-effectiveness analysis assessing the non-attenuated form of parent-focused programme to be important because the existing evidence was based on clinical evidence that had not distinguished between different intensities of programme delivery.

The objective of the analysis was to assess whether the intervention cost was offset by the potential savings incurred due to improvement in the behaviour of children whose parents were offered a parent-focused programme. The population for the analysis consisted of parents of children and young people between the age of 3 and 11 years who were diagnosed as having conduct disorder. The perspective adopted in the main analysis was that of NHS and PSS, as recommended by NICE (2009c). A secondary analysis was also conducted, adopting a wider perspective because the GDG considered other costs, such as education and crime, to be significant and expected them to be reduced greatly following the successful treatment of a person with conduct disorder.

Estimation of QALYs was not undertaken in the analysis due to the limitations of the available health utilities data, which have been discussed in Section 7.3.1.

## Economic modelling methods

*Interventions assessed*
The model compared the non-attenuated form of parenting programme delivered to parents of children between the ages of 3 to 11 years old with no treatment. The GDG considered the Incredible Years programme (Webster-Stratton, 1998) to be a comprehensive form of the non-attenuated type of parenting programme. Because there was no identified differential effect between group and individual therapy from the guideline meta-analysis, no separate analysis between group versus individual programme was conducted; group therapy consumes fewer resources (because therapists' time is spread over more families) and therefore is more cost-effective than individual therapy. Thus, the economic analysis assessed the group parenting programme.

*Model structure*
The starting population consisted of a cohort of children aged 3 years with a conduct disorder whose parents were offered either parent-focused programme or no treatment. The model structure and model states are the same as in the child-focused programme (see Section 7.3.1 and Figure 11). The assumptions and baseline CBCL T-scores also remained the same as in child-focused programme.

*Clinical input parameters*
From the meta-analysis of clinical evidence, the effect size reported as SMD was estimated to be 0.50 (95% CI, 0.38 to 0.63) at post-treatment. This estimate was based on parent-rated antisocial behaviour outcomes, demonstrating an overall moderate effect relative to no treatment.

*Time horizon*
Evidence regarding the natural history of conduct disorder as well as the sustained treatment effect of parent-focused programme is rather weak. None of the longitudinal studies have sufficient data to allow for modelling long-term transitions between the states of conduct disorder, conduct problems and no conduct problems (Cohen et al., 1993; Fergusson et al., 1995). Because of a lack of good quality data on the natural history of conduct disorder, the model adopted a 9-year time horizon where children were offered an intervention when they were 3 years old and then followed-up to 12 years of age. This time period covers the age range of children and young people to whom the intervention is expected to be offered to (3 to 12 years old).

*Cost data*
**Intervention cost**
A comprehensive estimate of the cost of the Incredible Years programme in groups of 12 families delivered by two therapists was reported in Curtis (2011) as £1,209 per

family. The comparator in this analysis is no treatment and therefore its intervention cost is zero.

**Estimation of costs of states relating to conduct disorder**

The method used for estimating the costs associated with conduct disorder, conduct problems and no conduct problem is the same as in the child-focused programme (see Section 7.3.1). However, because the population in parent-focused programmes starts from the younger age of 3 years, there was no associated cost of crime until the age of 10 years. See Table 77 for a summary of the costs of the conduct disorder, conduct problems and no conduct problems states.

*Discounting*
Discounting was applied at an annual rate of 3.5%, as recommended by NICE (2009d); prices were expressed in 2011 UK pounds and uplifted, when necessary, using the Hospital and Community Health Service Pay and Price Index (Curtis, 2011).

*Data analysis and presentation of the results*
The difference in the mean costs, within the time horizon, between the treated and untreated groups was estimated in order to determine the extent of cost savings that resulted from an improvement in the behaviour state of the target population. The results are presented in two parts: the main analysis, where NHS and PSS costs alone were considered, and the secondary analysis, where wider costs to other sectors were considered. Sensitivity analysis was conducted for the secondary analysis, to test the impact of potential uncertainty around the rate of relapse, cost of intervention and cost of crime by varying the base case value by 50%. In addition to deterministic analysis, a probabilistic analysis in which input parameters were assigned probabilistic distributions rather than being expressed as point estimates was undertaken. Probability distributions around the cost data and treatment effect, as shown in both Table 78 and Table 83, were generated

**Table 83:  Other input parameters and their distributions for the analysis of parent-focused interventions**

| Parameter | Distribution | Point estimate | Probability distribution | Reference and comment |
|---|---|---|---|---|
| Effect size (parent-focused versus no treatment) | Normal | 0.50 | 95% CI, 0.38 to 0.63 | Meta-analysis |
| Cost of parent-focused intervention | Gamma | £1,209 | Alpha = 2.04 Beta = 592.41 | Curtis (2011) |

using gamma distribution for cost parameters and normal distribution for effect sizes. Subsequently, 10,000 iterations of the economic model were run, each drawing random values out of the distributions fitted onto the model input parameters. Mean costs for the treated and untreated groups were calculated by averaging across 10,000 iterations. Results of probabilistic analysis are also presented in the form of cost-effectiveness acceptability curves, which show the probability of the intervention being cost-effective at different levels of willingness-to-pay per person with conduct disorder that improved to having no conduct problem following treatment.

## Economic modelling results

### Results of analysis

A parent-focused programme compared with no treatment resulted in a reduction in the proportion of children and young with conduct disorder from 100% before treatment to 43% after treatment, because a proportion of children improved to conduct problems or no conduct problems (26% and 31%, respectively) (see Table 84). In the cost analysis, this improvement in the behaviour state resulted in a net cost of £71 for the NHS and PSS (Table 85) and an overall net saving of up to £770 per child over a 9-year period when a wider perspective is considered (Table 86). For the three sectors considered, 57% of the total savings (£1,979) fall under the NHS and PSS while 40% and 3% fall under education and the criminal justice system,

#### Table 84: Estimated proportion of children in each conduct state after parent-focused intervention

| Health state | Proportion at post-treatment |
|---|---|
| Conduct disorder | 0.43 |
| Conduct problems | 0.26 |
| No conduct problems | 0.31 |

#### Table 85: Results of main economic analysis of parent-focused intervention for children with conduct disorder

| Cost component | Parent focused + treatment as usual | Treatment as usual | Incremental cost |
|---|---|---|---|
| Intervention cost | £1,209 | – | £1,209 |
| NHS and PSS cost | £9,199 | £10,337 | −£1,138 |
| Total cost | **£10,408** | **£10,337** | **£71** |

286

**Table 86: Results of secondary economic analysis of parent-focused intervention for children with conduct disorder**

| Cost component | Parent-focused + treatment as usual | Treatment as usual | Incremental cost |
|---|---|---|---|
| Intervention cost | £1,209 | – | £1,209 |
| NHS and PSS cost | £9,199 | £10,337 | −£1,138 |
| Education cost | £6,388 | £7,179 | −£791 |
| Crime cost | £18,009 | £18,059 | −£50 |
| **Total cost (deterministic)** | **£34,805** | **£35,575** | **−£770** |
| **Total incremental cost (probabilistic)** | | | **−767** |

respectively. The smallest proportion of savings falls under the criminal justice system, which is consistent with the child population considered in the model (3 to 11 years) where crime costs are expected to be incurred by those who are 10 years old and above.

From the results of the sensitivity analysis shown in Table 87, the model results were robust across alternative scenarios tested; that is, provision of the intervention always results in cost-savings. The results of probabilistic analysis were essentially the same with deterministic estimates. Further to the sensitivity analysis, Figure 13 shows that the probability of parent-focused programmes being cost-effective compared with no treatment is 60% at zero willingness-to-pay per extra child with conduct disorder improved to having no conduct problems following treatment, and the cost-effectiveness increases with increasing levels of willingness-to-pay.

**Table 87: Sensitivity analysis of parent-focused programmes**

| Variable | Value | Net cost |
|---|---|---|
| Relapse rate | 25% | −£3,206 |
| Relapse rate | 75% | −£108 |
| Intervention cost | 50% higher | −£165 |
| Intervention cost | 50% lower | −£1,374 |
| Crime cost | 50% lower | −£745 |

**Figure 13:  Probability of parent-focused programmes being cost-effective at different levels of willingness-to-pay per child with conduct disorder improved to having no conduct problems**

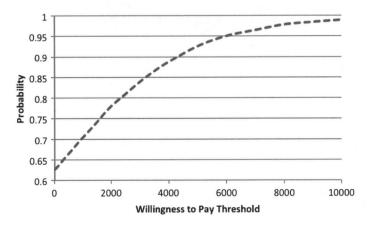

## Discussion – limitations of analysis

*Discussion*

The analysis was based on evidence from meta-analysis and also on various assumptions about relapse rates and the persistence of the condition in those that were not offered treatment. The analysis was focused on estimating the savings to be achieved by reducing the chance of conduct disorder persisting over time. When only considering the NHS and PSS costs in the main analysis, the parent-focused programme was shown to result in a net cost of £71 over a 9-year period. However, when a wider perspective was considered, there was an overall net saving of £770. In general, the results suggest that the use of a parent-focused programme is potentially a cost-effective programme when compared with no treatment in children with conduct disorder.

The analysis model considered the potential impact of relapse after treatment. Given that there is limited data available to model the relapse rate for those whose conduct problems improved after treatment, an assumption of a 50% relapse rate was made. For individuals with conduct problems after treatment it was assumed that they could relapse to conduct disorder and that those with no conduct problems after treatment could also relapse to conduct disorder; that is, all states could change to the worst health state following relapse. This is a conservative approach because it is possible that an individual with no conduct problems could develop conduct problems, but not conduct disorder. However, there is no data to determine the differential relapse from no conduct problems to conduct problems, or from no conduct problems to conduct disorder. Recovery was not considered in the analysis due to a lack of data on differential recovery from conduct disorder to conduct problems or no conduct problems, and from conduct problems to no conduct problems.

In comparison with the net savings of £4,660 to the public sector from the parenting programme by Bonin and colleagues (2011), the net savings in this analysis are considerably lower. This could be due to the longer time horizon of 20 years, the inclusion of crime from the age of 5 years and the assumption of a 0% relapse rate in Bonin and colleagues (2011). However, the results are similar in that the programme is associated with potentially significant savings to the public sector, even with a relapse rate of 50% or more.

*Limitations of the analysis*
The limitations of this model are similar to that of the child-focused model. The first limitation is the arbitrary cut-off points of the CBCL scores and, second, the assumption of a normal distribution of children and young people's CBCL scores around this scale. There is the possibility of a loss of information as a result of the cut-off points. However, this was essential in order to estimate the percentage of children in different health states and subsequently attach costs associated with different health states relating to conduct disorder.

*Overall conclusions from the economic evidence*
Standard (non-attenuated) parent-focused interventions for parents with children and young people with a conduct disorder are cost effective compared with no treatment.

### 7.3.3 Family-focused programmes

*Systematic literature review*
The systematic literature review of economic evidence on family-focused programmes for children and young people with conduct disorder identified two existing studies that met the inclusion criteria (see Chapter 3 for details of the inclusion criteria). Both studies were conducted in the US (Barnoski, 2004; Dembo et al., 2000).

The study by Barnoski (2004) assessed the cost-savings associated with functional family therapy and aggression replacement training versus a waitlist control for young people aged 13 to 17 years with a moderate-to-high risk of juvenile re-offending. Programme costs and criminal justice costs were considered. The study assessed whether the reduction in the rate of crime as a result of the intervention would result in any savings over an 18-month period. Functional family therapy yielded a 38% reduction in the rate of recidivism compared with waitlist control, while aggression replacement training resulted in a 24% reduction in the rate of recidivism when compared with waitlist control. The overall costs avoided were $22,448 and $8,684 for functional family therapy and aggression replacement training, respectively, compared with waitlist control. In terms of benefit–cost ratio estimation, functional family therapy and aggression replacement training were assessed and resulted in a saving of around $11 and $12 per $1 spent on functional family therapy and aggression replacement training, respectively.

Similarly, Dembo and colleagues (2000) assessed the net cost savings of family empowerment intervention compared with extended services intervention for juvenile offenders aged 11 to 18 years. With the primary outcome being the number of new arrests over a 12-month period, family empowerment intervention resulted in 43%

fewer arrests compared with extended services intervention. Intervention and crime costs were considered in the analysis. The net cost saving from avoiding crime costs over a 2-year time horizon was estimated to be $1,302 per youth offender for family empowerment intervention compared with extended services intervention.

Overall, the economic evidence on family therapy indicates that such programmes are potentially cost-effective. However, both studies considered were conducted in the US and, other than family empowerment intervention, the assessed interventions may not be commonly available in the NHS.

No further economic modelling was developed for family-focused intervention because it was not considered to be an area of high priority by the GDG.

### 7.3.4    Multi-component programmes

*Systematic literature review*

Existing economic evidence on individual and group psychosocial interventions for children and young people with conduct disorders was scarce. A systematic review of economic literature identified four studies (Caldwell et al., 2006; Foster et al., 2006; Foster et al., 2007; Robertson et al., 2001) that met the inclusion criteria as described in Chapter 3. All studies were conducted in the US and were partial economic evaluation studies looking at the programme costs and associated downstream cost savings.

Foster and colleagues (2006) reported a long-term cost-effectiveness analysis, comparing the Fast Track intervention with a matched control that followed-up children in kindergarden who screened positive for conduct problems for up to 10 years. The Fast Track programme targeted multiple critical determinants of development such as parenting, peer relations, and social-cognitive and cognitive skills. During the programme, all families were offered parent training with home visits, academic tutoring and social skills training. Only the cost of intervention was considered in the analysis. The mean cost of the intervention was estimated to be $58,283 per child and $0 for the control group in 2004 US dollars. The ICER was estimated for each of the three primary outcomes: $3,481,433 for the extra number of conduct disorders averted; $423,480 for the extra number of index crimes avoided; and $736,010 for the extra number of acts of interpersonal violence avoided. In uncertainty analysis, the Fast Track programme was not cost effective at a willingness-to-pay threshold of $50,000 for each of the outcomes considered in the analysis. However, the authors reported that if the high-risk group (defined based on a high index of crime and poverty in a given community) was considered, the programme had a 69% probability of being cost effective for conduct disorder outcome measures, a 57% probability for index crime outcome measures and 0% for interpersonal violence outcome measures.

Foster and colleagues (2007) assessed the cost-effectiveness of six multi-components of a parent–child–teacher training programme (child training, parent training, child training plus parent training, parent training plus teacher training, child training plus teacher training and child training plus parent training plus teacher training) against a no treatment comparator, delivered to children aged 3 to 8 years who had had conduct problems for more than 6 months. Taking the payers' perspective, costs included were programme costs alone; the behaviour problem outcome measures were the Preschool Behaviour Questionnaire and Dyadic Parent-Child Interaction Coding System – Revised. The result of the estimate was reported as the cost per child treated. The base-case ICER was not given, but it was reported that for the Preschool Behaviour Questionnaire outcome and at a willingness-to-pay level of $3,000 and above, parent training plus teacher training was more cost-effective with the probability of being cost-effective ranging from about 60 to 80%. However, for the Dyadic Parent-Child Interaction Coding System – Revised outcome, the most cost-effective option was reported to be parent training plus child training plus teacher training, with the probability of being cost-effective at $3,000 and above ranging from about 50 to 65%. The evaluation adopted a short-term horizon that was not specified.

Caldwell and colleagues (2006) performed a cost analysis of an intensive juvenile corrective service program versus usual juvenile corrective service delivered to unmanageable juvenile delinquent boys in the Mendota Juvenile Treatment Centre, Madison, Wisconsin. The experimental group received a decompression treatment model using aggression replacement training and cognitive behavioural treatment delivered by a psychiatric nurse. With the primary outcome as the rate of recidivism, the program was found to significantly reduce the number of offences committed by the target population over a 4.5-year time horizon. The perspective of the analysis was that of the criminal justice system. The mean total costs (programme costs and downstream costs) in 2001 US dollars were estimated to be $173,012 per participant in the experimental group and $216,388 per participant in the control group, with a resultant net saving of $43,376. The authors estimated the potential cost saving per $1 invested in the programme to be about $7.18 over the course of the 4.5-year period.

In the study by Robertson and colleagues (2001), juvenile offenders aged 11 to 17 years who were referred to youth courts for delinquent activities were either offered intensive supervision monitoring or cognitive-behavioural treatment as a new intervention. These experiment groups were compared with regular probation control in terms of the programme costs and downstream costs resulting from recidivism. The primary outcome was the rate of recidivism. The method of cost analysis was a regression method using the rate of recidivism resulting from each intervention group as an explanatory variable. Cognitive behavioural treatment was found to result in a net reduction in local justice expenditure of about $1,435 per offender while intensive supervision monitoring did not result in any significant difference in criminal justice system expenditures when compared with regular probation services. The estimated cost saved per $1 invested in cognitive behavioural treatment was $1.96.

Other than the programme of Foster and colleagues (2007), none of the above experimental programmes are generally available through the NHS. Due to the variation in the cost-effectiveness between the parent, child and teacher programme in Foster and colleagues' (2007) study coupled with the different outcome measure, the outcome of different combinations of the programme is uncertain. Also, given the non-availability of the other programmes outside the US, there could be considerable uncertainty and limitations in implementing such programmes in the UK.

No further economic modelling was developed for multi-component intervention because it was not considered to be an area of high priority by the GDG.

### 7.3.5    Multimodal interventions

*Systematic literature review*

From the systematic review of economic evidence on multimodal interventions for children and young people with conduct disorders, three studies (Klietz et al., 2010; Olsson, 2010a; Olsson, 2010b) which met the inclusion criteria given in Chapter 3 were identified. None of these studies were conducted in the UK.

A cost analysis study of a US multimodal intervention by Klietz and colleagues (2010) evaluated the potential cost savings of multisystemic therapy compared with individual therapy delivered to juvenile offenders aged between 11.8 and 15.2 years. The outcome measure that informed the extent of crime costs averted was the rate of recidivism, while the costs included were that of the intervention and the potential downstream costs associated with criminal activities by the juvenile offenders. Multisystemic therapy was shown to be more effective, reducing the rate of recidivism by 50%, compared with the individual therapy recidivism reduction rate of about 19%. Notwithstanding the high cost of multisystemic therapy ($8,827 more than individual therapy) per participant, multisystemic therapy was found to demonstrate potential savings of about $9.51 to $23.59 per $1. This was due to the huge potential cost savings arising from crime avoidance.

In Sweden, two separate studies (Olsson, 2010a; Olsson, 2010b) using the effectiveness data from a single trial reporting outcomes at two different time points (7 months and 2 years, respectively) evaluated the costs associated with a multisystemic therapy programme delivered to individuals aged 12 to 17 years with a clinical diagnosis of conduct disorder. The comparator for these analyses was treatment as usual. The costs considered were treatment, placement and non-placement costs. In addition to these costs, productivity loss was included in the later study. Crime costs were not included. The primary outcome was antisocial behaviour. The result showed no significant difference between the effects of the intervention and its comparator, and that the intervention group had a positive incremental cost at both time points, which at 7 months was $5,038 and at 2 years was 44,500 Swedish krona. As a result, multisystemic therapy was considered not to be cost-effective in the Swedish setting. These results contrast with that of Klietz and colleagues (2010) conducted in the US.

The US and Swedish studies of multisystemic therapy programmes discussed above reported different conclusions. While both studies were based on good quality trials, there may be many reasons for this disparity, one being the difference in the comparator used in the trials and the populations selected. In the US study the control arm was individual therapy, which was described as being representative of usual community outpatient treatment for juvenile offenders with potential variations in the therapists' strategies. However, in the Swedish study, the comparator was described as social service care delivered by the social welfare administration, the precise content of which was dependent on the social worker and families concerned. Also, in the US study the population was juvenile offenders, but in the Swedish study the population comprised youth with a clinical diagnosis of conduct disorder who were not necessarily offenders. As such, the resulting impact of care can be expected to be different.

*Economic modelling*
**Introduction – objective of economic modelling**
From the systematic review of the clinical evidence on multimodal interventions, multisystemic therapy was found to be more clinically effective compared with treatment as usual for young people with conduct disorder. On the basis of significant differences in the economic results from studies conducted in the US and Sweden, and the potentially huge resources involved in the delivery of the programmes, the GDG considered that a further cost-effectiveness analysis in a UK setting was necessary.

The objective of the analysis was to assess whether the intervention costs would be off-set by the potential savings accrued by improving the behaviour of adolescents with conduct disorder. The population under analysis was adolescents between 10 and 17 years old who had been diagnosed with conduct disorder, many of whom may have already been in contact with the criminal justice system. The perspective adopted was that of the NHS and PSS in the main analysis, as recommended by NICE (2009c). A secondary analysis was also conducted adopting a wider perspective because the GDG considered other costs, such as education and crime, to be significant and expected them to reduce greatly following the successful treatment of a person with conduct disorder.

Estimation of QALYs was not undertaken in the analysis due to the poor quality of the available data on health utilities, as discussed in Section 7.3.1.

**Economic modelling methods**

*Interventions assessed*
The type of multimodal intervention assessed in this analysis was multisystemic therapy. It was compared with care as usual, of which youth offending was identified by the GDG as a comparable usual service for this group. Multisystemic therapy was specifically developed for working with conduct-disordered adolescents (Henggeler et al., 1998). Further details on multisystemic therapy are given in Section 7.2.1.

*Model structure*
The starting population consisted of a cohort of adolescents aged 10 years with a diagnosis of conduct disorder. The model structure and model states were the same as those in the economic model of child-focused programme (see Section 7.3.1). The assumptions and baseline CBCL T-scores also remained the same as in the model of child-focused programme.

*Clinical input parameters*

From the meta-analysis of clinical evidence, the effect size reported as the SMD was estimated to be 0.47 (95% CI, 0.21, 0.74) at post-treatment. This estimate was based on the parent-rated antisocial behaviour outcome, demonstrating an overall moderate effect relative to treatment as usual. The full details on the methods used to estimate the magnitude of change in the baseline CBCL scores are the same as those used for child-focused interventions, as discussed in Section 7.3.1.

*Time horizon*

The model adopted an 8-year time horizon, to represent a young person receiving an intervention at age 10 years and then being followed-up to 18 years old. This age range of 10 to 18 years represents those at whom the intervention was targeted. Because there was no strong evidence of a sustained treatment effect, an annual relapse rate of 50% was assumed over the remaining years after treatment.

*Cost data*

**Estimation of intervention cost**

The cost of multisystemic therapy and treatment as usual were estimated using information on resource use from Butler and colleagues (2011), and the expert opinion of the GDG. A YOT was taken to be representative of the treatment as usual offered to this population. The details of the resource use and cost of multisystemic therapy and treatment as usual are given in Table 88 and Table 89, respectively. Multisystemic therapy was estimated to last for an average of 20 weeks, during which period nine families were seen by a team of three therapists and one supervisor with each session lasting 90 minutes (based on the expert opinion of the GDG members). Other than the family visits, telephone support was made available to each family 24 hours a day, 7 days a week. Given the specialised nature of multisystemic therapy, the therapists were offered training, with booster training at intervals. The estimated cost per family was £7,312. This was close to the estimate of £7,000 that was reported in the costing report for antisocial personality disorder, based on discussions with experts and on costs provided by the Department of Health (NICE, 2009d).

**Estimation of costs of states relating to conduct disorder**

The methods used to estimate the costs associated with conduct disorder, conduct problems and no conduct problem states were the same as those used for the child-focused programme (see Section 7.3.1 for a summary of the costs of the conduct disorder, conduct problems and no conduct problem states).

*Discounting*

Discounting was applied at an annual rate of 3.5% as recommended by NICE (2009d); prices were expressed in 2011 UK pounds and uplifted, when necessary, using the Hospital and Community Health Service Pay and Price Index (Curtis, 2011).

**Table 88: Cost of multisystemic therapy programme**

| Resource use | Description | Unit cost | Total cost | Source |
|---|---|---|---|---|
| Staff costs | Three therapists (NHS Band 7 equivalent), with each therapist visiting three families every week for a 1.5-hour session for a total of 20 weeks (total 270 hours); 30 minutes' travel time each way per visit (180 hours); 1 hour of telephone support each week per family (180 hours). 630 hours in total for nine families. | £83 per hour | £52,290 | Resource use: expert opinion. Unit cost: Curtis (2011) |
| Supervision costs | 1-hour weekly joint supervision of three therapists by a supervisor (NHS Band 8c equivalent) for 20 weeks (20 hours); 45 minutes' travel time each way per week (30 hours). 50 hours in total for nine families. | £135 per hour | £6,750 | Resource use: expert opinion. Unit cost: (Curtis, 2011) |
| Travel costs | 180 visits by three therapists for nine families. 20 visits by a supervisor for joint therapist's supervision. 200 visits in total for nine families. | £1.54 per visit | £308 | Resource use: expert opinion. Unit cost: (Webster-Stratton, 1998) |
| Consultation costs | Weekly consultation via telephone with a multisystemic therapy expert. 20 consultations in total per nine families. | £100 per consultation | £2,000 | Unit cost: expert opinion |
| Audit costs | Twice-yearly implementation review by experts at £1000 per review. For a 20-week period, there is 0.769 potential review for nine families. | £1000 per review | £769 | Unit cost: expert opinion |

*Continued*

295

**Table 88:** *(Continued)*

| Resource use | Description | Unit cost | Total cost | Source |
|---|---|---|---|---|
| Training costs | One-off initial training: £6,000 per therapist. Assuming that the impact of the training lasts for 5 years in 20-week periods, there will be 0.231 equivalent therapists' training cost for nine families. | £6,000 | £1,386 | Unit cost: expert opinion |
| Booster training sessions | Four booster therapist training sessions per year at £500 for each therapist. There will be 4.62 therapists' booster training sessions over a 20-week period for nine families | £500 | £2,310 | Unit cost: expert opinion |
| **Total cost for nine families** | | | **£65,813** | |
| **Cost per family** | | | **£7,312** | |

**Table 89: Cost of treatment as usual (YOT)**

| Resource use | Description | Unit cost (£) | Total cost (£) | Source |
|---|---|---|---|---|
| Staff costs | One facilitator (social worker equivalent) with 21 professional appointments lasting for 90 minutes. Total of 31.5 hours. | 74 (client-related work including qualification cost) | £2,331 | Resource use: expert opinion Unit costs: (Curtis, 2011) |
| **Cost per family** | | | **£2,331** | |

*Data analysis and presentation of the results*

The difference in the mean costs over the time horizon of analysis between the treated and untreated groups was estimated, in order to determine the extent of cost savings due to improvement in the behaviour state of the target population. The results are presented in two parts: the main analysis, where NHS and PSS costs were considered only, and the secondary analysis, where wider costs to other sectors were considered. Sensitivity analysis was conducted for the secondary analysis to test the impact of potential uncertainty around the rate of relapse, cost of intervention and cost of crime by varying the base case value by 50%. In addition to deterministic analysis, a probabilistic analysis in which input parameters were assigned probabilistic distributions rather than being expressed as point estimates was undertaken. Probability distributions around the cost data and treatment effect (as shown in both Table 78 and Table 90) were generated using gamma distribution for cost parameters and normal distribution for effect sizes. Subsequently, 10,000 iterations of the economic model were run, each drawing random values out of the distributions fitted onto the model input parameters. Mean costs and QALYs for the two groups (intervention and control) were calculated by averaging across 10,000 iterations. Results of probabilistic analysis are also presented in the form of cost-effectiveness acceptability curve, which show the probability of the intervention being cost-effective at different levels of willingness-to-pay per person with conduct disorder that improved to having no conduct problems following treatment.

**Economic modelling results**

*Results of analysis*

The multimodal programme compared with treatment as usual resulted in a reduction in the proportion of adolescents with conduct disorder from 100% before

**Table 90:  Other input parameters and their distributions for the
analysis of multimodal interventions**

| Parameter | Distribution | Point estimate | Probability distribution | Reference and comment |
|---|---|---|---|---|
| Effect size (multimodal versus treatment as usual) | Normal | 0.47 | 95% CI, 0.21 to 0.74 | Meta-analysis |
| Cost of multimodal intervention | Gamma | £7.312 | Alpha = 2.04 Beta = 3,582.96 | See Table 88 |
| Cost of treatment as usual (YOT) | Gamma | £2,331 | Alpha = 2.04 Beta = 1,142.19 | See Table 89 |

treatment to 47% after treatment, because a proportion of children improved to a
better behaviour state of either conduct problems or no conduct problems (13% and
40%, respectively) (see Table 91). In the cost analysis, this improvement in behaviour state resulted in a mean net cost of £3,867 for the NHS and PSS in the main
analysis (Table 92), and an overall mean net saving of up to £7,125 over an 8-year
period when a wider perspective was considered (Table 93). Out of £12,106 of the
total savings, 9% fall under health and social services, 6% under education and 85%
under criminal justice services.

The sensitivity analysis results in Table 94 show that the model was robust
across different scenarios; that is, cost-savings were incurred under all estimates.
The results of the probabilistic analysis were essentially the same with the deterministic estimates. Further to the sensitivity analysis above, Figure 14 shows that
the probability of multimodal intervention being cost-effective is 77% at zero
willingness-to-pay per additional adolescent with conduct disorder improved to
having no conduct problems following treatment, and increases with increasing levels of willingness-to-pay.

**Table 91:  Estimated proportion of adolescents in each health state
after multisystemic therapy**

| Health state | Proportion at post-treatment |
|---|---|
| Conduct disorder | 0.47 |
| Conduct problems | 0.13 |
| No conduct problems | 0.40 |

**Table 92: Results of main economic analysis of multisystemic therapy for adolescents with conduct disorder**

| Cost component | Child focused + treatment as usual | Treatment as usual (YOT) | Incremental cost |
|---|---|---|---|
| Intervention cost | £7,312 | 2,331 | £4,981 |
| NHS and PSS cost | £8,226 | £9,340 | −£1,114 |
| Total cost | **£15,538** | **£11,671** | **£3,867** |

**Table 93: Results of secondary economic analysis of multisystemic therapy for adolescents with conduct disorder**

| Cost component | Multisystemic therapy | Treatment as usual (YOT) | Incremental cost |
|---|---|---|---|
| Intervention cost | £7,312 | £2,331 | £4,981 |
| NHS and PSS cost | £8,226 | £9,340 | −£1,114 |
| Education cost | £5,712 | £6,486 | −£774 |
| Crime cost | £72,920 | £83,138 | −£10,218 |
| **Total cost (deterministic)** | **£94,170** | **£101,295** | −**£7,125** |
| **Total incremental cost (probabilistic)** | | | −7,124 |

**Table 94: Sensitivity analysis for the analysis of multisystemic therapy**

| Variable | Value | Net cost |
|---|---|---|
| Relapse rate | 25% | −£16,079 |
| Relapse rate | 75% | −£3,294 |
| Intervention cost | 50% higher | −£3,469 |
| Intervention cost | 50% lower | −£10,781 |
| Crime cost | 50% lower | −£2,016 |

**Figure 14: Probability of multisystemic therapy being cost-effective at different levels of willingness-to-pay per adolescent with conduct disorder improved to having no conduct problems**

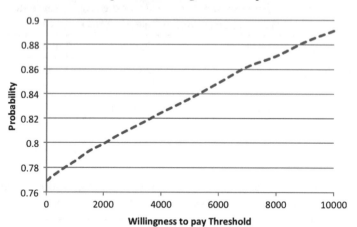

## Discussion – limitations of the analysis

*Discussion*

The analysis was based on evidence from the meta-analysis, as well as on various assumptions about relapse rates and the persistence of the condition in young people who were not offered treatment. The analysis focused on estimating the savings that could be made by reducing the chance of conduct disorder persisting over time. Limiting the perspective to NHS and PSS in the main analysis, multimodal interventions are shown to result in a net cost of £3,867 over an 8-year period. However, when a wider perspective is considered, there is an overall net saving of £7,125. An intervention that is not cost saving is not necessarily not cost effective. Because the main costs are other costs to the public sector incurred by this population, as shown by Scott and colleagues (2001), which are highly important, the GDG considered the total NHS and PSS costs, overall cost-savings and clinical outcomes, and concluded that the interventions were cost-effective.

The model considered the potential impact of relapse after treatment. Given that there was limited data available to model the relapse rate for those with improved states after treatment of conduct problems, the assumption of a 50% relapse rate was made. For those with conduct problems after treatment, it was assumed that they could relapse to conduct disorder; those with no conduct problems after treatment were also assumed to relapse to conduct disorder – that is, all individuals who relapsed changed to the worst state. This is still conservative because there is the possibility that children and young people who show no conduct problems could relapse to having conduct problems and not to conduct disorder. However, there is no data to determine such differential relapse from no conduct problems to conduct problems, or no conduct problems to conduct disorder. Recovery was not considered in the analysis due to a lack of data on differential recovery from conduct disorder to conduct problems or no conduct problems, or from conduct problems to no problems.

As discussed in the child-focused programme (see Section 7.3.1), it is possible that the overall net saving estimated in this analysis may be an under-estimate of the potential benefit of multisystemic therapy, given that the crime cost used in the analysis is less than that reported in the Ministry of Justice technical paper on the cost of young offenders (National Audit Office, 2011). In comparison with the net savings of £4,660 estimated by Bonin and colleagues (2011) over a 20-year period from a parenting programme offered to children at the age of 5 years, savings from multisystemic therapy (£7,125) over a shorter period of 8 years are significantly more. Such significant savings may be expected because the target population is mainly adolescents with a severe form of conduct disorder, who are likely to be in contact with the criminal justice system.

*Limitations of the analysis*
The limitations of this model are similar to those of the child-focused model (see Section 7.3.1). The first limitation is the arbitrary cut-off points of the CBCL scores and, second, the assumption of a normal distribution of children and young people's CBCL scores around this scale. There is potentially a loss of information as a result of the cut-off points. However, this was essential in order to estimate the percentage of children in different health states and subsequently attach costs associated with different health states relating to conduct disorder.

*Overall conclusion from economic evidence*
Multimodal interventions (multisystemic therapy) for young people with a conduct disorder are cost-effective compared with treatment as usual.

## 7.4    FROM EVIDENCE TO RECOMMENDATIONS

### 7.4.1    Relative value placed on the outcomes considered:

Due to a large number of child outcomes the GDG decided to focus on the following, which were considered to be critical:
- agency contact (for example residential care, criminal justice system)
- antisocial behaviour (at home, at school, in the community)
- drug/alcohol use
- educational attainment (that is, the highest level of education completed)
- offending behaviour
- school exclusion due to antisocial behaviour.

### 7.4.2    Trade-off between clinical benefits and harms

In younger children (<11 years old) with a conduct disorder (or at high risk, based on symptoms or contact with the criminal justice system), the GDG considered there to be reasonable evidence that the benefits of parent-focused interventions outweigh the minimal risk of harm (for example from stigmatisation). Based on the evidence, the GDG also concluded that first-line treatment should utilise group-based manualised interventions. The recommendations replace those made in the NICE technology appraisal guidance 102 (NICE, 2006) on parent-training programmes. Changes to the wording were made to conform to current NICE style and be consistent with the evidence-base. Although the evidence base for foster carer-focused interventions was much smaller, the GDG felt that these programmes should be recommended given the evidence supporting parent-focused interventions.

It should be noted that the NICE clinical practice guideline 77 (NCCMH, 2010) on antisocial personality disorder recommends that additional interventions targeted specifically at the parents of children with conduct problems (such as interventions for parental, marital or interpersonal problems) should not be provided routinely alongside parent-training programmes because they are unlikely to have an impact on the child's conduct problems. This topic was outside the scope of the present guideline and, therefore, this recommendation remains valid.

In older children (9 to 14 years old) with a conduct disorder (or at high risk, based on symptoms or contact with the criminal justice system), the GDG felt there was reasonable evidence that the benefits of child-focused interventions outweighed the minimal risk of harm. The recommendation differs somewhat from that made in the antisocial personality disorder guideline in that the recommendation is not conditional on traits of the child or the families engagement in a parent-training programme. The antisocial personality disorder guideline also recommended that for children who have residual problems following cognitive problem-solving skills training, consideration should be given to anger control or social problem-solving skills training, depending on the nature of the residual problems. Based on the updated evidence base, which included seven more trials, the GDG did not support this recommendation. However, the GDG recognised that individual parent and child training programmes would be appropriate for children aged between 3 and 11 years with severe and complex needs.

In young people (11+ years old) with a conduct disorder (or at high risk, based on symptoms or contact with the criminal justice system), the GDG felt there was sufficient evidence that the benefits of multimodal interventions outweighed the minimal risk of harm. It should be noted that the recommendation made here is broader than that made in the antisocial personality disorder guideline due to the larger evidence base. It should also be noted that the antisocial personality disorder guideline made additional recommendations for parent-focused, family-focused and foster carer-focused interventions for this age group. However, for parent-focused interventions only two of the 54 trials included in the current meta-analysis were conducted with parents of children over 10 years old. None of the foster carer-focused interventions were conducted specifically in this age group, and for family-focused interventions the evidence was inconclusive. Therefore, the GDG felt that the focus should be on providing evidence-based multimodal interventions.

The GDG felt the evidence did not currently support a recommendation for interventions given separately to parents and to teachers, classroom-based interventions, multi-component interventions or non-violent resistance. Evidence from trials comparing two different interventions (head-to-head) supported this conclusion.

### 7.4.3    Trade-off between net health benefits and resource use

Parent-focused interventions, child-focused interventions and multimodal interventions are all cost-effective and, therefore, the GDG agreed that there was sufficient evidence to conclude that net health benefits outweighed the resource use. The GDG also agreed that, for efficient resource use, group programmes should be offered first. More complex situations may require individual and/or combined programmes.

### 7.4.4    Quality of the evidence

For parent-focused interventions, the evidence ranged from moderate to high quality. Reasons for downgrading concerned either a lack of evidence or heterogeneity. In the latter case, some of the between-study variance could be explained by method of delivery (group versus individual) and the underlying principles used to develop the intervention. Importantly, the evidence was consistent between parent- and observer-rated outcomes.

For child-focused interventions, the evidence ranged from low to moderate quality. Reasons for downgrading concerned either a lack of evidence or heterogeneity. In the latter case, some of the between-study variance could be explained by the setting (where the intervention was delivered) and format of the intervention (group or individual). Despite low quality evidence for some outcomes (particularly at follow-up), the evidence across outcome raters was consistent.

For multimodal interventions, the evidence ranged from low to high quality. Reasons for downgrading concerned issues to do with imprecision of the effect. There was insufficient evidence to explore the reasons for this, but evidence across outcome raters was consistent.

### 7.4.5    Other considerations

When drafting the recommendations, the GDG discussed the need for training and staff supervision to effectively deliver the recommended interventions and to work safely with children and young people with a conduct disorder. Drawing on expert opinion, two recommendations were drafted that covered these issues.

### 7.5    RECOMMENDATIONS

### 7.5.1    Clinical practice recommendations

*Working safely and effectively with children and young people*
7.5.1.1    Health and social care professionals working with children and young people who present with behaviour suggestive of a conduct disorder, or who have conduct disorder, should be trained and competent and able to work with different levels of learning ability, cognitive capacity, emotional maturity and developmental levels.

*Staff supervision*

7.5.1.2    Health and social care services should ensure that staff supervision is built into the routine working of the service, is properly resourced within local systems and is monitored. Supervision should:

- make use of direct observation (for example recordings of sessions) and routine outcome measures
- support adherence to the specific intervention
- focus on outcomes
- be regular and apply to the whole caseload.

*Treatment and indicated prevention*

In this guideline indicated prevention refers to interventions targeted to high-risk individuals who are identified as having detectable signs or symptoms that may lead to the development of conduct disorders but who do not meet diagnostic criteria for conduct disorders when offered an intervention.

The interventions in recommendations 7.5.1.3 to 7.5.1.14 are suitable for children and young people who have a diagnosis of oppositional defiant disorder or conduct disorder, are in contact with the criminal justice system for antisocial behaviour, or have been identified as being at high risk of a conduct disorder using established rating scales of antisocial behaviour (for example the Child Behavior Checklist and the Eyberg Child Behavior Inventory).

**Parent training programmes**

7.5.1.3    Offer a group parent training programme to the parents of children and young people aged between 3 and 11 years who:

- have been identified as being at high risk of developing oppositional defiant disorder or conduct disorder **or**
- have oppositional defiant disorder or conduct disorder **or**
- are in contact with the criminal justice system because of antisocial behaviour.

7.5.1.4    Group parent training programmes should involve both parents if this is possible and in the best interests of the child or young person, and should:

- typically have between ten and 12 parents in a group
- be based on a social learning model, using modelling, rehearsal and feedback to improve parenting skills
- typically consist of ten to 16 meetings of 90 to 120 minutes' duration
- adhere to the developer's manual[56] and employ all of the necessary materials to ensure consistent implementation of the programme.

7.5.1.5    Offer an individual parent training programme to the parents of children and young people aged between 3 and 11 years who are not able to participate in a group parent training programme and whose child:

---

[56] The manual should have been positively evaluated in a randomised controlled trial.

- has been identified as being at high risk of developing oppositional defiant disorder or conduct disorder **or**
- has oppositional defiant disorder or conduct disorder **or**
- is in contact with the criminal justice system because of antisocial behaviour.

7.5.1.6 Individual parent training programmes should involve both parents if this is possible and in the best interests of the child or young person, and should:
- be based on a social learning model using modelling, rehearsal and feedback to improve parenting skills
- typically consist of up to eight to ten meetings of 60 to 90 minutes' duration
- adhere to the developer's manual[57] and employ all of the necessary materials to ensure consistent implementation of the programme.

**Parent and child training programmes for children with complex needs**

7.5.1.7 Offer individual parent and child training programmes to children and young people aged between 3 and 11 years if the problems are severe and complex and they:
- have been identified as being at high risk of developing oppositional defiant disorder or conduct disorder **or**
- have oppositional defiant disorder or conduct disorder **or**
- are in contact with the criminal justice system because of antisocial behaviour.

7.5.1.8 Individual parent and child training programmes should involve both parents, foster carers or guardians if this is possible and in the best interests of the child or young person, and should:
- be based on a social learning model using modelling, rehearsal and feedback to improve parenting skills
- consist of up to ten meetings of 60 minutes' duration
- adhere to the developer's manual[58] and employ all of the necessary materials to ensure consistent implementation of the programme.

**Foster carer/guardian training programmes**

7.5.1.9 Offer a group foster carer/guardian training programme to foster carers and guardians of children and young people aged between 3 and 11 years who:
- have been identified as being at high risk of developing oppositional defiant disorder or conduct disorder **or**
- have oppositional defiant disorder or conduct disorder **or**

---

[57]The manual should have been positively evaluated in a randomised controlled trial.
[58]The manual should have been positively evaluated in a randomised controlled trial.

- are in contact with the criminal justice system because of antisocial behaviour.

7.5.1.10  Group foster carer/guardian training programmes should involve both of the foster carers or guardians if this is possible and in the best interest of the child or young person, and should:
- modify the intervention to take account of the care setting in which the child is living
- typically have between eight and 12 foster carers of guardians in a group
- be based on a social learning model using modelling, rehearsal and feedback to improve parenting skills
- typically consist of between 12 and 16 meetings of 90 to 120 minutes' duration
- adhere to the developer's manual[59] and employ all of the necessary materials to ensure consistent implementation of the programme.

7.5.1.11  Offer an individual foster carer/guardian training programme to the foster carers or guardians of children and young people aged between 3 and 11 years who are not able to participate in a group programme and whose child:
- has been identified as being at high risk of developing oppositional defi-ant disorder or conduct disorder **or**
- has oppositional defiant disorder or conduct disorder **or**
- is in contact with the criminal justice system because of antisocial behaviour.

7.5.1.12  Individual foster carer/guardian training programmes should involve both of the foster carers if this is possible and in the best interests of the child or young person, and should:
- modify the intervention to take account of the care setting in which the child is living
- be based on a social learning model using modelling, rehearsal and feedback to improve parenting skills
- consist of up to ten meetings of 60 minutes' duration
- adhere to the developer's manual[60] and employ all of the necessary materials to ensure consistent implementation of the programme.

**Child-focused programmes**

7.5.1.13  Offer group social and cognitive problem-solving programmes to children and young people aged between 9 and 14 years who:
- have been identified as being at high risk of developing oppositional defiant disorder or conduct disorder **or**
- have oppositional defiant disorder or conduct disorder **or**
- are in contact with the criminal justice system because of antisocial behaviour

---

[59]The manual should have been positively evaluated in a randomised controlled trial.
[60]The manual should have been positively evaluated in a randomised controlled trial.

7.5.1.14   Group social and cognitive problem solving programmes should be adapted to the children's or young people's developmental level and should:
- be based on a cognitive–behavioural problem-solving model
- use modelling, rehearsal and feedback to improve skills
- typically consist of ten to 18 weekly meetings of 2 hours' duration
- adhere to the developer's manual[61] and employ all of the necessary materials to ensure consistent implementation of the programme.

**Multimodal interventions**

7.5.1.15   Offer multimodal interventions, for example, multisystemic therapy) to children and young people aged between 11 and 17 years for the treatment of conduct disorder.
7.5.1.16   Multimodal interventions should involve the child or young person and their parents and carers and should:
- have an explicit and supportive family focus
- be based on a social learning model with interventions provided at individual, family, school, criminal justice and community levels
- be provided by specially trained case managers
- typically consist of three to four meetings per week over a 3- to 5-month period
- adhere to the developer's manual[62] and employ all of the necessary materials to ensure consistent implementation of the programme.

**7.5.2     Research recommendations**

7.5.2.1   What is the effectiveness of parent training programmes for conduct disorders in children and young people aged 12 years and over?
7.5.2.2   What is the effectiveness of interventions to maintain the benefits of treatment and prevent relapse after successful treatment for a conduct disorder?
7.5.2.3   What is the efficacy of combining treatment for mental health problems in parents with treatment for conduct disorders in their children?

---

[61]The manual should have been positively evaluated in a randomised controlled trial.
[62]The manual should have been positively evaluated in a randomised controlled trial.

# 8    PHARMACOLOGICAL AND PHYSICAL TREATMENT INTERVENTIONS FOR CONDUCT DISORDERS

## 8.1    INTRODUCTION

Pharmacological and physical treatments generally have a less prominent role in the treatment of mental disorders in children and young people than in adults with mental disorders. For certain disorders such as ADHD, medication (principally methylphenidate) has a central role in the treatment of the disorder (NICE, 2009b); in other disorders in childhood and adolescence such as schizophrenia (NICE, 2013) and depression (NICE, 2005), medication can also play an important part in treatment. For a range of other child and adolescent disorders, including conduct disorders, medication has had less evidence to support its use and has not had a prominent role; psychosocial interventions have been the best supported treatment. Currently in the UK, only risperidone is licensed for the short-term symptomatic treatment (up to 6 weeks) of persistent aggression in conduct disorder in children from the age of 5 years.

However, sometimes medication is used on its own and in combination with psychological interventions for the treatment of conduct disorder, but this is more common in the US than the UK (Turgay, 2004). A range of psychotropic medications has been used including stimulants, lithium and antipsychotics, in particular risperidone. Prescribed medication tends to be used in more severe forms of conduct disorder and is targeted at specific symptoms such as hyperactivity, impulsivity and aggression, in particular explosive aggression that is destructive and dangerous. Use is more common in older children, and in inpatient and residential settings, and will often only be offered after other interventions have been of no or limited benefit. The mechanisms of action of medication in conduct disorder, with the exception of those coexistent symptoms of hyperactivity, are not well understood. But as conduct disorder is a condition in which biological phenomena such as genetic predisposition and atypical brain maturation or physiologically-based emotional dysregulation can make a significant contribution, medication may act to correct or ameliorate some of these factors.

Comorbidities such as ADHD and depression are common in children and young people with a conduct disorder and medication may be used to treat the comorbid condition. This is probably the most common indication for the use of medication in children and young people with conduct disorders.

Again, in contrast to other childhood disorders such as autism and ADHD, other physical treatments such as restricted diets, dietary supplements and physical activity have not been much used in the treatment of conduct disorders as there has been little or no evidence to support their use.

In developing the reviews below the GDG was also mindful of the potential harms associated with the use of medication: for example the development of prolactinaemia and marked weight gain with the use of risperidone, and the wide range of side effects associated with lithium and antipsychotic drugs.

This chapter considers the evidence that has emerged for the specific treatment of conduct disorder (with and without a coexisting disorder). The treatment and management of coexisting conditions is considered in other guidance. In addition, studies of children and young people with subaverage IQ (defined for the purpose of the guideline as a mean IQ of less than 60) were not included in this review.

## 8.2 CLINICAL EVIDENCE REVIEW

### 8.2.1 Interventions

The following interventions were considered in the review of pharmacological and physical interventions.

*Pharmacological interventions*
Individual drugs were grouped for the purposes of the guideline into the following categories:

● antidepressant drugs (for example citalopram, fluoxetine)
● antihypertensive drugs (for example clonidine)
● antimanic and anticonvulsant drugs (for example carbamazepine, divalproex, lithium)
● antipsychotics (for example risperidone, aripiprazole, haloperidol, thioridazine)
● central nervous system stimulant drugs (for example methylphenidate, dexamphetamine)
● selective norepinephrine reuptake inhibitor drugs (for example atomoxetine)
● other drugs (naltrexone, guanfacine).

*Physical interventions*
Individual physical interventions were grouped for the purposes of the guideline into the following categories:

● diet
● holding therapy
● physical activity
● food additives
● dietary supplements (for example fish oils).

### 8.2.2 Clinical review protocol

A summary of the review protocol, including the review questions, information about the databases searched and the eligibility criteria used for this section of the guideline, can be found in Table 95 (a complete list of review questions can be found in Appendix 5; further information about the search strategy can be found in Appendix 7; the full review protocols can be found in Appendix 15).

**Table 95: Clinical review protocol for the review of pharmacological and physical interventions**

| Component | Description |
|---|---|
| Review questions* | • For children and young people with conduct disorders, what are the benefits and potential harms associated with pharmacological interventions? (RQ-E4)<br>• For children and young people with conduct disorders, what are the benefits and potential harms associated with physical interventions (for example diet)? (RQ-E5)<br>• For children and young people with conduct disorders, should interventions found to be safe and effective be modified in any way in light of coexisting conditions (such as ADHD, depression, anxiety disorders, attachment insecurity) or demographics (such as age, particular black and minority ethnic groups, or gender)? (RQ-E7) |
| Objectives | • To evaluate the clinical effectiveness and safety of pharmacological and physical interventions for conduct disorders<br>• To evaluate if any modifications should be made to interventions to take into account co-existing conditions or demographic variation. |
| Population | Children and young people (aged 18 years and younger), including looked-after children and those in contact with the criminal justice system, diagnosed with a conduct disorder, including oppositional defiant disorder or persistent offending/symptoms of conduct problems (conduct disorder and oppositional defiant disorder are characterised by repetitive and persistent patterns of antisocial, aggressive or defiant behaviour that amounts to significant and persistent violations of age-appropriate social expectations). Studies of children and young people with subaverage IQ (defined for the purpose of the guideline as a mean IQ of less than 60) were excluded. |
| Interventions | • Pharmacological interventions (for example antipsychotic drugs)<br>• Physical interventions (for example diet). |
| Comparison | Treatment as usual, placebo, other active interventions. |

*Continued*

**Table 95:** (*Continued*)

| Component | Description |
|---|---|
| Critical outcomes | Child outcomes:<br>• antisocial behaviour (at home, at school, in the community)**<br>• offending behaviour<br>• school exclusion due to antisocial behaviour<br>• educational attainment (that is, the highest level of education completed)<br>• agency contact (for example residential care, criminal justice system)<br>• sexual behaviour<br>• drug/alcohol use. |
| Electronic databases | Mainstream databases:<br>• Embase, MEDLINE, PreMEDLINE, PsycINFO.<br><br>Topic specific databases and grey literature databases (see search strategy in Appendix 7)[†]. |
| Date searched | Inception to June 2012. |
| Study design | RCT |

*Under 'Review questions', the review question reference (for example RQ-A1) can be used to cross-reference against the full review protocol in Appendix 15.
**RCT.
[†]In addition to electronic databases, the following Cochrane review was hand-reference searched: Loy and colleagues (2012).

### 8.2.3 Studies considered[63]

Twenty-eight RCTs (N = 2,789) met the eligibility criteria for this review: AMAN2002 (Aman et al., 2002), BANGS2008 (Bangs et al., 2008), BARZMAN2006 (Barzman et al., 2006), BLADER2009 (Blader et al., 2009), BUITELAAR2001 (Buitelaar et al., 2001), CAMPBELL1982 (Campbell et al., 1982) , CAMPBELL1995 (Campbell et al., 1995), CONNERS1963 (Conners & Eisenberg, 1963), CONNERS1971 (Conners et al., 1971), CONNOR2008 (Connor et al., 2008), CONNOR2010 (Connor et al., 2010), CUEVA1996 (Cueva et al., 1996), DELLAGNELLO2009 (Dell'Agnello et al., 2009), DITTMANN2011 (Dittmann et al., 2011), DONOVAN2000 (Donovan et al., 2000), FINDLING2000 (Findling et al., 2000), HAZELL2003 (Hazell & Stuart, 2003), HAZELL2006 (Hazell et al., 2006), KAPLAN2004 (Kaplan et al.,

---

[63] Here and elsewhere in the guideline, each study considered for review is referred to by a study ID in capital letters (primary author and date of study publication, except where a study is in press or only submitted for publication, then a date is not used).

2004), KLEIN1997 (Klein et al., 1997), MALONE2000 (Malone et al., 2000), NEWCORN2005 (Newcorn et al., 2005), REYES2006 (Reyes et al., 2006), RIFKIN1997 (Rifkin et al., 1997), RIGGS2007 (Riggs et al., 2007), SNYDER2002 (Snyder et al., 2002), SPENCER2006 (Spencer et al., 2004) and STEINER2003 (Steiner et al., 2003). Of these, all were published in peer-reviewed journals between 1963 and 2011. In addition, 127 studies were excluded from the review. Further information about both included and excluded studies can be found in Appendix 16c.

Of the 28 eligible trials, 18 (N = 1,666) included sufficient data to be included in the set of meta-analyses comparing a pharmacological intervention with placebo. All other eligible trials did not report any critical outcomes and, therefore, are not described further. No trials were found that examined the efficacy of physical interventions. For the purposes of the guideline, pharmacological interventions were categorised as antihypertensive drugs, antipsychotic drugs, antimanic and anticonvulsant drugs, central nervous system stimulant drugs and selective norepinephrine reuptake inhibitor drugs. Table 96 and Table 97 provide an overview of the trials included in each category.

### 8.2.4 Clinical evidence for the review of a pharmacological intervention versus placebo

The critical outcome of antisocial behaviour was sub-categorised according to the person who rated the outcome: (a) observer rated, (b) researcher/clinician rated, (c) peer rated, (d) teacher rated and (e) parent rated. No other critical outcomes were reported in adequate numbers to be included in meta-analyses.

Because within each category there was a paucity of evidence from the included RCTs relating to adverse effects of each drug, information has been quoted from the *British National Formulary for Children* (BNFC) *2011–2012* (Paediatric Formulary Committee, 2011). In most cases these data have not been collected from children and young people with conduct disorder. In addition, where available, evidence from observational studies, as well as RCTs, included in three recent systematic reviews (Maayan & Correll, 2011; Scotto Rosato et al., 2012; Zuddas et al., 2011) was used to quantify the absolute risk using the number needed to harm (NNH). Maayan and Correll (2011) reviewed evidence for weight gain and metabolic risks associated with the use of antipsychotic drugs in children and young people (from 43 studies, including six focusing on conduct disorders). Scotto Rosato and colleagues (2012) reviewed evidence for adverse events associated with the use of antipsychotic, stimulant and mood stabiliser drugs in children and young people (from 29 studies, including 24 focusing on conduct disorders/disruptive behaviour disorders). Zuddas and colleagues (2011) reviewed evidence for adverse events associated with the use of antipsychotic drugs in children and young people with non-psychotic disorders (from 32 studies, including seven focusing on conduct disorders).

Summary of findings tables are used below to summarise the evidence. The forest plots and associated GRADE evidence profiles can be found in Appendix 17 and Appendix 18, respectively.

**Table 96:  Study information table for trials included in the meta-analysis of pharmacological interventions (antihypertensive, antimanic and anticonvulsant drugs) versus placebo**

| | Antihypertensive drugs | Antimanic and anticonvulsant drugs |
|---|---|---|
| Total no. of trials (N) | 1 RCT (67) | 6 RCTs (196) |
| Study ID | HAZELL2003 | BLADER2009<br>CAMPBELL1995<br>CUEVA1996<br>DONOVAN2000<br>MALONE2000<br>RIFKIN1997 |
| Country | Australia (k = 1) | US (k = 6) |
| Year of publication | 2003 | 1996 to 2009 (k = 5) |
| Mean age of children/young people | 9.9 years | 8.5 to 15.2 years |
| Gender of children/young people (% female) | 0 to 25% (k = 1) | 0 to 25% (k = 5)<br>26 to 50% (k = 0)<br>51 to 75% (k = 1)<br>76 to 100% (k = 0) |
| Ethnicity of children/young people (% white) | 0 to 25% (k = 0)<br>26 to 50% (k = 0)<br>51 to 75% (k = 0)<br>76 to 100% (k = 0)<br>Not reported (k = 1) | 0 to 25% (k = 4)<br>26 to 50% (k = 0)<br>51 to 75% (k = 1)<br>76 to 100% (k = 0)<br>Not reported (k = 1) |
| Conduct disorder diagnosis | Conduct disorder/oppositional defiant disorder (k = 1) | Conduct disorder/oppositional defiant disorder (k = 6) |
| Coexisting ADHD | 100% (k = 1) | 0% (k = 4)<br>1 to 25% (k = 1)<br>26 to 50% (k = 0)<br>51 to 75% (k = 0)<br>76 to 100% (k = 1) |
| Timepoint (weeks) | Post-treatment: 6 (k = 1) | Post-treatment: 2 to 8 (k = 6) |
| Comparisons | Clonidine (0.1 to 0.2 mg/day) versus placebo (k = 1) | Carbamazepine (683 mg/day) versus placebo (k = 1)<br>Divalproex (567 to 1,500 mg/day) versus placebo (k = 2)<br>Lithium (1,248 to 1,425 mg/day) versus placebo (k = 3) |

**Table 97: Study information table for trials included in the meta-analysis of pharmacological interventions (antimanic drugs, central nervous system stimulant drugs, selective norepinephrine reuptake inhibitor drugs) versus placebo**

| | Antipsychotic drugs | Central nervous system stimulant drugs | Selective norepinephrine reuptake inhibitor drugs |
|---|---|---|---|
| Total no. of trials (N) | 5 RCTs (621) | 2 RCTs (203) | 4 RCTs (578) |
| Study ID | AMAN2002<br>BUITELAAR2001<br>FINDLING2000<br>REYES2006<br>SNYDER2002 | KLEIN1997<br>SPENCER2006 | BANGS2008<br>DELLAGNELLO2009<br>KAPLAN2004<br>NEWCORN2005 |
| Country | Canada (k = 1)<br>Germany (k = 1)<br>Netherlands (k = 1)<br>US (k = 3) | US (k = 2) | Australia/multiple<br>European (k = 1)<br>Italy (k = 1)<br>US (k = 2) |
| Year of publication | 2000 to 2009 | 1997 to 2006 | 2004 to 2009 |
| Mean age of children/young people | 8.4 to 13.9 years | 10.2 to 10.6 years | 9.5 to 11.2 years |
| Gender of children/young people (% female) | 0 to 25% (k = 5) | 0 to 25% (k = 1)<br>26 to 50% (k = 1)<br>51 to 75% (k = 0)<br>76 to 100% (k = 0) | 0 to 25% (k = 4)<br>26 to 50% (k = 0)<br>51 to 75% (k = 0)<br>76 to 100% (k = 0) |

| | | | |
|---|---|---|---|
| Ethnicity of children/young people (% white) | 0 to 25% (k = 0)<br>26 to 50% (k = 0)<br>51 to 75% (k = 1)<br>76 to 100% (k = 1)<br>Not reported (k = 3) | 0 to 25% (k = 0)<br>26 to 50% (k = 0)<br>51 to 75% (k = 2)<br>76 to 100% (k = 0)<br>Not reported (k = 0) | 0 to 25% (k = 0)<br>26 to 50% (k = 0)<br>51 to 75% (k = 1)<br>76 to 100% (k = 0)<br>Not reported (k = 3) |
| Conduct disorder diagnosis | Conduct disorder (k = 1)<br>Conduct disorder/oppositional defiant disorder (k = 4) | Conduct disorder (k = 1)<br>Oppositional defiant disorder (k = 1) | Oppositional defiant disorder (k = 4) |
| Coexisting ADHD | 0 (k = 1)<br>1 to 25% (k = 0)<br>26 to 50% (k = 0)<br>51 to 75% (k = 3)<br>76 to 100% (k = 1) | 0% (k = 0)<br>1 to 25% (k = 0)<br>26 to 50% (k = 0)<br>51 to 75% (k = 1)<br>76 to 100% (k = 1) | 0% (k = 0)<br>1 to 25% (k = 0)<br>26 to 50% (k = 0)<br>51 to 75% (k = 0)<br>76 to 100% (k = 4) |
| Timepoint (weeks) | Post-treatment: 6 to 26 (k = 5) | Post-treatment: 4 to 5 (k = 2) | Post-treatment: 8 to 9 (k = 4) |
| Comparisons | Risperidone (0.5 to 2.9 mg/day) versus placebo (k = 5) | Methylphenidate (1 mg/kg/day) versus placebo (k = 1)<br>Mixed amphetamine salts (30 mg/day) versus placebo (k = 1) | Atomoxetine (0.5 to 1.6 mg/kg/day) versus placebo (k = 4) |

315

*Antihypertensive drugs (clonidine)*

Moderate quality evidence from one trial with 67 participants showed that antihypertensive drugs when compared with placebo reduced antisocial behaviour when rated by teachers at post-treatment, measured using a continuous outcome (Table 98). In the same trial, when the outcome was rated by parents, the intervention was shown to be effective (moderate quality evidence) when measured using both continuous and dichotomous outcomes, although only the latter was statistically significant. In this trial, 100% of the participants had coexisting ADHD.

With regard to adverse effects of clonidine, the BNFC[64] gives a number of cautions, including 'must be withdrawn gradually to avoid hypertensive crisis; mild to moderate bradyarrhythmia; constipation; polyneuropathy; Raynaud's syndrome or other occlusive peripheral vascular disease; history of depression'. In addition, the following side effects are listed: 'constipation, nausea, dry mouth, vomiting, postural hypotension, dizziness, sleep disturbances, headache, malaise, drowsiness, depression, sexual dysfunction'. Less common side effects are also listed (see the BNFC 2011–2012 for more information) (Paediatric Formulary Committee, 2011).

*Antimanic (carbamazepine) and anticonvulsant drugs (divalproex sodium/lithium)*

These drugs have different modes of action and therefore were analysed separately.

For carbamazepine, moderate quality evidence from one trial with 22 participants was inconclusive with regard to whether the drug, when compared with placebo, reduced antisocial behaviour when rated by researchers/clinicians at post-treatment, measured using either a continuous or dichotomous outcome (Table 99).

For divalproex, moderate quality evidence from one trial with 27 participants (parent-rated outcome) was inconclusive with regard to whether the drug, when compared with placebo, reduced antisocial behaviour at post-treatment using a continuous outcome measure (Table 99). However, moderate quality from one trial with 20 participants (researcher-/clinician-rated outcome) and one trial with 27 participants (parent-rated outcome) demonstrated improved response/remission at post-treatment using dichotomous outcomes. In the two trials, one included 20% of participants with ADHD and the other included 100% with ADHD.

For lithium, moderate quality evidence from one trial with 40 participants (researcher-/clinician-rated outcome) was inconclusive with regard to whether the drug when compared with placebo reduced antisocial behaviour at post-treatment using a continuous outcome measure (Table 99). However, moderate quality evidence from three trials with 116 participants (researcher-/clinician-rated outcome) showed that lithium improved treatment response at post-treatment using a dichotomous outcome measure.

With regard to adverse effects of carbamazepine, the BNFC gives a number of cautions, including advice that 'children or their carers should be told how to recognise signs of blood, liver, or skin disorders, and advised to seek immediate medical attention if symptoms such as fever, rash, mouth ulcers, bruising, or bleeding develop'. In addition, the following side effects are listed: 'dry mouth, nausea, vomiting, oedema, ataxia, dizziness, drowsiness, fatigue, headache, hyponatraemia (leading in

---

[64] www.bnf.org

**Table 98: Summary of findings table for antihypertensive drugs compared with placebo (post-treatment)**

**Patient or population:** children and young people with conduct disorders (post-treatment)
**Intervention:** antihypertensive drugs
**Comparison:** placebo

| Outcomes | Illustrative comparative risks* (95% CI) | | Relative effect (95% CI) | No. of participants (studies) | Quality of the evidence (GRADE) |
|---|---|---|---|---|---|
| | Assumed risk | Corresponding risk | | | |
| | Placebo | Antihypertensive drugs | | | |
| **Teacher-rated antisocial behaviour (continuous outcome)** Any valid rating scale | – | The mean teacher-rated antisocial behaviour (continuous outcome) in the intervention groups was **0.68 standard deviations lower** (1.17 to 0.19 lower) | – | 67 (1) | ⊕⊕⊕⊝ **moderate**[1] |
| **Parent-rated antisocial behaviour (continuous outcome)** Any valid rating scale | – | The mean parent-rated antisocial behaviour (continuous outcome) in the intervention groups was **0.31 standard deviations lower** (0.80 lower to 0.18 higher) | – | 67 (1) | ⊕⊕⊕⊝ **moderate**[1] |
| **Parent-rated antisocial behaviour (dichotomous outcome)** Conners Parent Rating Scale – conduct problems – no. achieving 38% reduction from baseline | – | | **RR 0.55** (0.36 to 0.82) | 66 (1) | ⊕⊕⊕⊝ **moderate**[1] |

[1]OIS (for dichotomous outcomes, OIS = 300 events; for continuous outcomes, OIS = 400 participants) not met.

**Table 99: Summary of findings table for antimanic and anticonvulsant drugs compared with placebo (post-treatment)**

**Patient or population:** children and young people with conduct disorders (post-treatment)
**Intervention:** antimanic drugs
**Comparison:** placebo

| Outcomes | Illustrative comparative risks (95% CI) | | Relative effect (95% CI) | No. of participants (studies) | Quality of the evidence (GRADE) |
|---|---|---|---|---|---|
| | Assumed risk | Corresponding risk | | | |
| | Placebo | Antimanic/anticonvulsant drugs | | | |
| **Researcher-/clinician-rated antisocial behaviour (continuous outcome)/carbamazepine** Any valid rating scale | – | The mean researcher-/clinician-rated antisocial behaviour (continuous outcome)/carbamazepine in the intervention groups was **0.01 standard deviations lower** (0.81 lower to 0.79 higher) | | 22 (1) | ⊕⊕⊕⊝ **moderate**[1] |
| **Parent-rated antisocial behaviour (continuous outcome)/divalproex** Any valid rating scale | – | The mean parent-rated antisocial behaviour (continuous outcome)/divalproex in the intervention groups was **0.26 standard deviations lower** (1.00 lower to 0.48 higher) | | 27 (1) | ⊕⊕⊕⊝ **moderate**[1] |
| **Researcher-/clinician-rated antisocial behaviour (continuous outcome)/lithium** Any valid rating scale | – | The mean researcher-/clinician-rated antisocial behaviour (continuous outcome) in the intervention groups was **0.56 standard deviations lower** (1.19 lower to 0.07 higher) | | 40 (1) | ⊕⊕⊕⊝ **moderate**[1] |

| | | | | |
|---|---|---|---|---|
| Researcher-/clinician-rated antisocial behaviour (dichotomous outcome)/carbamazepine Response | — | RR 0.40 (0.10 to 1.64) | 22 (1) | ⊕⊕⊕⊝ moderate[1] |
| Researcher-/clinician-rated antisocial behaviour (dichotomous outcome)/divalproex Response | | RR 0.24 (0.08 to 0.71) | 20 (1) | ⊕⊕⊕⊝ moderate[1] |
| Parent-rated antisocial behaviour (dichotomous outcome)/divalproex Remission (Retrospective-Modified Overt Aggression Scale – total score <10) | — | RR 0.51 (0.27 to 0.97) | 27 (1) | ⊕⊕⊕⊝ moderate[1] |
| Researcher-/clinician-rated antisocial behaviour (dichotomous outcome)/lithium Response | | RR 0.60 (0.36 to 1.00) | 116 (3) | ⊕⊕⊕⊝ moderate[1] |

[1]OIS (for dichotomous outcomes, OIS = 300 events; for continuous outcomes, OIS = 400 participants) not met.

319

rare cases to water intoxication), blood disorders (including eosinophilia, leucopenia, thrombocytopenia, haemolytic anaemia, and aplastic anaemia), dermatitis, urticarial'. Less common side effects are also listed (see the BNFC for more information). Scotto Rosata and colleagues (2012) reported that carbamazepine compared with placebo had a NNH of five for weight gain.

With regard to adverse effects of divalproex sodium, which consists of a compound of sodium valproate and valproic acid, the BNFC gives a number of cautions on the use of sodium valproate, including 'monitor liver function before therapy and during first 6 months especially in children most at risk'. In addition, the following side effects are listed: 'nausea, gastric irritation, diarrhoea; weight gain; hyperammonaemia, thrombocytopenia; transient hair loss (regrowth may be curly)'. Less common side effects are also listed (see the BNFC for more information). Scotto Rosata and colleagues (2012) reported that valproate compared with placebo had a NNH of eight for weight gain.

With regard to adverse effects of lithium carbonate, the BNFC gives a number of cautions, including: 'measure renal function and thyroid function every 6 months on stabilised regimens and advise children and carers to seek attention if symptoms of hypothyroidism develop (females are at greater risk) for example lethargy, feeling cold'. In addition, the following side effects are listed:

> *gastro-intestinal disturbances, fine tremor, renal impairment (particularly impaired urinary concentration and polyuria), polydipsia, leucocytosis; also weight gain and oedema (may respond to dose reduction); hyperparathyroidism and hypercalcaemia reported; signs of intoxication are blurred vision, increasing gastro-intestinal disturbances (anorexia, vomiting, diarrhoea), muscle weakness, increased central nervous system disturbances (mild drowsiness and sluggishness increasing to giddiness with ataxia, coarse tremor, lack of coordination, dysarthria), and require withdrawal of treatment; with severe overdosage (serum-lithium concentration above 2 mmol per litre) hyperreflexia and hyperextension of limbs, convulsions, toxic psychoses, syncope, renal failure, circulatory failure, coma, and occasionally, death; goitre, raised antidiuretic hormone concentration, hypothyroidism, hypokalaemia, ECG [electrocardiogram] changes, and kidney changes may also occur.*

Scotto Rosata and colleagues (2012) reported that lithium compared with placebo had a NNH of three for weight gain and ten for sedation.

*Antipsychotic drugs (risperidone)*
Moderate quality evidence from three trials with 387 participants showed that antipsychotic drugs, when compared with placebo, reduced antisocial behaviour when rated by parents at post-treatment using a continuous outcome measure (Table 100). Two trials with 280 participants also reported moderate quality evidence favouring the intervention when rated by researchers/clinicians using a dichotomous outcome. However, this was not clearly supported by researcher-/clinician- or teacher-rated continuous outcomes (moderate quality evidence from two trials with 56 participants and one trial with 38 participants, respectively). Out of the five trials, four included participants with coexisting ADHD (the proportion with ADHD ranged from 59 to 76%).

**Table 100: Summary of findings table for antipsychotic drugs compared with placebo (post-treatment)**

**Patient or population:** children and young people with conduct disorders (post-treatment)
**Intervention:** antipsychotic drugs
**Comparison:** placebo

| Outcomes | Illustrative comparative risks (95% CI) | | Relative effect (95% CI) | No. of participants (studies) | Quality of the evidence (GRADE) |
| --- | --- | --- | --- | --- | --- |
| | **Assumed risk** Placebo | **Corresponding risk** Antipsychotic drugs | | | |
| **Researcher-/clinician-rated antisocial behaviour (continuous outcome)** Any valid rating scale | – | The mean researcher-/clinician-rated antisocial behaviour (continuous outcome) in the intervention groups was **0.31 standard deviations lower** (1.15 lower to 0.52 higher) | | 56 (2) | ⊕⊕⊕⊝ **moderate**[1] |
| **Teacher-rated antisocial behaviour (continuous outcome)** Any valid rating scale | – | The mean teacher-rated antisocial behaviour (continuous outcome) in the intervention groups was **0.13 standard deviations higher** (0.50 lower to 0.76 higher) | | 38 (1) | ⊕⊕⊕⊝ **moderate**[1] |
| **Parent-rated antisocial behaviour (continuous outcome)** Any valid rating scale | – | The mean parent-rated antisocial behaviour (continuous outcome) in the intervention groups was **0.49 standard deviations lower** (0.69 to 0.30 lower) | | 387 (3) | ⊕⊕⊕⊝ **moderate**[1] |
| **Researcher-/clinician-rated antisocial behaviour (dichotomous outcome)** Clinical Global Impression – Improvement – much/very much improved/symptom recurrence | | | **RR 0.57** (0.44 to 0.73) | 280 (2) | ⊕⊕⊕⊝ **moderate**[1] |

[1]OIS (for dichotomous outcomes, OIS = 300 events; for continuous outcomes, OIS = 400 participants) not met.

With regard to adverse effects of risperidone, the BNFC gives a number of cautions, including 'hyperprolactinaemia, prolactin-dependent tumours; dehydration; family history of sudden cardiac death (perform an electrocardiogram); avoid in acute porphyria'. In addition, the following side effects are listed: 'gastro-intestinal disturbances (including diarrhoea, constipation, nausea and vomiting, dyspepsia, abdominal pain), dry mouth; dyspnoea; drowsiness, asthenia, tremor, sleep disturbances, agitation, anxiety, headache; urinary incontinence; hyperprolactinaemia (less commonly galactorrhoea, menstrual disturbances, gynaecomastia); arthralgia, myalgia; abnormal vision; epistaxis; rash'. Other less common side effects are also listed (see the BNFC for more information). Evidence from systematic reviews suggests that risperidone compared with placebo had a NNH of about eight for weight gain, about nine for prolactinemia, about ten for sedation, somnolence or drowsiness, and about 12 for tremor/extrapyramidal symptoms. A NNH for neurological side effects could not be estimated. Furthermore, Zuddas and colleagues (2011) suggest that in children the potential weight gain induced by second-generation antipsychotic drugs 'is comparable to that seen in adults, with the exception of a greater potential risk for risperidone'.

### Central nervous system stimulant drugs (methylphenidate/mixed amphetamine salts)

Moderate quality evidence from one trial with 47 participants (observer-rated outcome), two trials with 135 participants (teacher-rated outcome) and one trial with 74 participants (parent-rated outcome) showed that central nervous system stimulants, when compared with placebo, reduced antisocial behaviour at post-treatment using a continuous outcome measure (Table 101). In these trials, 69 to 79% of the participants had coexisting ADHD (it should be noted that methylphenidate and dexamfetamine are indicated for use in children with ADHD) (Paediatric Formulary Committee, 2011).

With regard to the adverse effects of methylphenidate, the BNFC gives a number of cautions, including:

> *monitor for psychiatric disorders; anxiety or agitation; tics or a family history of Tourette syndrome; drug or alcohol dependence; epilepsy (discontinue if increased seizure frequency); avoid abrupt withdrawal'. In addition, the following side-effects are listed: 'abdominal pain, nausea, vomiting, diarrhoea, dyspepsia, dry mouth, anorexia, reduced weight gain; tachycardia, palpitation, arrhythmias, changes in blood pressure; tics (very rarely Tourette syndrome), insomnia, nervousness, asthenia, depression, irritability, aggression, headache, drowsiness, dizziness, movement disorders; fever, arthralgia; rash, pruritus, alopecia; growth restriction.*

Less common side effects are also listed (see the BNFC for more information).

With regard to adverse effects of mixed amphetamine salts (listed in the BNFC as dexamphetamine sulphate), the BNFC gives a number of cautions, including:

> *anorexia; mild hypertension (contra-indicated if moderate or severe); psychosis or bipolar disorder; monitor for aggressive behaviour or hostility during initial treatment; history of epilepsy (discontinue if convulsions occur); tics and*

**Table 101: Summary of findings table for central nervous system stimulant drugs compared with placebo (post-treatment)**

**Patient or population:** children and young people with conduct disorders (post-treatment)
**Intervention:** central nervous system stimulants
**Comparison:** placebo

| Outcomes | Illustrative comparative risks (95% CI) | | No. of participants (studies) | Quality of the evidence (GRADE) |
| --- | --- | --- | --- | --- |
| | **Assumed risk** | **Corresponding risk** | | |
| | **Placebo** | **Central nervous system stimulants** | | |
| **Observer-rated antisocial behaviour (continuous outcome)** Any valid rating scale | – | The mean observer-rated antisocial behaviour (continuous outcome) in the intervention groups was **0.88 standard deviations lower** (1.47 to 0.29 lower) | 47 (1) | ⊕⊕⊕⊖ **moderate**[1] |
| **Teacher-rated antisocial behaviour (continuous outcome)** Any valid rating scale | – | The mean teacher-rated antisocial behaviour (continuous outcome) in the intervention groups was **0.93 standard deviations lower** (1.51 to 0.35 lower) | 135 (2) | ⊕⊕⊕⊖ **moderate**[1] |
| **Parent-rated antisocial behaviour (continuous outcome)** Any valid rating scale | – | The mean parent-rated antisocial behaviour (continuous outcome) in the intervention groups was **0.47 standard deviations lower** (0.94 lower to 0.00 higher) | 74 (1) | ⊕⊕⊕⊖ **moderate**[1] |

[1]OIS (for dichotomous outcomes, OIS = 300 events; for continuous outcomes, OIS = 400 participants) not met.

> *Tourette syndrome (use with caution) – discontinue if tics occur; susceptibility to angle-closure glaucoma; avoid abrupt withdrawal; data on safety and efficacy of long-term use not complete; acute porphyria.*

In addition, the following side effects are listed:

> *nausea, diarrhoea, dry mouth, abdominal cramps, anorexia (increased appetite also reported), weight loss, taste disturbance, ischaemic colitis, palpitation, tachycardia, chest pain, hypertension, hypotension, cardiomyopathy, myocardial infarction, cardiovascular collapse, cerebral vasculitis, stroke, headache, restlessness, depression, hyperreflexia, hyperactivity, impaired concentration, ataxia, anxiety, aggression, dizziness, confusion, sleep disturbances, dysphoria, euphoria, irritability, nervousness, malaise, obsessive-compulsive behaviour (OCD), paranoia, psychosis, panic attack, tremor, convulsions, neuroleptic malignant syndrome, anhedonia, growth restriction in children, hyperpyrexia, renal impairment, sexual dysfunction, acidosis, rhabdomyolysis, mydriasis, visual disturbances, alopecia, rash, sweating, urticaria; central stimulants have provoked choreoathetoid movements and dyskinesia, tics and Tourette syndrome in predisposed individuals (see also Cautions).*

Less common side effects are also listed (see the BNFC for more information).

*Selective norepinephrine reuptake inhibitor drugs (atomoxetine)*
Moderate quality evidence from one trial with 137 participants (teacher-rated outcome) and high quality evidence from four trials with 497 participants (parent-rated outcome) showed that atomoxetine, when compared with placebo, reduced antisocial behaviour at post-treatment when measured using a continuous outcome (Table 102). In one trial with 221 participants (researcher-/clinician-rated outcome), moderate quality evidence was inconclusive. In all trials, 100% of the participants had coexisting ADHD (it should be noted that atomoxetine is indicated for use in children with ADHD, see the BNFC 2011–2012[65]).

With regard to adverse effects of atomoxetine, the BNFC gives a number of cautions, including 'cardiovascular disease including hypertension and tachycardia; structural cardiac abnormalities; QT-interval prolongation (avoid concomitant use of drugs that prolong QT interval[66]); psychosis or mania; history of seizures; aggressive behaviour, hostility, or emotional lability; susceptibility to angle-closure glaucoma'. In addition, the following side effects are listed,

> *anorexia, dry mouth, nausea, vomiting, abdominal pain, constipation, dyspepsia, flatulence; palpitation, tachycardia, increased blood pressure, postural hypotension, hot flushes; sleep disturbance, dizziness, headache, fatigue, lethargy, depression, psychotic or manic symptoms, aggression, hostility, emotional*

---

[65] www.bnf.org
[66] The period from the start of the Q wave to the end of the T wave (duration of ventricular electrical activity).

**Table 102: Summary of findings table for selective norepinephrine (noradrenaline) reuptake inhibitor drug compared with placebo (post-treatment)**

**Patient or population:** children and young people with conduct disorders (post-treatment)
**Intervention:** atomoxetine
**Comparison:** placebo

| Outcomes | Illustrative comparative risks (95% CI) | | No. of participants (studies) | Quality of the evidence (GRADE) |
|---|---|---|---|---|
| | Assumed risk | Corresponding risk | | |
| | Placebo | Selective norepinephrine reuptake inhibitor drugs (atomoxetine) | | |
| **Researcher-/clinician-rated antisocial behaviour (continuous outcome)** Any valid rating scale | – | The mean researcher-/clinician-rated antisocial behaviour (continuous outcome) in the intervention groups was **0.16 standard deviations lower** (0.45 lower to 0.13 higher) | 221 (1) | ⊕⊕⊕⊝ **moderate**[1] |
| **Teacher-rated antisocial behaviour (continuous outcome)** Any valid rating scale | – | The mean teacher-rated antisocial behaviour (continuous outcome) in the intervention groups was **1.12 standard deviations lower** (1.53 to 0.71 lower) | 137 (1) | ⊕⊕⊕⊝ **moderate**[1] |
| **Parent-rated antisocial behaviour (continuous outcome)** Any valid rating scale | – | The mean parent-rated antisocial behaviour (continuous outcome) in the intervention groups was **0.40 standard deviations lower** (0.60 to 0.20 lower) | 497 (4) | ⊕⊕⊕⊕ **high** |

[1]OIS (for dichotomous outcomes, OIS = 300 events; for continuous outcomes, OIS = 400 participants) not met.

*lability, drowsiness, anxiety, irritability, tremor, rigors; urinary retention, prostatitis, sexual dysfunction, menstrual disturbances; mydriasis, conjunctivitis; dermatitis, pruritus, rash, sweating.*

Less common side effects are also listed (see the BNFC for more information).

### 8.2.5    Clinical evidence summary

Within each intervention category there were relatively few trials providing appropriate data that could be included in the review, but what data were available on the benefit of treatment were graded as moderate quality. Most evidence exists for drugs commonly used to treat psychosis (risperidone) and ADHD (methylphenidate, mixed amphetamine salts and atomoxetine). In both cases, the majority of trials included participants with coexisting ADHD. The strongest evidence of benefit also exists for these drugs, with medium to large effects on teacher- and parent-rated outcomes. However, all drugs reviewed carry important cautions for use and risk of adverse events (Paediatric Formulary Committee, 2011). In particular, risperidone, lithium, valproate and carbamazepine are all associated with an increased risk of weight gain (Maayan & Correll, 2011; Scotto Rosato et al., 2012; Zuddas et al., 2011).

Risperidone is the only drug licensed for use in the UK with a specific indication concerning conduct disorder. Specifically, it is indicated for short-term treatment (up to 6 weeks) of persistent aggression in conduct disorder (under specialist supervision) (Paediatric Formulary Committee, 2011). It is not recommended in children less than 5 years of age. Although licensed, there is a recognised need for further research concerning both the efficacy and tolerability of risperidone, and the Pediatric European Risperidone Studies project is currently underway to address this need[67].

Methylphenidate, dexamfetamine and atomoxetine are indicated for use in children and young people (aged 6 to 18 years) with ADHD (Paediatric Formulary Committee, 2011).

No RCT evidence was found to support the use of other antipsychotic drugs that are sometimes prescribed for conduct disorders, such as aripiprazole. Finally, no RCT evidence for non-pharmacological physical interventions was identified in this review.

### 8.3    HEALTH ECONOMIC EVIDENCE

### 8.3.1    Systematic literature review

No studies assessing the cost effectiveness of pharmacological interventions for children and young people with conduct disorder were identified by the systematic search of the economic literature undertaken for this guideline. Details on the methods used for the systematic search of the economic literature are described in Chapter 3.

---

[67]www.pers-project.com/

No further economic modelling was developed for pharmacological interventions because this was not considered to be an area of high priority by the GDG.

## 8.4     FROM EVIDENCE TO RECOMMENDATIONS

*Relative value placed on the outcomes considered*
The GDG focused their consideration of the evidence on the outcomes that they considered critical to understanding their impact on conduct disorder, which included antisocial behaviour (at home, at school and in the community), offending behaviour, school exclusion due to antisocial behaviour, educational attainment (that is, the highest level of education completed) and agency contact (for example residential care, criminal justice system).

*Trade-off between clinical benefits and harms*
After carefully reviewing the evidence, the GDG took the view that the evidence of benefit does not outweigh the known and potential harms associated with drug treatment for the routine management of behavioural problems in children and young people with a conduct disorder. However, drawing both on the evidence reviewed in this chapter and their expert knowledge and experience, the GDG judged that in young people with conduct disorder who have significant problems with explosive anger and emotional dysregulation, the benefits of antipsychotic medication (risperidone) may outweigh the risk of harm. Treatment should normally be limited to the short-term management of severely aggressive behaviour.

For children and young people with oppositional defiant disorder or conduct disorder and coexisting ADHD the GDG concluded that treatment with methylphenidate or atomoxetine outweighs the potential risk of harm. The GDG also noted that NICE clinical guideline 72, *Attention Deficit Hyperactivity Disorder* (NICE, 2009b) should be consulted for advice about the general treatment and management of ADHD.

*Quality of the evidence*
The available evidence for the benefit of drug treatment is generally of moderate quality. However, within each intervention category, there is a paucity of evidence (for example, at most, data from only four studies with 497 participants were combined in a single meta-analysis). Because of the paucity of data, evidence about side effects was taken from the BNFC, most of which was collected from young people with diagnoses other than conduct disorder. It was not possible to grade the quality of this evidence.

*Other considerations*
The GDG had concerns about the potential misuse of the medication reviewed in this chapter and took the view that a child and adolescent psychiatrist with experience of pharmacological treatment for behavioural disorders should initiate any pharmacological treatment for conduct disorder. This should not normally be commenced until

psychosocial interventions have been given a thorough trial and should only be done after a careful assessment for the presence of any comorbid disorders. In rare circumstances, for example when behavioural problems are very severe or there is an immediate need to manage a severe behavioural problem, a thorough trial of a psychosocial intervention may not be possible. The psychiatrist should discuss medication options with the young person and family including a discussion of side effects and measures to minimise these.

Given the potential seriousness of the side effects associated with the use of the psychotropic medication in children and young people, the psychiatrist should ensure that a proper assessment of a young person's physical health is carried out, including baseline and follow-up measurements of height, weight, blood pressure, liver function, fasting blood sugar, lipids, and other measurements such as renal and liver function, as indicated by the particular side effect profile of the drug prescribed.

The GDG drew on the *Schizophrenia* guideline (NICE, 2009e) regarding the use of antipsychotic medication because the following review questions were judged to be relevant:

● For people with first-episode or early schizophrenia, what are the benefits and downsides of continuous oral antipsychotic drug treatment when compared with another oral antipsychotic drug at the initiation of treatment (when administered within the recommended dose range [BNF 54])?

● For people with an acute exacerbation or recurrence of schizophrenia, what are the benefits and downsides of continuous oral antipsychotic drug treatment when compared with another oral antipsychotic drug (when administered within the recommended dose range [BNF 54])?

● For people with schizophrenia that is in remission, what are the benefits and downsides of continuous oral antipsychotic drug treatment when compared with another antipsychotic drug (when administered within the recommended dose range [BNF 54])?

After reviewing the guideline, the GDG decided to adapt one recommendation using the methods set out in Chapter 3. The original recommendation is listed in Table 103 in column one, the original evidence base in column two, and the adapted recommendation is in column three. The rationale for adaptation is provided in column four. In column one the numbers refer to the recommendations in the *Schizophrenia* guideline (NICE, 2009e). In column three the numbers in brackets following the recommendation refer to Section 8.5 in this guideline.

## 8.5 RECOMMENDATIONS

### 8.5.1 Clinical practice recommendations

8.5.1.1    Do not offer pharmacological interventions for the routine management of behavioural problems in children and young people with oppositional defiant disorder or conduct disorder.

**Table 103: Recommendations from *Schizophrenia* for inclusion**

| Original recommendation from *Schizophrenia* | Evidence base of existing recommendation | Recommendation following adaptation for this guideline | Reasons for adaptation |
|---|---|---|---|
| 1.2.4.3 Treatment with antipsychotic medication should be considered an explicit individual therapeutic trial. Include the following:<br>• Record the indications and expected benefits and risks of oral antipsychotic medication, and the expected time for a change in symptoms and appearance of side effects.<br>• At the start of treatment give a dose at the lower end of the licensed range and slowly titrate upwards within the dose range given in the British National Formulary or SPC.<br>• Justify and record reasons for dosages outside the range given in the BNF or SPC. | • Nine RCTs with a total of 1,801 participants with first-episode or early schizophrenia (including people with a recent onset of schizophrenia and people who have never been treated with antipsychotic medication). [*Schizophrenia*, Chapter 6, Section 6.2]<br>• 72 RCTs involving 16,556 participants with an acute exacerbation or recurrence of schizophrenia. [*Schizophrenia*, Chapter 6, Section 6.3]<br>• 17 RCTs including 3,535 participants with schizophrenia in remission. [*Schizophrenia*, Chapter 6, Section 6.4] | Treatment with risperidone[68] should be carefully evaluated, and include the following:<br>• Record the indications and expected benefits and risks, and the expected time for a change in symptoms and appearance of side effects.<br>• At the start of treatment give a dose at the lower end of the licensed range and slowly titrate upwards within the dose range given in the *British National Formulary for Children* (BNFC) or the summary of product characteristics (SPC).<br>• Justify and record reasons for dosages above the range given in the BNFC or SPC. | This recommendation was adapted to make it relevant for the short-term management of severely aggressive behaviour in young people with conduct disorder; only risperidone is licensed for use in children and young people with a conduct disorder therefore only this drug is recommended. The original recommendation has therefore been adapted to take account of this, including reference to the BNFC, rather than the adult BNF.<br>The GDG also judged that it was prudent to provide further specificity around dosing and monitoring in young people, including weight and height, fasting blood glucose, HbA$_{1c}$, blood lipid and prolactin levels. |

*Continued*

329

**Table 103:** *(Continued)*

| Original recommendation from *Schizophrenia* | Evidence base of existing recommendation | Recommendation following adaptation for this guideline | Reasons for adaptation |
|---|---|---|---|
| • Monitor and record the following regularly and systematically throughout treatment, but especially during titration:<br>– efficacy, including changes in symptoms and behaviour<br>– side effects of treatment, taking into account overlap between certain side effects and clinical features of schizophrenia, for example the overlap between akathisia and agitation or anxiety<br>– adherence<br>– physical health.<br>• Record the rationale for continuing, changing or stopping medication, and the effects of such changes.<br>• Carry out a trial of the medication at optimum dosage for 4–6 weeks. | | • Monitor and record systematically throughout treatment, but especially during titration:<br>– efficacy, including changes in symptoms and behaviour<br>– the emergence of movement disorders<br>– weight and height (weekly)<br>– fasting blood glucose, glycosylated haemoglobin (HBA$_{1C}$)<br>– adherence to medication<br>– physical health, including warning parents or carers and the young people about symptoms and signs of neuroleptic malignant syndrome<br>– record the rationale for continuing or stopping treatment and the effects of these decisions [8.5.1.6] | |

[68]At the time of publication (February 2013) some preparations of risperidone did not have a UK marketing authorisation for this indication in young people and no preparations were authorised for use in children aged under 5 years. The prescriber should consult the summary of product characteristics for the individual risperidone and follow relevant professional guidance, taking full responsibility for the decision. Informed consent should be obtained and documented. See the General Medical Council's 'Good practice in prescribing medicines – guidance for doctors' for further information (http:// www.gmc-uk.org/guidance/ethical_guidance/prescriptions_faqs.asp).

8.5.1.2    Offer methylphenidate or atomoxetine, within their licensed indications, for the management of ADHD in children and young people with oppositional defiant disorder or conduct disorder, in line with *Attention Deficit Hyperactivity Disorder* (NICE clinical guideline 72).

8.5.1.3    Consider risperidone[69] for the short-term management of severely aggressive behaviour in young people with a conduct disorder who have problems with explosive anger and severe emotional dysregulation and who have not responded to psychosocial interventions.

8.5.1.4    Provide young people and their parents or carers with age-appropriate information and discuss the likely benefits and possible side effects of risperidone[70] including:

● metabolic (including weight gain and diabetes)
● extrapyramidal (including akathisia, dyskinesia and dystonia)
● cardiovascular (including prolonging the QT interval)
● hormonal (including increasing plasma prolactin)
● other (including unpleasant subjective experiences).

8.5.1.5    Risperidone[71] should be started by an appropriately qualified healthcare professional with expertise in conduct disorders and should be based on a comprehensive assessment and diagnosis. The healthcare professional should undertake and record the following baseline investigations:

● weight and height (both plotted on a growth chart)
● waist and hip measurements
● pulse and blood pressure
● fasting blood glucose, glycosylated haemoglobin ($HbA_{1c}$), blood lipid and prolactin levels
● assessment of any movement disorders
● assessment of nutritional status, diet and level of physical activity.

---

[69]At the time of publication (2013) some preparations of risperidone did not have a UK marketing authorisation for this indication in young people and no preparations were authorised for use in children aged under 5 years. The prescriber should consult the summary of product characteristics for the individual risperidone and follow relevant professional guidance, taking full responsibility for the decision. Informed consent should be obtained and documented. See the General Medical Council's 'Good practice in prescribing and managing medicines and devices' for further information.

[70]At the time of publication (2013) some preparations of risperidone did not have a UK marketing authorisation for this indication in young people and no preparations were authorised for use in children aged under 5 years. The prescriber should consult the summary of product characteristics for the individual risperidone and follow relevant professional guidance, taking full responsibility for the decision. Informed consent should be obtained and documented. See the General Medical Council's 'Good practice in prescribing and managing medicines and devices' for further information.

[71]At the time of publication (2013) some preparations of risperidone did not have a UK marketing authorisation for this indication in young people and no preparations were authorised for use in children aged under 5 years. The prescriber should consult the summary of product characteristics for the individual risperidone and follow relevant professional guidance, taking full responsibility for the decision. Informed consent should be obtained and documented. See the General Medical Council's 'Good practice in prescribing and managing medicines and devices' for further information.

8.5.1.6    Treatment with risperidone[72] should be carefully evaluated, and include the following:

- Record the indications and expected benefits and risks, and the expected time for a change in symptoms and appearance of side effects.
- At the start of treatment give a dose at the lower end of the licensed range and slowly titrate upwards within the dose range given in the *British National Formulary for Children* (BNFC) or the summary of product characteristics (SPC).
- Justify and record reasons for dosages above the range given in the BNFC or SPC.
- Monitor and record systematically throughout treatment, but especially during titration:
  - efficacy, including changes in symptoms and behaviour
  - the emergence of movement disorders
  - weight and height (weekly)
  - fasting blood glucose, $HbA_{1c}$, blood lipid and prolactin levels
  - adherence to medication
  - physical health, including warning parents or cares and the young person about symptoms and signs of neuroleptic malignant syndrome.
- Record the rationale for continuing or stopping treatment and the effects of these decisions[73].

8.5.1.7    Review the effects of risperidone[74] after 3–4 weeks and discontinue it if there is no indication of a clinically important response at 6 weeks.

### 8.5.2    Research recommendations

8.5.2.1    For children and young people with a conduct disorder and coexisting depression, are selective serotonin reuptake inhibitor antidepressant drugs when used in combination with a psychosocial intervention for conduct disorders effective and cost-effective at reducing antisocial behaviour?

---

[72] At the time of publication (2013) some preparations of risperidone did not have a UK marketing authorisation for this indication in young people and no preparations were authorised for use in children aged under 5 years. The prescriber should consult the summary of product characteristics for the individual risperidone and follow relevant professional guidance, taking full responsibility for the decision. Informed consent should be obtained and documented. See the General Medical Council's 'Good practice in prescribing and managing medicines and devices' for further information.

[73] Adapted from *Schizophrenia* (NICE clinical guideline 82).

[74] At the time of publication (2013) some preparations of risperidone did not have a UK marketing authorisation for this indication in young people and no preparations were authorised for use in children aged under 5 years. The prescriber should consult the summary of product characteristics for the individual risperidone and follow relevant professional guidance, taking full responsibility for the decision. Informed consent should be obtained and documented. See the General Medical Council's 'Good practice in prescribing and managing medicines and devices' for further information.

# 9    SUMMARY OF RECOMMENDATIONS

## 9.1    GENERAL PRINCIPLES OF CARE

*Working safely and effectively with children and young people*

9.1.1.1    Health and social care professionals working with children and young people who present with behaviour suggestive of a conduct disorder, or who have a conduct disorder, should be trained and competent to work with children and young people of all levels of learning ability, cognitive capacity, emotional maturity and development.

9.1.1.2    Health and social care professionals should ensure that they:
- can assess capacity and competence, including 'Gillick competence', in children and young people of all ages **and**
- understand how to apply legislation, including the Children Act (1989), the Mental Health Act (1983; amended 1995 and 2007) and the Mental Capacity Act (2005), in the care and treatment of children and young people.

9.1.1.3    Health and social care providers should ensure that children and young people:
- can routinely receive care and treatment from a single team or professional
- are not passed from one team to another unnecessarily
- do not undergo multiple assessments unnecessarily[75].

9.1.1.4    When providing assessment or treatment interventions for children and young people, ensure that the nature and content of the intervention is suitable for the child or young person's developmental level.

9.1.1.5    Consider children and young people for assessment according to local safeguarding procedures if there are concerns regarding exploitation or self-care, or if they have been in contact with the criminal justice system[76].

*Establishing relationships with children and young people and their parents or carers*

9.1.1.6    Be aware that many children and young people with a conduct disorder may have had poor or punitive experiences of care and be mistrustful or dismissive of offers of help as a result.

9.1.1.7    Develop a positive, caring and trusting relationship with the child or young person and their parents or carers to encourage their engagement with services.

---

[75]Adapted from *Service User Experience in Adult Mental Health* (NICE clinical guidance 136).
[76]Adapted from *Service User Experience in Adult Mental Health* (NICE clinical guidance 136).

9.1.1.8    Health and social care professionals working with children and young people should be trained and skilled in:
- negotiating and working with parents and carers **and**
- managing issues relating to information sharing and confidentiality as these apply to children and young people.

9.1.1.9    If a young person is 'Gillick competent' ask them what information can be shared before discussing their condition with their parents or carers.

9.1.1.10   When working with children and young people with a conduct disorder and their parents or carers:
- make sure that discussions take place in settings in which confidentiality, privacy and dignity are respected
- be clear with the child or young person and their parents or carers about limits of confidentiality (that is, which health and social care professionals have access to information about their diagnosis and its treatment and in what circumstances this may be shared with others)[77].

9.1.1.11   When coordinating care and discussing treatment decisions with children and young people and their parents or carers, ensure that:
- everyone involved understands the purpose of any meetings and why information might need to be shared between services **and**
- the right to confidentiality is respected throughout the process.

*Working with parents and carers*

9.1.1.12   If parents or carers are involved in the treatment of young people with a conduct disorder, discuss with young people of an appropriate developmental level, emotional maturity and cognitive capacity how they want them to be involved. Such discussions should take place at intervals to take account of any changes in circumstances, including developmental level, and should not happen only once[78].

9.1.1.13   Be aware that parents and carers of children and young people with a conduct disorder might feel blamed for their child's problems or stigmatised by their contact with services. When offering or providing interventions such as parent training programmes, directly address any concerns they have and set out the reasons for and purpose of the intervention.

9.1.1.14   Offer parents and carers an assessment of their own needs including:
- personal, social and emotional support **and**
- support in their caring role, including emergency plans **and**
- advice on practical matters such as childcare, housing and finances, and help to obtain support.

*Communication and information*

9.1.1.15   When communicating with children and young people with a conduct disorder and their parents or carers:

---

[77]Adapted from *Service User Experience in Adult Mental Health* (NICE clinical guidance 136).
[78]Adapted from *Service User Experience in Adult Mental Health* (NICE clinical guidance 136).

- take into account the child or young person's developmental level, emotional maturity and cognitive capacity, including any learning disabilities, sight or hearing problems, or delays in language development or social communication difficulties
- use plain language if possible and clearly explain any clinical language; adjust strategies to the person's language ability, for example, breaking up information, checking back, summarising and recapping
- check that the child or young person and their parents or carers understand what is being said
- use communication aids (such as pictures, symbols, large print, braille, different languages or sign language) if needed.

9.1.1.16    When giving information to children and young people with a conduct disorder and their parents or carer, ensure you are:
- familiar with local and national sources (organisations and websites) of information and/or support for children and young people with a conduct disorder and their parents or carers
- able to discuss and advise how to access these resources
- able to discuss and actively support children and young people and their parents or carers to engage with these resources[79].

9.1.1.17    When communicating with a child or young person use diverse media, including letters, phone calls, emails or text messages, according to their preference[80].

*Culture, ethnicity and social inclusion*

9.1.1.18    When working with children and young people with a conduct disorder and their parents or carers:
- take into account that stigma and discrimination are often associated with using mental health services
- be respectful of and sensitive to children and young people's gender, sexual orientation, socioeconomic status, age, background (including cultural, ethnic and religious background) and any disability
- be aware of possible variations in the presentation of mental health problems in children and young people of different genders, ages, cultural, ethnic, religious or other diverse backgrounds[81].

9.1.1.19    When working with children and young people and their parents or carers who have difficulties speaking or reading English:
- provide and work proficiently with interpreters if needed
- offer a list of local education providers who can provide English language teaching.

---

[79]Adapted from *Service User Experience in Adult Mental Health* (NICE clinical guidance 136).
[80]Adapted from *Service User Experience in Adult Mental Health* (NICE clinical guidance 136).
[81]Adapted from *Service User Experience in Adult Mental Health* (NICE clinical guidance 136).

*Summary of recommendations*

9.1.1.20    Health and social care professionals working with children and young people with a conduct disorder and their parents or carers should have competence in:

- assessment skills and using explanatory models of conduct disorder
for people from different cultural, ethnic, religious or other diverse
backgrounds
- explaining the possible causes of different mental health problems, and
care, treatment and support options
- addressing cultural, ethnic, religious or other differences in treatment
expectations and adherence
- addressing cultural, ethnic, religious or other beliefs about biological,
social and familial influences on the possible causes of mental health
problems
- conflict management and conflict resolution[82].

*Staff supervision*

9.1.1.21    Health and social care services should ensure that staff supervision is built
into the routine working of the service, is properly resourced within local
systems and is monitored. Supervision should:

- make use of direct observation (for example, recordings of sessions) and
routine outcome measures
- support adherence to the specific intervention
- focus on outcomes
- be regular and apply to the whole caseload.

*Transfer and discharge*

9.1.1.22    Anticipate that withdrawal and ending of treatments or services, and transition from one service to another, may evoke strong emotions and reactions
in children and young people with a conduct disorder and their parents or
carers. Ensure that:

- such changes, especially discharge and transfer from CAMHS to adult
services, are discussed and planned carefully beforehand with the child
or young person and their parents or carers, and are structured and
phased
- children and young people and their parents or carers are given comprehensive information about the way adult services work and the nature of
any potential interventions provided
- any care plan supports effective collaboration with social care and other
care providers during endings and transitions, and includes details of
how to access services in times of crisis
- when referring a child or young person for an assessment in other services (including for psychological interventions), they are supported

---

[82]Adapted from *Service User Experience in Adult Mental Health* (NICE clinical guidance 136).

during the referral period and arrangements for support are agreed beforehand with them[83].

9.1.1.23   For young people who continue to exhibit antisocial behaviour or meet criteria for a conduct disorder while in transition to adult services (in particular those who are still vulnerable, such as those who have been looked after or who have limited access to care) refer to *Antisocial Personality Disorder* (NICE clinical guideline 77). For those who have other mental health problems refer to other NICE guidance for the specific mental health problem.

## 9.2     SELECTIVE PREVENTION

In this guideline selective prevention refers to interventions targeted to individuals or to a subgroup of the population whose risk of developing a conduct disorder is significantly higher than average, as evidenced by individual, family and social risk factors. Individual risk factors include low school achievement and impulsiveness; family risk factors include parental contact with the criminal justice system and child abuse; social risk factors include low family income and little education.

9.2.2.1   Offer classroom-based emotional learning and problem-solving programmes for children aged typically between 3 and 7 years in schools where classroom populations have a high proportion of children identified to be at risk of developing oppositional defiant disorder or conduct disorder as a result of any of the following factors:
● low socioeconomic status
● low school achievement
● child abuse or parental conflict
● separated or divorced parents
● parental mental health or substance misuse problems
● parental contact with the criminal justice system.

9.2.2.2   Classroom-based emotional learning and problem-solving programmes should be provided in a positive atmosphere and consist of interventions intended to:
● increase children's awareness of their own and others' emotions
● teach self-control of arousal and behaviour
● promote a positive self-concept and good peer relations
● develop children's problem-solving skills.
Typically the programmes should consist of up to 30 classroom-based sessions over the course of one school year.

---

[83]Adapted from *Service User Experience in Adult Mental Health* (NICE clinical guidance 136).

## 9.3 IDENTIFICATION AND ASSESSMENT

*Initial assessment of children and young people with a possible conduct disorder*

9.3.1.1 Adjust delivery of initial assessment methods to:
- the needs of children and young people with a suspected conduct disorder **and**
- the setting in which they are delivered (for example, health and social care, educational settings or the criminal justice system).

9.3.1.2 Undertake an initial assessment for a suspected conduct disorder if a child or young person's parents or carers, health or social care professionals, school or college, or peer group raise concerns about persistent antisocial behaviour.

9.3.1.3 Do not regard a history of a neurodevelopmental condition (for example, attention deficit hyperactivity disorder [ADHD]) as a barrier to assessment.

9.3.1.4 For the initial assessment of a child or young person with a suspected conduct disorder, consider using the Strengths and Difficulties Questionnaire (completed by a parent, carer or teacher).

9.3.1.5 Assess for the presence of the following significant complicating factors:
- a coexisting mental health problem (for example, depression, post-traumatic stress disorder)
- a neurodevelopmental condition (in particular ADHD and autism)
- a learning disability or difficulty
- substance misuse in young people.

9.3.1.6 If any significant complicating factors are present refer the child or young person to a specialist CAMHS for a comprehensive assessment.

9.3.1.7 If no significant complicating factors are present consider direct referral for an intervention.

*Comprehensive assessment*

9.3.1.8 A comprehensive assessment of a child or young person with a suspected conduct disorder should be undertaken by a health or social care professional who is competent to undertake the assessment and should:
- offer the child or young person the opportunity to meet the professional on their own
- involve a parent, carer or other third party known to the child or young person who can provide information about current and past behaviour
- if necessary involve more than one health or social care professional to ensure a comprehensive assessment is undertaken.

9.3.1.9 Before starting a comprehensive assessment, explain to the child or young person how the outcome of the assessment will be communicated to them. Involve a parent, carer or advocate to help explain the outcome.

9.3.1.10 The standard components of a comprehensive assessment of conduct disorders should include asking about and assessing the following:

- core conduct disorders symptoms including:
    - patterns of negativistic, hostile, or defiant behaviour in children aged under 11 years
    - aggression to people and animals, destruction of property, deceitfulness or theft and serious violations of rules in children aged over 11 years
- current functioning at home, at school or college and with peers
- parenting quality
- history of any past or current mental or physical health problems.

9.3.1.11  Take into account and address possible coexisting conditions such as:
- learning difficulties or disabilities
- neurodevelopmental conditions such as ADHD and autism
- neurological disorders including epilepsy and motor impairments
- other mental health problems (for example, depression, post-traumatic stress disorder and bipolar disorder)
- substance misuse
- communication disorders (for example, speech and language problems).

9.3.1.12  Consider using formal assessment instruments to aid the diagnosis of coexisting conditions, such as:
- the Child Behavior Checklist for all children and young people
- the Strengths and Difficulties Questionnaire for all children or young people
- the Connors Rating Scales – Revised for a child or young person with suspected ADHD
- a validated measure of autistic behaviour for a child or young person with a suspected autism spectrum disorder (see *Autism: Recognition, Referral and Diagnosis of Children and Young People on the Autism Spectrum* [NICE clinical guideline 128])
- a validated measure of cognitive ability for a child or young person with a suspected learning disability
- a validated reading test for a child or young person with a suspected reading difficulty.

9.3.1.13  Assess the risks faced by the child or young person and if needed develop a risk management plan for self-neglect, exploitation by others, self-harm or harm to others.

9.3.1.14  Assess for the presence or risk of physical, sexual and emotional abuse in line with local protocols for the assessment and management of these problems.

9.3.1.15  Conduct a comprehensive assessment of the child or young person's parents or carers, which should cover:
- positive and negative aspects of parenting, in particular any use of coercive discipline
- the parent–child relationship
- positive and negative adult relationships within the child or young person's family, including domestic violence

- parental wellbeing, encompassing mental health, substance misuse (including whether alcohol or drugs were used during pregnancy) and criminal behaviour.

9.3.1.16 Develop a care plan with the child or young person and their parents or carers that includes a profile of their needs, risks to self or others, and any further assessments that may be needed. This should encompass the development and maintenance of the conduct disorder and any associated behavioural problems, any coexisting mental or physical health problems and speech, language and communication difficulties, in the context of:
- any personal, social, occupational, housing or educational needs
- the needs of parents or carers
- the strengths of the child or young person and their parents or carers.

## 9.4 IDENTIFYING EFFECTIVE TREATMENT AND CARE OPTIONS

9.4.1.1 When discussing treatment or care interventions with a child or young person with a conduct disorder and, if appropriate, their parents or carers, take account of:
- their past and current experience of the disorder
- their experience of, and response to, previous interventions and services
- the nature, severity and duration of the problem(s)
- the impact of the disorder on educational performance
- any chronic physical health problem
- any social or family factors that may have a role in the development or maintenance of the identified problem(s)
- any coexisting conditions[84].

9.4.1.2 When discussing treatment or care interventions with a child or young person and, if appropriate, their parents or carers, provide information about:
- the nature, content and duration of any proposed intervention
- the acceptability and tolerability of any proposed intervention
- the possible impact on interventions for any other behavioural or mental health problem
- the implications for the continuing provision of any current interventions[85].

9.4.1.3 When making a referral for treatment or care interventions for a conduct disorder, take account of the preferences of the child or young person and, if appropriate, their parents or carers when choosing from a range of evidence-based interventions[86].

---

[84]Adapted from *Common Mental Health Disorders* (NICE clinical guideline 123).
[85]Adapted from *Common Mental Health Disorders* (NICE clinical guideline 123).
[86]Adapted from *Common Mental Health Disorders* (NICE clinical guideline 123).

**9.5      PSYCHOSOCIAL INTERVENTIONS – TREATMENT AND INDICATED PREVENTION**

In this guideline indicated prevention refers to interventions targeted to high-risk individuals who are identified as having detectable signs or symptoms that may lead to the development of conduct disorders but who do not meet diagnostic criteria for conduct disorders when offered an intervention.

The interventions in recommendations 9.5.1.1–9.5.1.12 are suitable for children and young people who have a diagnosis of oppositional defiant disorder or conduct disorder, are in contact with the criminal justice system for antisocial behaviour, or have been identified as being at high risk of a conduct disorder using established rating scales of antisocial behaviour (for example, the Child Behavior Checklist and the Eyberg Child Behavior Inventory).

*Parent training programmes*

9.5.1.1    Offer a group parent training programme to the parents of children and young people aged between 3 and 11 years who:
● have been identified as being at high risk of developing oppositional defiant disorder or conduct disorder or
● have oppositional defiant disorder or conduct disorder or
● are in contact with the criminal justice system because of antisocial behaviour.

9.5.1.2    Group parent training programmes should involve both parents if this is possible and in the best interests of the child or young person, and should:
● typically have between 10 and 12 parents in a group
● be based on a social learning model, using modelling, rehearsal and feedback to improve parenting skills
● typically consist of 10 to 16 meetings of 90 to 120 minutes' duration
● adhere to a developer's manual[87] and employ all of the necessary materials to ensure consistent implementation of the programme.

9.5.1.3    Offer an individual parent training programme to the parents of children and young people aged between 3 and 11 years who are not able to participate in a group parent training programme and whose child:
● has been identified as being at high risk of developing oppositional defiant disorder or conduct disorder or
● has oppositional defiant disorder or conduct disorder or
● is in contact with the criminal justice system because of antisocial behaviour.

9.5.1.4    Individual parent training programmes should involve both parents if this is possible and in the best interests of the child or young person, and should:
● be based on a social learning model using modelling, rehearsal and feedback to improve parenting skills
● typically consist of 8 to 10 meetings of 60 to 90 minutes' duration

---

[87]The manual should have been positively evaluated in a randomised controlled trial.

- adhere to a developer's manual[88] and employ all of the necessary materials to ensure consistent implementation of the programme.

*Parent and child training programmes for children with complex needs*

9.5.1.5    Offer individual parent and child training programmes to children and young people aged between 3 and 11 years if their problems are severe and complex and they:
- have been identified as being at high risk of developing oppositional defiant disorder or conduct disorder **or**
- have oppositional defiant disorder or conduct disorder **or**
- are in contact with the criminal justice system because of antisocial behaviour.

9.5.1.6    Individual parent and child training programmes should involve both parents, foster carers or guardians if this is possible and in the best interests of the child or young person, and should:
- be based on a social learning model using modelling, rehearsal and feedback to improve parenting skills
- consist of up to 10 meetings of 60 minutes' duration
- adhere to a developer's manual[89] and employ all of the necessary materials to ensure consistent implementation of the programme.

*Foster carer/guardian training programmes*

9.5.1.7    Offer a group foster carer/guardian training programme to foster carers and guardians of children and young people aged between 3 and 11 years who:
- have been identified as being at high risk of developing oppositional defiant disorder or conduct disorder **or**
- have oppositional defiant disorder or conduct disorder **or**
- are in contact with the criminal justice system because of antisocial behaviour.

9.5.1.8    Group foster carer/guardian training programmes should involve both of the foster carers or guardians if this is possible and in the best interests of the child or young person, and should:
- modify the intervention to take account of the care setting in which the child is living
- typically have between 8 and 12 foster carers or guardians in a group
- be based on a social learning model using modelling, rehearsal and feedback to improve parenting skills
- typically consist of between 12 and 16 meetings of 90 to 120 minutes' duration
- adhere to a developer's manual[90] and employ all of the necessary materials to ensure consistent implementation of the programme.

---

[88] The manual should have been positively evaluated in a randomised controlled trial.
[89] The manual should have been positively evaluated in a randomised controlled trial.
[90] The manual should have been positively evaluated in a randomised controlled trial.

9.5.1.9    Offer an individual foster carer/guardian training programme to the foster
           carers or guardians of children and young people aged between 3 and 11
           years who are not able to participate in a group programme and whose
           child:
           ● has been identified as being at high risk of developing oppositional defi-
             ant disorder or conduct disorder **or**
           ● has oppositional defiant disorder or conduct disorder **or**
           ● is in contact with the criminal justice system because of antisocial
             behaviour.

9.5.1.10   Individual foster carer/guardian training programmes should involve both
           of the foster carers if this is possible and in the best interests of the child or
           young person, and should:
           ● modify the intervention to take account of the care setting in which the
             child is living
           ● be based on a social learning model using modelling, rehearsal and
             feedback to improve parenting skills
           ● consist of up to 10 meetings of 60 minutes' duration
           ● adhere to a developer's manual[91] and employ all of the necessary materi-
             als to ensure consistent implementation of the programme.

*Child-focused programmes*

9.5.1.11   Offer group social and cognitive problem-solving programmes to children
           and young people aged between 9 and 14 years who:
           ● have been identified as being at high risk of developing oppositional
             defiant disorder or conduct disorder **or**
           ● have oppositional defiant disorder or conduct disorder **or**
           ● are in contact with the criminal justice system because of antisocial
             behaviour.

9.5.1.12   Group social and cognitive problem-solving programmes should be
           adapted to the children's or young people's developmental level and should:
           ● be based on a cognitive–behavioural problem-solving model
           ● use modelling, rehearsal and feedback to improve skills
           ● typically consist of 10 to 18 weekly meetings of 2 hours' duration
           ● adhere to a developer's manual[92] and employ all of the necessary materi-
             als to ensure consistent implementation of the programme.

*Multimodal interventions*

9.5.1.13   Offer multimodal interventions, for example, multisystemic therapy, to
           children and young people aged between 11 and 17 years for the treatment
           of conduct disorder.

9.5.1.14   Multimodal interventions should involve the child or young person and
           their parents and carers and should:

---

[91] The manual should have been positively evaluated in a randomised controlled trial.
[92] The manual should have been positively evaluated in a randomised controlled trial.

- have an explicit and supportive family focus
- be based on a social learning model with interventions provided at individual, family, school, criminal justice and community levels
- be provided by specially trained case managers
- typically consist of 3 to 4 meetings per week over a 3 to 5-month period
- adhere to a developer's manual[93] and employ all of the necessary materials to ensure consistent implementation of the programme.

## 9.6 PHARMACOLOGICAL INTERVENTIONS

9.6.1.1 Do not offer pharmacological interventions for the routine management of behavioural problems in children and young people with oppositional defiant disorder or conduct disorder.

9.6.1.2 Offer methylphenidate or atomoxetine, within their licensed indications, for the management of ADHD in children and young people with oppositional defiant disorder or conduct disorder, in line with *Attention Deficit Hyperactivity Disorder* (NICE clinical guideline 72).

9.6.1.3 Consider risperidone[94] for the short-term management of severely aggressive behaviour in young people with a conduct disorder who have problems with explosive anger and severe emotional dysregulation and who have not responded to psychosocial interventions.

9.6.1.4 Provide young people and their parents or carers with age-appropriate information and discuss the likely benefits and possible side effects of risperidone[95] including:

- metabolic (including weight gain and diabetes)
- extrapyramidal (including akathisia, dyskinesia and dystonia)
- cardiovascular (including prolonging the QT interval)
- hormonal (including increasing plasma prolactin)
- other (including unpleasant subjective experiences).

---

[93] The manual should have been positively evaluated in a randomised controlled trial.

[94] At the time of publication (2013) some preparations of risperidone did not have a UK marketing authorisation for this indication in young people and no preparations were authorised for use in children aged under 5 years. The prescriber should consult the summary of product characteristics for the individual risperidone and follow relevant professional guidance, taking full responsibility for the decision. Informed consent should be obtained and documented. See the General Medical Council's 'Good practice in prescribing and managing medicines and devices' for further information.

[95] At the time of publication (2013) some preparations of risperidone did not have a UK marketing authorisation for this indication in young people and no preparations were authorised for use in children aged under 5 years. The prescriber should consult the summary of product characteristics for the individual risperidone and follow relevant professional guidance, taking full responsibility for the decision. Informed consent should be obtained and documented. See the General Medical Council's 'Good practice in prescribing and managing medicines and devices' for further information.

9.6.1.5    Risperidone[96] should be started by an appropriately qualified healthcare professional with expertise in conduct disorders and should be based on a comprehensive assessment and diagnosis. The healthcare professional should undertake and record the following baseline investigations:
- weight and height (both plotted on a growth chart)
- waist and hip measurements
- pulse and blood pressure
- fasting blood glucose, glycosylated haemoglobin ($HbA_{1c}$), blood lipid and prolactin levels
- assessment of any movement disorders
- assessment of nutritional status, diet and level of physical activity.

9.6.1.6    Treatment with risperidone[97] should be carefully evaluated, and include the following:
- Record the indications and expected benefits and risks, and the expected time for a change in symptoms and appearance of side effects.
- At the start of treatment give a dose at the lower end of the licensed range and slowly titrate upwards within the dose range given in the *British National Formulary for Children* (BNFC) or the summary of product characteristics (SPC).
- Justify and record reasons for dosages above the range given in the BNFC or SPC.
- Monitor and record systematically throughout treatment, but especially during titration:
  - efficacy, including changes in symptoms and behaviour
  - the emergence of movement disorders
  - weight and height (weekly)
  - fasting blood glucose, $HbA_{1c}$, blood lipid and prolactin levels
  - adherence to medication
  - physical health, including warning parents or carers and the young person about symptoms and signs of neuroleptic malignant syndrome.
- Record the rationale for continuing or stopping treatment and the effects of these decisions[98].

---

[96]At the time of publication (2013) some preparations of risperidone did not have a UK marketing authorisation for this indication in young people and no preparations were authorised for use in children aged under 5 years. The prescriber should consult the summary of product characteristics for the individual risperidone and follow relevant professional guidance, taking full responsibility for the decision. Informed consent should be obtained and documented. See the General Medical Council's 'Good practice in prescribing and managing medicines and devices' for further information.

[97]At the time of publication (2013) some preparations of risperidone did not have a UK marketing authorisation for this indication in young people and no preparations were authorised for use in children aged under 5 years. The prescriber should consult the summary of product characteristics for the individual risperidone and follow relevant professional guidance, taking full responsibility for the decision. Informed consent should be obtained and documented. See the General Medical Council's 'Good practice in prescribing and managing medicines and devices' for further information.

[98]Adapted from *Schizophrenia* (NICE clinical guideline 82).

9.6.1.7    Review the effects of risperidone[99] after 3–4 weeks and discontinue it if there is no indication of a clinically important response at 6 weeks.


**9.7        ORGANISATION AND DELIVERY OF CARE**

*Improving access to services*
9.7.1.1    Health and social care professionals, managers and commissioners should collaborate with colleagues in educational settings to develop local care pathways that promote access to services for children and young people with a conduct disorder and their parents and carers by:
- supporting the integrated delivery of services across all care settings
- having clear and explicit criteria for entry to the service
- focusing on entry and not exclusion criteria
- having multiple means (including self-referral) of access to the service
- providing multiple points of access that facilitate links with the wider care system, including educational and social care services and the community in which the service is located[100].

9.7.1.2    Provide information about the services and interventions that constitute the local care pathway, including the:
- range and nature of the interventions provided
- settings in which services are delivered
- processes by which a child or young person moves through the pathway
- means by which progress and outcomes are assessed
- delivery of care in related health and social care services[101].

9.7.1.3    When providing information about local care pathways for children and young people with a conduct disorder and their parents and carers:
- take into account the person's knowledge and understanding of conduct disorders and their care and treatment
- ensure that such information is appropriate to the communities using the pathway[102].

9.7.1.4    Provide all information about services in a range of languages and formats (visual, verbal and aural) and ensure that it is available in a range of settings throughout the whole community to which the service is responsible[103].

---

[99]At the time of publication (2013) some preparations of risperidone did not have a UK marketing authorisation for this indication in young people and no preparations were authorised for use in children aged under 5 years. The prescriber should consult the summary of product characteristics for the individual risperidone and follow relevant professional guidance, taking full responsibility for the decision. Informed consent should be obtained and documented. See the General Medical Council's 'Good practice in prescribing and managing medicines and devices' for further information.

[100]Adapted from *Common Mental Health Disorders* (NICE clinical guideline 123).

[101]From *Common Mental Health Disorders* (NICE clinical guideline 123).

[102]Adapted from *Common Mental Health Disorders* (NICE clinical guideline 123).

[103]From *Common Mental Health Disorders* (NICE clinical guideline 123).

9.7.1.5    Health and social care professionals, managers and commissioners should collaborate with colleagues in educational settings to develop local care pathways that promote access for a range of groups at risk of under-utilising services, including:
● girls and young women
● black and minority ethnic groups
● people with a coexisting condition (such as ADHD or autism)[104].

9.7.1.6    Support access to services and increase the uptake of interventions by:
● ensuring systems are in place to provide for the overall coordination and continuity of care
● designating a professional to oversee the whole period of care (for example, a staff member in a CAMHS or social care setting)[105].

9.7.1.7    Support access to services and increase the uptake of interventions by providing services for children and young people with a conduct disorder and their parents and carers, in a variety of settings. Use an assessment of local needs as a basis for the structure and distribution of services, which should typically include delivery of:
● assessment and interventions outside normal working hours
● assessment and interventions in the person's home or other residential settings
● specialist assessment and interventions in accessible community-based settings (for example, community centres, schools and colleges and social centres) and if appropriate, in conjunction with staff from those settings
● both generalist and specialist assessment and intervention services in primary care settings[106].

9.7.1.8    Health and social care professionals, managers and commissioners should collaborate with colleagues in educational settings to look at a range of services to support access to and uptake of services. These could include:
● crèche facilities
● assistance with travel
● advocacy services[107].

*Developing local care pathways*
9.7.1.9    Local care pathways should be developed to promote implementation of key principles of good care. Pathways should be:
● negotiable, workable and understandable for children and young people with a conduct disorder and their parents and carers as well as professionals

---

[104]Adapted from *Common Mental Health Disorders* (NICE clinical guideline 123).
[105]Adapted from *Common Mental Health Disorders* (NICE clinical guideline 123).
[106]Adapted from *Common Mental Health Disorders* (NICE clinical guideline 123).
[107]Adapted from *Common Mental Health Disorders* (NICE clinical guideline 123).

- accessible and acceptable to all people in need of the services served by the pathway
- responsive to the needs of children and young people with a conduct disorder and their parents and carers
- integrated so that there are no barriers to movement between different levels of the pathway
- focused on outcomes (including measures of quality, service user experience and harm)[108].

9.7.1.10 Responsibility for the development, management and evaluation of local care pathways should lie with a designated leadership team, which should include health and social care professionals, managers and commissioners. The leadership team should work in collaboration with colleagues in educational settings and take particular responsibility for:
- developing clear policy and protocols for the operation of the pathway
- providing training and support on the operation of the pathway
- auditing and reviewing the performance of the pathway[109].

9.7.1.11 Health and social care professionals, managers and commissioners should work with colleagues in educational settings to design local care pathways that promote a model of service delivery that:
- has clear and explicit criteria for the thresholds determining access to and movement between the different levels of the pathway
- does not use single criteria such as symptom severity or functional impairment to determine movement within the pathway
- monitors progress and outcomes to ensure the most effective interventions are delivered[110].

9.7.1.12 Health and social care professionals, managers and commissioners should work with colleagues in educational settings to design local care pathways that promote a range of evidence-based interventions in the pathway and support children and young people with a conduct disorder and their parents and carers in their choice of interventions[111].

9.7.1.13 All staff should ensure effective engagement with parents and carers, if appropriate, to:
- inform and improve the care of the child or young person with a conduct disorder
- meet the needs of parents and carers[112].

9.7.1.14 Health and social care professionals, managers and commissioners should work with colleagues in educational settings to design local care pathways that promote the active engagement of all populations served by the pathway. Pathways should:

---

[108]Adapted from *Common Mental Health Disorders* (NICE clinical guideline 123).
[109]Adapted from *Common Mental Health Disorders* (NICE clinical guideline 123).
[110]Adapted from *Common Mental Health Disorders* (NICE clinical guideline 123).
[111]Adapted from *Common Mental Health Disorders* (NICE clinical guideline 123).
[112]Adapted from *Common Mental Health Disorders* (NICE clinical guideline 123).

- offer prompt assessments and interventions that are appropriately adapted to the cultural, gender, age and communication needs of children and young people with a conduct disorder and their parents and carers
- keep to a minimum the number of assessments needed to access interventions[113].

9.7.1.15 Health and social care professionals, managers and commissioners should work with colleagues in educational settings to design local care pathways that respond promptly and effectively to the changing needs of all populations served by the pathways. Pathways should have in place:

- clear and agreed goals for the services offered to children and young people with a conduct disorder and their parents and carers
- robust and effective means for measuring and evaluating the outcomes associated with the agreed goals
- clear and agreed mechanisms for responding promptly to changes in individual needs[114].

9.7.1.16 Health and social care professionals, managers and commissioners should work with colleagues in educational settings to design local care pathways that provide an integrated programme of care across all care settings. Pathways should:

- minimise the need for transition between different services or providers
- allow services to be built around the pathway and not the pathway around the services
- establish clear links (including access and entry points) to other care pathways (including those for physical healthcare needs)
- have designated staff who are responsible for the coordination of people's engagement with the pathway[115].

9.7.1.17 Health and social care professionals, managers and commissioners should work with colleagues in educational settings to ensure effective communication about the functioning of the local care pathway. There should be protocols for:

- sharing information with children and young people with a conduct disorder, and their parents and carers, about their care
- sharing and communicating information about the care of children and young people with other professionals (including GPs)
- communicating information between the services provided within the pathway
- communicating information to services outside the pathway[116].

9.7.1.18 Health and social care professionals, managers and commissioners should work with colleagues in educational settings to design local care pathways

---

[113]Adapted from *Common Mental Health Disorders* (NICE clinical guideline 123).
[114]Adapted from *Common Mental Health Disorders* (NICE clinical guideline 123).
[115]Adapted from *Common Mental Health Disorders* (NICE clinical guideline 123).
[116]Adapted from *Common Mental Health Disorders* (NICE clinical guideline 123).

that have robust systems for outcome measurement in place, which should be used to inform all involved in a pathway about its effectiveness. This should include providing:

- individual routine outcome measurement systems
- effective electronic systems for the routine reporting and aggregation of outcome measures
- effective systems for the audit and review of the overall clinical and cost effectiveness of the pathway[117].

---

[117]Adapted from *Common Mental Health Disorders* (NICE clinical guideline 123).

# 10   APPENDICES

*Appendices*

# APPENDIX 1:
# SCOPE FOR THE DEVELOPMENT OF THE
# CLINICAL GUIDELINE

## GUIDELINE TITLE

Conduct disorders and antisocial behaviour in children and young people: recognition, intervention and management[118]

## SHORT TITLE

Conduct disorders in children and young people

## THE REMIT

The Department of Health has asked NICE and the Social Care Institute for Excellence (SCIE): 'To produce a clinical guideline on the recognition, identification and management of conduct disorder (including oppositional defiance disorder) in children and young people.'

## CLINICAL NEED FOR THE GUIDELINE

### Epidemiology

a. Conduct disorders are characterised by repetitive and persistent patterns of antisocial, aggressive or defiant behaviour that amounts to significant and persistent violations of age-appropriate social expectations. The current World Health Organization classification of the disorders (ICD-10) identifies two subgroups: conduct disorder and oppositional defiant disorder. Conduct disorder is more common in older children (11 to 12 years and older) and oppositional defiant disorder is more common in those aged 10 years or younger. The major distinction between the disorders is the extent and the severity of the antisocial behaviour. Isolated

---

[118] The guideline title was changed during development to *Antisocial Behaviour and Conduct Disorders in Children and Young People: Recognition, Intervention and Management.*

antisocial or criminal acts are not sufficient to support a diagnosis of conduct disorder or oppositional defiant disorder.

b. Conduct disorders are the most common mental health disorder in children and young people. The Office of National Statistics surveys of 1999 and 2004 reported that the prevalence of conducts disorders and associated impairment was 5% among children and young people. The prevalence without impairment was not much larger, because conduct disorders nearly always have a significant impact on functioning and quality of life. The first survey demonstrated that conduct disorders have a steep social class gradient, with a three to fourfold increase in the social classes D and E compared with social class A. The second survey found that almost 40% of looked-after children, those who have been abused and/or those on child protection/safeguarding registers, between 5 and 17 years old, have conduct disorders.

c. The prevalence of conduct disorders increases throughout childhood and they are more common in boys than girls. For example, 7% of boys and 3% of girls aged 5 to 10 years have conduct disorders; for children aged 11 to 16 years the number rises to 8% for boys and 5% for girls.

d. Conduct disorders commonly coexist with other mental health disorders, for example 46% of boys and 36% of girls have at least one other coexisting mental health disorder. The coexistence of conduct disorders with attention deficit hyperactivity disorder (ADHD) is particularly high and in some groups more than 40% of people with a diagnosis of conduct disorder also have a diagnosis of ADHD. The presence of conduct disorder in childhood is also associated with a significantly increased rate of mental health disorders in adult life, including antisocial personality disorder (up to 50% of children and young people with a conduct disorder may go on to develop antisocial personality disorder). The prevalence of conduct disorders varies between ethnic groups, being lower than average in some groups (for example, south Asians) but higher in other groups (for example, African-Caribbeans).

e. A diagnosis of a conduct disorder is strongly associated with poor educational performance, social isolation, drug and alcohol misuse and increased contact with the criminal justice system. This association continues into adult life with poorer educational and occupational outcomes, involvement with the criminal justice system (as high as 50% in some groups) and a high level of mental health disorder (at some point in their lives 90% of people with antisocial personality disorder will have another mental disorder).

**Current practice**

a. Conduct disorders are the most common reason for referral of young children to child and adolescent mental health services (CAMHS). Children with conduct disorders also comprise a considerable proportion of the work of the health and social care system. For example, 30% of a typical GP's child consultations are for conduct disorders, 45% of community child health referrals are for behaviour disturbances, and psychiatric disorders are a factor in 28% of all paediatric outpatient referrals. In addition, social care services have significant involvement with children and young people with conduct disorders, with more vulnerable or disturbed children often being placed with a foster family or, in a small number of cases, in residential care. The demands on the educational system are also considerable and include the provision of special needs education. The criminal justice system also has significant involvement with older children with conduct disorders.

b.  Multiple agencies may be involved in the care and treatment of children with conduct disorders, which presents a major challenge for current services in the effective coordination of care across agencies.

c.  Several interventions have been developed for children with conduct disorder and related problems. These have been covered in 'Parent-training/education programmes in the management of children with conduct disorders', NICE technology appraisal guidance 102 and 'Antisocial personality disorder: treatment, management and prevention', NICE clinical guideline 77 (2009). Other interventions focused on prevention, such as the Nurse Parent Partnership, have recently been implemented in the UK and are current being evaluated. Three themes are common to these interventions: a strong focus on working with parents and families, recognition of the importance of the wider social system in enabling effective interventions, and a focus on preventing or reducing the escalation of existing problems.

d.  Uptake of the majority of these interventions varies across the country. Parenting programmes are the best established; implementation of multisystemic approaches and early intervention programmes is more variable. In addition to the programmes developed specifically for children with conduct disorders, a number of children (and their families) are treated by both specialist CAMHS teams and general community-based services such as Sure Start.

e.  Identifying which of the above interventions and agencies are the most appropriate is challenging, especially for non-specialist health, social care and educational services. Further challenges arise when considering the use of preventive and early intervention programmes and identifying which vulnerable groups stand to gain from such interventions. Factors that may be associated with a higher risk of developing conduct disorders include parental factors such as parenting style and parental adjustment (the impact of any mental health disorder or personality factors that impact on a parent's ability to effectively function as a parent), environmental factors such as poverty and place of residence (for example, foster care), and the presence of other mental health disorders.

## THE GUIDELINE

The guideline development process is described in detail on the NICE website (see section 6, 'Further information').

This scope defines what the guideline will (and will not) examine, and what the guideline developers will consider. The scope is based on the referral from the Department of Health.

*Appendix 1*

The areas that will be addressed by the guideline are described in the following sections.

**Population**

a. Children and young people

**Groups that will be covered**

a. Children and young people (aged 18 years and younger) with a diagnosed or suspected conduct disorder, including looked-after children and those in contact with the criminal justice system.
b. Children and young people identified as being at significant risk of developing conduct disorders.
c. Consideration will be given to the specific needs of:
   ● children and young people with conduct disorders and coexisting conditions (such as ADHD, depression, anxiety disorders and attachment insecurity)
   ● children and young people from particular black or minority ethnic groups
   ● girls with a diagnosis of, or at risk of developing, conduct disorders
   ● looked-after children and young people
   ● children and young people in contact with the criminal justice system.

**Groups that will not be covered**

Recommendations will be not be made specifically for the following groups, although the parts of the guideline may be relevant to their care:
a. Adults (aged 19 and older).
b. Children and young people with coexisting conditions if conduct disorder is not a primary diagnosis.
c. Children and young people with psychosis.
d. Children and young people with autism spectrum conditions.
e. Primary drug and alcohol problems.
f. Children and young people with speech and language difficulties whose behavioural problems arise from the speech and language difficulties.

**Health and social care setting**

a. Primary, secondary and tertiary healthcare, and social care settings.
b. The criminal justice system and forensic services.
c. Children's services and educational settings.

d. Other settings in which NHS and social care services are funded or provided, or where NHS or social care professionals are working in multi-agency teams.
e. The guideline will also comment on and include recommendations about the interface between the NHS and social care and other sectors and services, such as education services, youth service settings, the criminal justice system and the voluntary sector.

**Areas to be considered**

*Key areas that will be covered*
a. The behaviours, signs or symptoms that should prompt healthcare, education and social care professionals and others working with children and young people, to consider the presence of a conduct disorder.
b. Validity, specificity and reliability of the components of diagnostic assessment after referral, including:
   ● the structure for assessment
   ● diagnostic thresholds
   ● assessment of risk.
c. Psychosocial interventions, including:
   ● individual and group psychological interventions
   ● parenting and family interventions (including family-based prevention models)
   ● social care (including interventions for looked-after children and young people), vocational, educational and community interventions, and work with peer groups
   ● multimodal interventions.
d. Pharmacological interventions, including antipsychotics and antidepressants. Note that guideline recommendations will normally fall within licensed indications; exceptionally, and only if clearly supported by evidence, use outside a licensed indication may be recommended. The guideline will assume that prescribers will use a drug's summary of product characteristics to inform decisions made with individual patients.
e. Physical interventions, such as diet.
f. The organisation, coordination and delivery of care, and care pathways for the components of treatment and management. This will include transition planning and will be based on an ethos of multi-agency and multi-professional working.

**Interventions that will not be covered**

Specific interventions for sexually abused or traumatised children and young people.
a. Specific interventions for children and young people with speech and language difficulties.
b. Preventive interventions for the general population.
c. Setting-based interventions (for example, school-based interventions) for those who are not at significant risk of developing a conduct disorder.

**Main outcomes**

a. Antisocial behaviour at home, at school and in the community (including offending behaviour).
b. Psychological, educational and social functioning as rated by the child or young person, professionals (including teachers) and parents.

**Economic aspects**

The guideline will take into account both clinical and cost effectiveness when making recommendations involving a choice between alternative interventions. A review of the economic evidence will be conducted and analyses will be carried out as appropriate. The preferred unit of effectiveness will be the quality-adjusted life year (QALY), but a different unit of effectiveness may be used depending on the availability of appropriate clinical and utility data for children and young people with conduct disorders and associated antisocial behaviours. Costs considered will be from an NHS and personal social services (PSS) perspective in the main analyses, and a criminal justice perspective may also be considered. Further detail on the methods can be found in 'The Guidelines Manual' (see Section 6, 'Further information').

**STATUS**

**Scope**

This is the final scope.

**Timing**

The development of the guideline recommendations will begin in April 2011.

**RELATED NICE GUIDANCE**

**NICE guidance to be updated**

Depending on the evidence, this guideline might update and replace parts of the following NICE guidance:
● Parent-Training/Education Programmes in the Management of Children with Conduct Disorders. NICE technology appraisal guidance 102 (2006). Available from www.nice.org.uk/guidance/TA102

**Other related NICE guidance**

- Promoting the Quality of Life of Looked-after Children and Young People. NICE public health guideline 28 (2010). Available from www.nice.org.uk/guidance/PH28
- Antisocial Personality Disorder. NICE clinical guideline 77 (2009). Available from www.nice.org.uk/guidance/CG77
- Attention Deficit Hyperactivity Disorder. NICE clinical guideline 72 (2008). Available from www.nice.org.uk/guidance/CG72

**FURTHER INFORMATION**

Information on the guideline development process is provided in:
- 'How NICE clinical guidelines are developed: an overview for stakeholders, the public and the NHS'
- 'The guidelines manual'.

These are available from the NICE website (www.nice.org.uk/GuidelinesManual). Information on the progress of the guideline will also be available from the NICE website (www.nice.org.uk).

# APPENDIX 2:

# DECLARATIONS OF INTERESTS BY GUIDELINE DEVELOPMENT GROUP MEMBERS

With a range of practical experience relevant to conduct disorders in children and young people in the GDG, members were appointed because of their understanding and expertise in conduct disorders in children and young people and support for their families/carers, including: scientific issues; health research; the delivery and receipt of healthcare, along with the work of the healthcare industry; and the role of professional organisations and organisations for people with conduct disorders in children and young people and their families/carers.

To minimise and manage any potential conflicts of interest, and to avoid any public concern that commercial or other financial interests have affected the work of the GDG and influenced guidance, members of the GDG must declare as a matter of public record any interests held by themselves or their families which fall under specified categories (see below). These categories include any relationships they have with the healthcare industries, professional organisations and organisations for people with conduct disorders in children and young people and their families/carers.

Individuals invited to join the GDG were asked to declare their interests before being appointed. To allow the management of any potential conflicts of interest that might arise during the development of the guideline, GDG members were also asked to declare their interests at each GDG meeting throughout the guideline development process. The interests of all the members of the GDG are listed below, including interests declared prior to appointment and during the guideline development process.

**Categories of interest**

**Paid employment**

**Personal pecuniary interest:** financial payments or other benefits from either the manufacturer or the owner of the product or service under consideration in this guideline, or the industry or sector from which the product or service comes. This includes holding a directorship, or other paid position; carrying out consultancy or fee paid work; having shareholdings or other beneficial interests; receiving expenses and hospitality over and above what would be reasonably expected to attend meetings and conferences.

**Personal family interest:** financial payments or other benefits from the healthcare industry that were received by a family member.

**Non-personal pecuniary interest:** financial payments or other benefits received by the GDG member's organisation or department, but where the GDG member has not personally received payment, including fellowships and other support provided by the healthcare industry. This includes a grant or fellowship or other payment to sponsor a post, or contribute to the running costs of the department; commissioning of research or other work; contracts with or grants from NICE.

**Personal non-pecuniary interest:** these include, but are not limited to, clear opinions or public statements made about individuals with conduct disorders, holding office in a professional organisation or advocacy group with a direct interest in conduct disorders, other reputational risks relevant to conduct disorders.

| GDG – Declarations of interest | |
|---|---|
| **Professor Stephen Scott** | |
| Employment | Professor of Child Health and Behaviour, Institute of Psychiatry, King's College London; Consultant Child and Adolescent Psychiatrist and Head, National Conduct Problems Clinic and National Adoption and Fostering Clinic, Maudsley Hospital, London |
| Personal pecuniary interest | Involved in the Systemic Therapy for at Risk Teens (START) trial, with Peter Fonagy being the principal investigator. The START trial is a national trial that aims to compare multisystemic therapy with standard care, to determine whether it is associated with improved long-term outcomes; however, is agnostic about the benefits of multisystemic therapy. |
| | Has a small contract with Social Finance to look at the effect of evidence-based interventions on helping families where children are in need/on edge of entering care. Social Finance is a company which will be setting up social impact bonds, and they act as a broker between investors, local authorities and third sector agencies that would deliver the interventions. |
| Personal family interest | None |

| Non-personal pecuniary interest | None |
|---|---|
| Personal non-pecuniary interest | None |
| Non-personal non-pecuniary interest | None |
| Action taken | None |
| **Ms Beth Anderson** | |
| Employment | Senior Research Analyst, SCIE, London |
| Personal pecuniary interest | None |
| Personal family interest | Sister's long-term partner is a consultant neurologist who is also a minor shareholder and non-executive director in PsychologyOnline, which provides online psychological services including cognitive behavioural therapy, treating over-18s only, and a major shareholder and non-executive director in two biotech companies, Vastrata Ltd and Largren Ltd. The current programmes of work cover: schizophrenia, insomnia, migraine and menorrhagia. |
| Non-personal pecuniary interest | Undertook part-time agency employment with RPM Ltd, an experimental marketing company whose clients include pharmaceutical and healthcare industry companies. Worked on non-healthcare related campaigns (food and drink industry; automotive industry) for the period July 2011 to February 2012. |
| Personal non-pecuniary interest | None |
| Action taken | None |
| **Ms Sara Barratt** | |
| Employment | Consultant Systematic Psychotherapist; Team Leader, Fostering, Adoption and Kinship Care Team, Tavistock Centre, London |
| Personal pecuniary interest | None |
| Personal family interest | None |

| | |
|---|---|
| Non-personal pecuniary interest | None |
| Personal non-pecuniary interest | None |
| Non-personal non-pecuniary interest | None |
| Action taken | None |
| **Mrs Maria Brewster** | |
| Employment | Service user and carer representative |
| Personal pecuniary interest | None |
| Personal family interest | None |
| Non-personal pecuniary interest | None |
| Personal non-pecuniary interest | None |
| Action taken | None |
| **Dr Barbara Compitus** | |
| Employment | General Practitioner |
| Personal pecuniary interest | None |
| Personal family interest | None |
| Non-personal pecuniary interest | None |
| Personal non-pecuniary interest | None |
| Action taken | None |
| **Dr Moira Doolan** | |
| Employment | Consultant Systemic Psychotherapist; Lead for Interventions: Helping Children Achieve and Safe Studies National Academy for Parenting Research, Institute of Psychiatry, King's College London |

| Personal pecuniary interest | Mentor in the Incredible Years Programme, which is an evidence-based programme likely to be considered as part of the guideline. No funding has been received from the Incredible Years Organisation in the last 12 months. |
| --- | --- |
| | Mentors can be asked to provide training by the Incredible Years head office, but this has not been done because it would have been a conflict of interest with the National Academy for Parenting Practitioners role. Any such request for the duration of guideline development, if accepted, would be declined. |
| | Two studies at the National Academy for Parenting Research, Institute of Psychiatry, King's College London, were also declared. The Helping Children Achieve study, which uses the Incredible Years' programme, and the Supporting Parents on Kids Education in Schools programme. A second study of adolescents' family experiences uses the functional family therapy model. |
| | Holds a small contract with Social Finance to look at the effect of evidence-based interventions on helping families where children are in need/on the edge of entering care. Social Finance is a company which will be setting up social impact bonds, and they act as a broker between investors, local authorities and third sector agencies that would deliver the interventions. |
| Personal family interest | None |
| Non-personal pecuniary interest | Was a member of the research team evaluating Incredible Years on three occasions and there is an outcome paper published on each of these studies. Is also currently involved in a fourth RCT of Incredible Years and an RCT of functional family therapy. |
| Personal non-pecuniary interest | None |
| Action taken | None |

| Professor Peter Fonagy | |
|---|---|
| Employment | Chief Executive, Anna Freud Centre, London; Freud Memorial Professor of Psychoanalysis, University College London |
| Personal pecuniary interest | Is the Principal Investigator for Systemic Therapy for at Risk Teens (START) trial. The START trial is a national trial that aims to compare multisystemic therapy with standard care.<br><br>Is the National Clinical Lead for Improving Access to Psychological Therapies programme. |
| Personal family interest | None |
| Non-personal pecuniary interest | None |
| Personal non-pecuniary interest | None |
| Action taken | None |
| **Professor Nick Gould** | |
| Employment | Consultant, SCIE; Emeritus Professor of Social Work, University of Bath; Professor of Social Work, Griffith University, Queensland, Australia |
| Personal pecuniary interest | Specialist member, Mental Health Tribunal Consultant, SCIE; Adviser, Griffiths University, Brisbane, Australia; Adviser, Chinese University of Hong Kong, Hong Kong; Consultant, University of East London. |
| Personal family interest | None |
| Non-personal pecuniary interest | None |
| Personal non-pecuniary interest | None |
| Action taken | None |

| **Dr Daphne Keen** | |
|---|---|
| Employment | Consultant Developmental Paediatrician |
| Personal pecuniary interest | None |
| Personal family interest | None |
| Non-personal pecuniary interest | None |
| Personal non-pecuniary interest | None |
| Action taken | None |
| **Dr Paul McArdle** | |
| Employment | Consultant and Senior Lecturer Child and Adolescent Psychiatry |
| Personal pecuniary interest | None |
| Personal family interest | None |
| Non-personal pecuniary interest | None |
| Personal non-pecuniary interest | None |
| Action taken | None |
| **Dr Paul Mitchell** | |
| Employment | Clinical Lead, Hindley Young Offender Institution Mental Health Team |
| Personal pecuniary interest | None |
| Personal family interest | None |
| Non-personal pecuniary interest | None |
| Personal non-pecuniary interest | None |
| Action taken | None |
| **Dr Jenny Taylor** | |
| Employment | Consultant Clinical Psychologist; Supervisor of the Hackney site of the Department of Health's Multisystemic Therapy National Research Trial |

| | |
|---|---|
| Personal pecuniary interest | Is currently Past Chair of the Clinical Division of the British Psychological Society for which my employers (the East London NHS Foundation Trust) receive 0.2 whole time equivalent backfill.<br><br>Managed a START trail site in Hackney. |
| Personal family interest | None |
| Non-personal pecuniary interest | None |
| Personal non-pecuniary interest | Is currently Past Chair of the Clinical Division of the British Psychological Society; involved in the national trial of multisystemic therapy. |
| Action taken | None |
| **Ms Philippa Williams** | |
| Employment | Service user and carer representative |
| Personal pecuniary interest | None |
| Personal family interest | None |
| Non-personal pecuniary interest | None |
| Personal non-pecuniary interest | None |
| Action taken | None |
| **Mr Tony Wootton** | |
| Employment | Retired Head Teacher, Millthorpe School, York |
| Personal pecuniary interest | None |
| Personal family interest | None |
| Non-personal pecuniary interest | None |
| Personal non-pecuniary interest | None |
| Action taken | None |

| NCCMH staff | |
|---|---|
| **Professor Stephen Pilling** | |
| Employment | Director, NCCMH |
| Personal pecuniary interest | Involved in the Systematic Therapy for At-Risk Teens (START). The START trial is a national trial that aims to compare multisystemic therapy with standard care. |
| Personal family interest | None |
| Non-personal pecuniary interest | None |
| Personal non-pecuniary interest | None |
| Action taken | None |
| **Dr Benedict Anigbogu** | |
| Employment | Health Economist |
| Personal pecuniary interest | None |
| Personal family interest | None |
| Non-personal pecuniary interest | None |
| Personal non-pecuniary interest | None |
| Action taken | None |
| **Ms Ruth Braidwood** | |
| Employment | Research Assistant |
| Personal pecuniary interest | None |
| Personal family interest | None |
| Non-personal pecuniary interest | None |
| Personal non-pecuniary interest | None |
| Action taken | None |
| **Ms Laura Gibbon** | |
| Employment | Project Manager |
| Personal pecuniary interest | None |

| Personal family interest | None |
|---|---|
| Non-personal pecuniary interest | None |
| Personal non-pecuniary interest | None |
| Action taken | None |

| **Ms Naomi Glover** | |
|---|---|
| Employment | Research Assistant |
| Personal pecuniary interest | None |
| Personal family interest | None |
| Non-personal pecuniary interest | None |
| Personal non-pecuniary interest | None |
| Action taken | None |

| **Ms Bronwyn Harrison** | |
|---|---|
| Employment | Research Assistant |
| Personal pecuniary interest | None |
| Personal family interest | None |
| Non-personal pecuniary interest | None |
| Personal non-pecuniary interest | None |
| Action taken | None |

| **Ms Flora Kaminski** | |
|---|---|
| Employment | Research Assistant |
| Personal pecuniary interest | None |
| Personal family interest | None |
| Non-personal pecuniary interest | None |
| Personal non-pecuniary interest | None |
| Action taken | None |

*Appendix 2*

| Ms Maryla Moulin | |
|---|---|
| Employment | Project Manager |
| Personal pecuniary interest | None |
| Personal family interest | None |
| Non-personal pecuniary interest | None |
| Personal non-pecuniary interest | None |
| Actions taken | None |

| Dr Rosa Nieto-Hernandez | |
|---|---|
| Employment | Systematic Reviewer |
| Personal pecuniary interest | None |
| Personal family interest | None |
| Non-personal pecuniary interest | None |
| Personal non-pecuniary interest | None |
| Action taken | None |

| Ms Melinda Smith | |
|---|---|
| Employment | Research Assistant |
| Personal pecuniary interest | None |
| Personal family interest | None |
| Non-personal pecuniary interest | None |
| Personal non-pecuniary interest | None |
| Action taken | None |

| Ms Sarah Stockton | |
|---|---|
| Employment | Senior Information Scientist, NCCMH |
| Personal pecuniary interest | None |
| Personal family interest | None |
| Non-personal pecuniary interest | None |

| Personal non-pecuniary interest | None |
|---|---|
| Action taken | None |

**Dr Clare Taylor**

| Employment | Senior Editor |
|---|---|
| Personal pecuniary interest | None |
| Personal family interest | None |
| Non-personal pecuniary interest | None |
| Personal non-pecuniary interest | None |
| Action taken | None |

**Dr Amina Yesufu-Udechuku**

| Employment | Systematic Reviewer |
|---|---|
| Personal pecuniary interest | None |
| Personal family interest | None |
| Non-personal pecuniary interest | None |
| Personal non-pecuniary interest | None |
| Action taken | None |

**Dr Craig Whittington**

| Employment | Associate Director and Senior Systematic Reviewer |
|---|---|
| Personal pecuniary interest | None |
| Personal family interest | None |
| Non-personal pecuniary interest | None |
| Personal non-pecuniary interest | None |
| Action taken | None |

# APPENDIX 3:

# STAKEHOLDERS AND EXPERTS WHO SUBMITTED COMMENTS IN RESPONSE TO THE CONSULTATION DRAFT OF THE GUIDELINE

## Stakeholders

Aneurin Bevan Health Board
Association for Family Therapy and Systemic Practice
Association for Rational Emotive Behaviour Therapy
Association of Child Psychotherapists
The Association of Educational Psychologists
British Association for Adoption and Fostering
The British Association of Play Therapists
British Psychological Society
Centre for Mental Health
Cochrane Collaboration's Developmental, Psychosocial and Learning Problems Group
College of Mental Health Pharmacy
Department for Education
NHS Direct
PartnershipProjects UK Ltd
Royal College of Paediatrics and Child Health
Royal College of Speech and Language Therapists
Welsh Government

## Experts

Professor Frances Gardner
Dr Robert J. McMahon
Professor Eric Taylor
Dr Carolyn Webster-Stratton

# APPENDIX 4:
# RESEARCHERS CONTACTED TO REQUEST INFORMATION ABOUT UNPUBLISHED OR SOON-TO-BE PUBLISHED STUDIES

Dr Terje Ogden
Professor Thomas Sexton

# APPENDIX 5:

# REVIEW QUESTIONS

---

**Prevention**

A1a: What selective prevention interventions for at risk individuals (including children/ young people or their parents/families/carers) reduce the likelihood of children and young people developing a conduct disorder?

A1b: What indicated prevention interventions for at risk individuals (including children/ young people or their parents/families/carers) reduce the likelihood of children and young people developing a conduct disorder?

---

**Access and the organisation and delivery of care**

B1: What are the barriers to access that prevent children and young people at risk of – or diagnosed with – conduct disorders from accessing services?

B2: Do methods designed to remove barriers to services increase the proportion and diversity of children and young people accessing treatment?

G1: What are the effective models for the delivery of care to children with conduct disorders, including:
  - the structure and design of care pathways
  - systems for the delivery of care (for example, case management)
  - specialist teams?

G2: What are the essential elements that assist in the transition into adulthood services for young people with conduct disorders?

G3: What are the effective ways of monitoring progress in conduct disorders?

G4: What components of an intervention, or the way in which it is implemented, and by whom, are associated with successful outcomes?

---

**Case identification**

C1: What concerns and behaviours (as expressed by the carer or exhibited by the child) should prompt any professional who comes into contact with a child or young person with possible conduct disorders to consider referral for further assessment?

C2: What are the most effective methods/instruments for case identification of conduct disorders in children and young people?

C3: What amendments, if any, need to be made to the agreed methods for case identification to take into account:
  - demographics (for example, particular cultural or minority ethnic groups, or girls)
  - the environment in which case identification takes place (for example, social care, education)?

---

**Assessment**

D1: In children and young people with possible conduct disorders, what are the key components of, and the most effective structure for, a diagnostic assessment?

To answer this question, consideration should be given to:
- the nature and content of the interview and observation, which should both include an early developmental history where possible
- formal diagnostic methods/psychological instruments for the assessment of core features of conduct disorders
- the assessment of risk
- the assessment of need
- the setting(s) in which the assessment takes place
- the role of the any informants
- gathering of independent and accurate information from informants.

D2: When making a diagnosis of conduct disorders in children and young people, what amendments (if any) need to be made to take into account coexisting conditions (such as ADHD, depression, anxiety disorders and attachment insecurity)?

D3: What amendments, if any, need to be made to take into account particular cultural or minority ethnic groups or sex?

**Interventions**

E1: For children and young people with conduct disorders, what are the benefits and potential harms associated with individual and group psychosocial interventions?

E2: For children and young people with conduct disorders, what are the benefits and potential harms associated with parenting and family interventions?

E3: For children and young people with conduct disorders, what are the benefits and potential harms associated with multimodal/multiple interventions?

E4: For children and young people with conduct disorders, what are the benefits and potential harms associated with pharmacological interventions?

E5: For children and young people with conduct disorders, what are the benefits and potential harms associated with physical interventions (for example diet)?

E6: For children and young people with conduct disorders, what are the benefits and potential harms associated with school behaviour management?

E7: For children and young people with conduct disorders, should interventions found to be safe and effective be modified in any way in light of coexisting conditions (such as ADHD, depression, anxiety disorders, attachment insecurity) or demographics (such as age, particular black and minority ethnic groups, or sex)?

**Experience of care**

F1: For children and young people with a conduct disorder, what can be done to improve the experience of the disorder, and the experience of care?*

(*The question will be structured using a matrix of service user experience, which includes issues concerning support for families and carers [see matrix of service user experience on page 376].)

| Matrix of service user experience (including experience of the disorder) | | | | | |
|---|---|---|---|---|---|
| Dimensions of person-centred care (adapted from Picker Institute, 2009)[119] | Key points on the pathway of care | | | | Themes that apply to all points on the pathway |
| | Access | Assessment | Treatment | Education | |
| **The relationship between individual service users and professionals** — Involvement in decisions and respect for preferences | | | | | |
| Clear, comprehensible information and support for self-care | | | | | |
| Emotional support, empathy and respect | | | | | |
| **The way that services and systems work** — Fast access to reliable health advice | | | | | |
| Effective treatment delivered by trusted professionals | | | | | |
| Attention to physical and environmental needs | | | | | |
| Involvement of, and support for, family and carers | | | | | |
| Continuity of care and smooth transitions | | | | | |
| Other themes | | | | | |

[119] http:// www.pickereurope.org/patientcentred

# APPENDIX 6:

# REVIEW PROTOCOL TEMPLATE

Completed forms can be found in Appendix 15: Review Protocols, on the CD-ROM.

| TOPIC | |
|---|---|
| **Review question(s)** | |
| **Chapter** | |
| **Objectives** | |
| **Criteria for considering studies for the review** | |
| • Population | |
| • Intervention | |
| • Comparison | |
| • Critical outcomes | |
| • Important, but not critical outcomes | |
| • Other outcomes | |
| • Study design | |
| • Include unpublished data? | |
| • Restriction by date? | |
| • Minimum sample size | |
| • Study setting | |
| **Search strategy** | |
| **Searching other resources** | |
| **The review strategy** | |

# APPENDIX 7:
# SEARCH STRATEGIES FOR THE IDENTIFICATION OF CLINICAL STUDIES

Search strategies can be found on the CD-ROM.

# APPENDIX 8:
# DATA EXTRACTION FORMS

An Excel-based data extraction tool, developed by NCCMH staff, was used to extract RCT evidence. See page 380 for an example of part of an uncompleted form (completed tables are presented in Appendix 16a and 16c).

Review Manager 5.1[120] was used to extract data for the review of case identification instruments (completed tables are presented in Appendix 16b).

Word-based forms were used to extract evidence about access to services and the experience of care (completed tables are presented in Chapter 4, Section 4.2.3).

---

[120]The Cochrane Collaboration. Review Manager (RevMan) [Computer programme]. Version 5.1. Copenhagen: The Nordic Cochrane Centre, The Cochrane Collaboration; 2011.

# Excel-based data extraction tool

# APPENDIX 9:

# METHODOLOGY CHECKLIST TEMPLATE FOR CLINICAL STUDIES AND REVIEWS

The methodological quality of each study was evaluated using NICE checklists (NICE, 2009b). The checklist template for systematic reviews is reproduced below. The checklists for RCTs were incorporated into the Excel data extraction tool described in Appendix 8. For other checklists and further information about how to complete each checklist, see *The Guidelines Manual* (NICE, 2009c).

Data captured from each checklist can be found in study characteristics tables in Appendix 16.

| **Study identification** *Include author, title, reference, year of publication* | |
|---|---|
| **Guideline topic:** | Review question no: |
| **Checklist completed by:** | |
| SCREENING QUESTIONS | |
| In a well-conducted, relevant systematic review: | *Circle one option for each question* |
| The review addresses an appropriate and clearly focused question that is relevant to the guideline review question | Yes    No    Unclear |
| The review collects the type of studies you consider relevant to the guideline review question | Yes    No    Unclear |
| The literature search is sufficiently rigorous to identify all the relevant studies | Yes    No    Unclear |
| Study quality is assessed and reported | Yes    No    Unclear |
| An adequate description of the methodology used is included, and the methods used are appropriate to the question | Yes    No    Unclear |

# APPENDIX 10:
# SEARCH STRATEGIES FOR THE IDENTIFICATION OF HEALTH ECONOMIC EVIDENCE

Search strategies can be found on the CD-ROM.

# APPENDIX 11:

# METHODOLOGY CHECKLIST TEMPLATE FOR ECONOMIC STUDIES

The methodological quality of each study was evaluated using a NICE checklist (NICE, 2009b), reproduced below. For information about how to complete the checklist, see *The Guidelines Manual* [NICE, 2009b].

Data captured from each checklist can be found in study characteristics tables in Appendix 19.

| Study identification<br>*Including author, title, reference, year of publication* | | | |
|---|---|---|---|
| **Guideline topic:** | | | **Question no:** |
| **Checklist completed by:** | | | |
| **Section 1: Applicability (relevance to specific guideline review question(s) and the NICE reference case). This checklist should be used first to filter out irrelevant studies.** | | **Yes/Partly/ No/Unclear/ NA** | **Comments** |
| 1.1 | Is the study population appropriate for the guideline? | | |
| 1.2 | Are the interventions appropriate for the guideline? | | |
| 1.3 | Is the healthcare system in which the study was conducted sufficiently similar to the current UK NHS context? | | |
| 1.4 | Are costs measured from the NHS and personal social services (PSS) perspective? | | |
| 1.5 | Are all direct health effects on individuals included? | | |
| 1.6 | Are both costs and health effects discounted at an annual rate of 3.5%? | | |
| 1.7 | Is the value of health effects expressed in terms of quality-adjusted life years (QALYs)? | | |

| 1.8 | Are changes in health-related quality of life (HRQoL) reported directly from patients and/or carers? | | |
|---|---|---|---|
| 1.9 | Is the valuation of changes in HRQoL (utilities) obtained from a representative sample of the general public? | | |
| 1.10 | Overall judgement: Directly applicable/ Partially applicable/Not applicable. There is no need to use section 2 of the checklist if the study is considered 'not applicable'. | | |

Other comments:

| **Section 2: Study limitations (the level of methodological quality) This checklist should be used once it has been decided that the study is sufficiently applicable to the context of the clinical guideline.** | **Yes/Partly/ No/Unclear/ NA** | **Comments** |
|---|---|---|
| 2.1 Does the model structure adequately reflect the nature of the health condition under evaluation? | | |
| 2.2 Is the time horizon sufficiently long to reflect all important differences in costs and outcomes? | | |
| 2.3 Are all important and relevant health outcomes included? | | |
| 2.4 Are the estimates of baseline health outcomes from the best available source? | | |
| 2.5 Are the estimates of relative treatment effects from the best available source? | | |
| 2.6 Are all important and relevant costs included? | | |
| 2.7 Are the estimates of resource use from the best available source? | | |
| 2.8 Are the unit costs of resources from the best available source? | | |
| 2.9 Is an appropriate incremental analysis presented or can it be calculated from the data? | | |

| 2.10 | Are all important parameters whose values are uncertain subjected to appropriate sensitivity analysis? | | |
|---|---|---|---|
| 2.11 | Is there no potential conflict of interest? | | |
| 2.12 | Overall assessment: Minor limitations/ Potentially serious limitations/Very serious limitations | | |
| Other comments: | | | |

# APPENDIX 12:

# RESEARCH RECOMMENDATIONS

## 1. PARENT TRAINING PROGRAMMES FOR CHILDREN AGED 12 YEARS AND OVER WITH A CONDUCT DISORDER

What is the effectiveness of parent training programmes for conduct disorders in children and young people aged 12 years and over?

*Why this is important*
The evidence for parent training programmes is well established for children with conduct disorders aged 11 years and younger, with well-developed models for the delivery of care. In contrast there is little evidence for these programmes in older children despite the recognition that parenting problems continue to play a part in the development and maintenance of conduct disorders.

This question should be answered using a randomised controlled trial (RCT) design reporting short- and medium-term outcomes, including cost effectiveness, over at least 18 months. Attention should be paid to the adaptation of parent training programmes to older children, and to training and supervision of staff delivering the programmes to ensure robust and generalisable results. The outcomes and acceptability of the intervention should be rated by parents, teachers and independent observers. The study needs to be large enough to determine the presence of clinically important effects, and mediators and moderators of response should also be investigated.

## 2. IMPROVING UPTAKE OF AND ENGAGEMENT WITH INTERVENTIONS FOR CONDUCT DISORDERS

What strategies are effective in improving uptake of and engagement with interventions for conduct disorders?

*Why this is important*
Effective interventions exist for conduct disorders but access to and uptake of services is limited. This question should be addressed by a programme of work that tests a number of strategies to improve uptake and engagement, including:
- A cluster RCT comparing validated case identification tools with standard methods of case identification in non-healthcare settings, to ascertain whether case identification tools improve identification and uptake.
- Development and evaluation of pathways into care, in collaboration with people who have been identified as low users of services, through a series of cohort studies, with the outcomes including uptake of and retention in services.
- Adapting existing interventions for conduct disorder in collaboration with children and young people with a conduct disorder and their parents or carers. Adaptations

could include changes in the settings in which interventions are delivered, the methods of delivery or the staff delivering the interventions. These interventions should be tested in an RCT of at least 18 months' duration that reports short- and medium-term outcomes, including cost effectiveness.

## 3. MAINTAINING THE BENEFITS OF TREATMENT AND PREVENTING RELAPSE AFTER SUCCESSFUL TREATMENT FOR CONDUCT DISORDER

What is the effectiveness of interventions to maintain the benefits of treatment and relapse after successful treatment for conduct disorders?

*Why this is important*
The long-term effectiveness of interventions for the treatment of conduct disorder is not well established, with evidence of the attenuation of the effect over time. Little attention has been paid to the prevention of relapse.
   This question should be addressed in two stages.
● New interventions to maintain treatment effects should be developed in collaboration with service users and may include the use of 'booster' sessions, self-help materials or support groups.
● An RCT of at least 4 years' duration should compare the new interventions with standard care and should report short-, medium- and long-term outcomes, including cost effectiveness. The outcomes and acceptability of the interventions should be rated by parents, teachers and independent observers. The study needs to be large enough to determine the presence of clinically important effects, and mediators and moderators of response should be investigated.

## 4. COMBINING TREATMENT FOR MENTAL HEALTH PROBLEMS IN PARENTS WITH TREATMENT FOR CONDUCT DISORDERS IN THEIR CHILDREN

What is the efficacy of combining the treatment for mental health problems in parents with treatment for conduct disorders in their children?

*Why this is important*
Parental mental health is a factor in the development and maintenance of conduct disorders. This suggests that interventions targeting parental mental health could improve child outcomes. Current evidence does not provide support for this. If successful, the research will have implications for future collaborations between adult mental health services and CAMHS.
   This question should be addressed in two stages. Systematic reviews should be carried out to establish:
● effective interventions for adults as part of a combined intervention
● effective interventions for children in combination with a parental intervention
● which groups of parents and children may benefit from a combined intervention.

The combined intervention should be tested in an RCT design. It should be compared with the best child-only intervention and report outcomes, including cost effectiveness, of at least 24 months' duration. The outcomes and acceptability of the intervention should be rated by parents, teachers and independent observers. The study should be large enough to determine the presence of clinically important effects, and mediators and moderators of response should be investigated.

## 5. CLASSROOM-BASED INTERVENTIONS FOR CONDUCT DISORDERS

**What is the efficacy of classroom-based interventions for conduct disorders**

*Why this is important*
Interventions to prevent or treat conduct disorders have been specially designed for delivery in schools. Classroom-based interventions provide access to treatment for children who may not have access otherwise and have a more direct impact on children's educational performance.

This question should be addressed in an RCT design of at least 24 months' duration. It should compare a new classroom-based intervention with standard care and should report short-, medium- and long-term outcomes, including cost effectiveness. The outcomes and acceptability of the intervention should be rated by parents, teachers and independent observers. The study needs to be large enough to determine the presence of clinically important effects, and mediators and moderators of response should be investigated.

# APPENDIX 13:
# EXPERIENCE OF CARE SUMMARY EVIDENCE MATRIX

| Dimensions of person-centred care (adapted from Picker Institute) | Key points on the pathway of care | | | |
|---|---|---|---|---|
| | Access | Assessment and diagnosis | Treatment (including prevention) | Educational settings |
| **The relationship between individual service users and professionals** — **Involvement in decisions and respect for preferences** | Important to consult with looked-after children and young people in service provision discussions (systematic review – DAVIES2008). | | Important to consult with looked-after children and young people in their individual discussions (systematic review – DAVIES2008). There was a sense of cultural dissonance in the Webster–Stratton programmes for some families (primary study – CHILDREN1ST2007). There were feelings that the Webster–Stratton programmes take a simplistic/idealistic approach and were not related to the complexity or the severity of what parents/carers are experiencing – not addressing 'bad behaviour' outside the home and so on. Parents/carers expressed a desire for the programmes to be modified to their needs and circumstances, and not run by the book (primary study – CHILDREN1ST2007). Parent/family intervention programmes need to be culturally appropriate (systematic review – LOCHMAN2000). | Effective school-based mental health interventions 'addressed student concerns about teachers' (systematic review – OLIVER2008; p. 785–6). |

| Dimensions of person-centred care (adapted from Picker Institute) | Key points on the pathway of care | | | |
| --- | --- | --- | --- | --- |
| | Access | Assessment and diagnosis | Treatment (including prevention) | Educational settings |
| **Clear, comprehensible information and support for self-care** | Parents/carers would like more information about community services and available transitional/vocational services. Possible solutions to this could be to provide a central location/office (for example, at school) that distributes comprehensive information on all community services; or distribute information via intensive case management or a community-based agency. In terms of transitional services, school personnel could work closely with parents to develop a comprehensive plan for each child, addressing both child and family needs (primary study – SODERLUND1995).<br><br>To address unmet need within the context of limited capacity, services need to deliver interventions innovatively, for example using 'self-administered programming' and taking advantage of media technology (systematic review – SHEPARD2009, p. 8). | | Children and young people like to know what is going to happen to them when they are referred to services – provision of information leaflet (primary study – CHILDREN1ST2007). | |

The relationship between individual service users and professionals

| The relationship between individual service users and professionals | | |
|---|---|---|
| **Emotional support, empathy and respect** | Building relationships (the sense of something being done, respect for confidentiality, staff interactions) may be just as important to children and young people as intervention type/techniques/theories used (systematic review – DAVIES2008).<br><br>Children and young people experienced ambivalence towards talking and had a preference for non-verbal communication for engagement in the therapy process (systematic review – DAVIES2008).<br><br>Authoritarian management style not appreciated by prison detainees (primary study – ASHKAR2008).<br><br>Children and young people and parents/carers attending CAMHS appreciated having relationships with staff; support, help and advice given; being listened to, given time; able to talk and express feelings. Attention to initial concerns/worries could be improved (primary study – BARBER2006).<br><br>Effective interventions address children and young people's concerns about family conflict, bereavement and/or peer group rejection (systematic review – OLIVER2008).<br><br>Besides the skills and practical help that multisystemic therapy offered, parents strongly valued the sense of having someone there for them to 'share what you're going through', feeling that multisystemic therapy 'becomes a support and a friend' (TIGHE2012). | Children and young people with behavioural problems experienced animosity from teachers. Teachers need to see pupil engagement as a collaborative process, rather than something threatening. It is important to cater to holistic needs and engage students in alternative ways of learning (systematic review – CEFAI2010).<br><br>Separating the child from the behaviour, and conveying this to parents/carers is important (primary study – JRF2007). |

391

| Dimensions of person-centred care (adapted from Picker Institute) | Key points on the pathway of care | | | |
| --- | --- | --- | --- | --- |
| | Access | Assessment and diagnosis | Treatment (including prevention) | Educational settings |
| **Fast access to reliable health advice** | Incarcerated young people report limited availability of services tacking criminogenic need and educational and vocational services but positive experience of those services reported by those able to access them (primary study – ASHKAR2008).

Children and young people and parents/carers attending CAMHS report that accessibility could be improved (primary study – BARBER2006).

Inconveniently located services are seen as the most prominent barrier to services. Meetings conducted at a location designated by the parent or at home; or a school-linked services approach could be helpful (primary study – SODERLUND1995).

Need exceeds capacity, which is a barrier to access (systematic review – SHEPARD2009). | | Intensive, longer-term, evidence-based interventions could benefit looked-after children and 'prevent further movement away from family and community' (systematic review – LANDSVERK2009, p. 53).

Interventions targeting the broader issues that have an impact on mental health – for example housing, finance, and so on – can help to improve access to services, and may be particularly useful for reaching marginalised children and young people (systematic review – OLIVER2008). | Teachers report behaviour management to take precedence over identifying mental health problems. Teachers perceive parents to be significant barriers to mental health services for children in that they often did not act on teachers' referrals or recommendations believing teachers to be the ones to resolve their child's problems. Other barriers to identification/access include lack of resources in the school, large class sizes, no zero tolerance policy for certain behaviours, a lack of parenting classes and too much bureaucracy (primary study – WILLIAMS2007)

Parents/carers resent the attitude that teachers take that parents/carers should be expected to help sort out a problem without understanding all the other problems they are facing (primary study – JRF2007). |
| **The way that services and systems work** | | | | |

| | **The way that services and systems work** |
|---|---|
| | There can be multi-level barriers (community, organisational, individual) to implementing parent/family interventions including: lack of agency or professional 'ownership' of programme; lack of training/support for staff; parents' 'disinterest, resistance and lack of involvement' (systematic review – LOCHMAN2000; p. 260). |
| | Accessibility of treatment, and 'the organizational and economic context of … service delivery' are critical to treatment effectiveness in adolescent drug users. (systematic review – FLANZER2005; p. 894). |
| | The lack of available support for adolescent drug users is costly both in terms of the financial impact on other services and on outcomes for the individual (systematic review – FLANZER2005). |

| Dimensions of person-centred care (adapted from Picker Institute) | Key points on the pathway of care | | | |
| --- | --- | --- | --- | --- |
| | Access | Assessment and diagnosis | Treatment (including prevention) | Educational settings |
| **Effective treatment delivered by trusted health professionals** | Staff expected to deliver parent/family skills interventions may benefit from training models that allow for initial training with ongoing follow-up work and access to support rather than a single, stand-alone session (systematic review – LOCHMAN2000). | | Services might look to capitalise on incarcerated young people's readiness for positive change by developing rehabilitative programming (offence-specific treatment, psychological treatment, counselling, education, vocational training, social skills training, anger management, and problem solving) during incarceration (primary study – ASHKAR2008).<br><br>Children and young people and parents/carers attending CAMHS appreciated crisis care. The specifics of treatment could be improved. Children and young people with conduct problems were less likely to be satisfied with services, therefore it is important to work with this group more in the future so that their needs are better understood and expectations met (primary study – BARBER2006).<br><br>Therapists value a wide range of treatment strategies when working with children and young people with disruptive behavioural problems and their parents/carers. Understanding their attitudes towards treatment techniques and content may improve how interventions are implemented. Interventions most valued for children and young people are those that focus on the parent/child/family relationship and problem-solving/social skills. | Interventions for girls with aggression need to be designed along the lines of preventing escalation of aggression (aggression in girls tends to begin as non-physical and leads to physical). Interventions that help girls use aggressive behaviours in positive ways can be useful. Girls' friendships are very much tied up in their aggression, so mentoring programmes that emphasise this affinity for attachment could be helpful (primary study – ADAMSHICK2010). |

The way that services and systems work

Interventions most valued for older children and young people are those that focus on problem-solving/social skills and improved communication. For parents/carers, interventions most valued are those that identify strengths and modelling or psychoeducation (the latter for parents/carers of older children and young people) (primary study – BROOKMAN-FRAZEE2009).

Child welfare service staff need to understand 'the importance of early intervention and treatment' (systematic review – LANDSVERK2009, p. 64).

Accessibility of treatment, and 'the organizational and economic context of . . . service delivery' are critical to treatment effectiveness (systematic review – FLANZER2009; p. 894).

Staff morale and expertise is critical to drug treatment programme success: professionals need expertise in both navigating the criminal justice system and in providing treatment/ therapy to young people (systematic review – FLANZER2005).

Families trusted the therapist, and felt 'heard and understood', and indicated that the non-blaming approach, in which the therapist was 'working together with me as opposed to against me' was crucial to their engagement (TIGHE2012, p. 5).

**The way that services and systems work**

| Dimensions of person-centred care (adapted from Picker Institute) | Key points on the pathway of care | | | |
|---|---|---|---|---|
| | Access | Assessment and diagnosis | Treatment (including prevention) | Educational settings |
| **Attention to physical and environmental needs** | | | Practical arrangements and physical surroundings are an important therapeutic feature for children and young people (systematic review – DAVIES2008).<br><br>Children and young people and parents/carers attending CAMHS reported that facilities could be improved (primary study – BARBER2006).<br><br>Important to engage in children and young people in becoming analytical about their behaviour and attitudes (primary study – JRF2007).<br><br>Parents may be more likely to engage with family-focused interventions that fit in with their schedules, for example those that are delivered in community settings and have meals, childcare and/or transport provided (systematic review – LOCHMAN2000; systematic review – SHEPARD2009).<br><br>Families appreciate flexibility of the multi-systemic therapy model around their schedule and being located in their family home (TIGHE2012). | Difficulty adapting to a rigid school environment, students need support and encouragement to have a voice at school (systematic review – CEFAI2010). |

**The way that services and systems work**

| Involvement of, and support for, family and carers | | It is important for local authorities to consult parents/carers and children and young people in relation to their preferred choices for educational provision after a permanent exclusion from school (primary study – JRF2007). |
| --- | --- | --- |
| | | Services that do not address family needs are recognised as a barrier. Educational programmes (to learning effective methods for managing children's behaviour) and recreational/respite programmes (providing help in finding recreational activities for children and tips for finding personal time for parents) may be beneficial to families (primary study – SODERLUND1995). |
| | | Parents/carers enjoy being with other adults who share similar difficulties, allowing their sense of isolation to decrease. Incorporating regular support groups and the opportunity to address their lack of confidence or self-esteem in treatment is welcomed (primary study – CHILDREN1ST2007). |
| | | Continuous positive reinforcement needed to engage and retain parents/carers in treatment (primary study – CHILDREN1ST2007). It is more difficult with children whose parents/carers cannot engage (primary study – JRF2007). |
| | | A non-judgemental and individualised approach where parents/carers are given the chance to work out their own strategies is appreciated (primary study – JRF2007). |
| | | Parents may be more likely to engage with family-focused interventions that enable them to share experiences and bond with other parents (systematic review – LOCHMAN2000). |
| | | High value was placed on the therapists' ability to connect with different family members, showing empathy, understanding and genuine care (TIGHE2012). |

**The way that services and systems work**

397

| Dimensions of person-centred care (adapted from Picker Institute) | Key points on the pathway of care | | | |
|---|---|---|---|---|
| | Access | Assessment and diagnosis | Treatment (including prevention) | Educational settings |
| **Continuity of care and smooth transitions** | For children and young people in care, unnecessary delays at entry to care may result in an increased risk of mental health problems (primary study – DEMOS2010). Staff working with looked-after children need to understand the range of mental health services and support available in the locality and how to access/refer to them (systematic review – LANDSVERK2009). | Services could consider standardising mental health assessment for children and young people entering care (systematic review – LANDSVERK 2009). | Children and young people and parents/carers attending CAMHS appreciate the flexibility of the service. Waiting time for first appointment could be improved (primary study – BARBER2006). Liaison with schools is important to the success of the programmes so that teachers can reinforce new learning and behaviour (primary study – CHILDREN1ST2007) For children and young people in care, placement stability can help mitigate emotional difficulties and challenging behaviour. Training carers to deal with emotional problems and mental health support can minimise the likelihood of placement breakdown. Adequate attention also needs to be given to support for children and young people when they are on the verge of leaving care and living independently (primary study – DEMOS2010). In terms of a community-level approach to antisocial behaviour there needs to be better coordination between projects and better integration of antisocial behaviour work within neighbourhood renewal strategies (primary study – JRF2005). | |

**The way that services and systems work**

398

It may be beneficial to incorporate programme delivery into existing community structures to encourage attendance from those unlikely to attend programmes in traditional mental health settings (systematic review – SHEPARD2009).

Case management approaches can help deliver integrated, coordinated, coherent care by 'establishing linkages across programmes and systems' (systematic review – FLANZER2005; p. 899).

Adolescent drug misuse services can fail as a result of an over-focus on criminal behaviour rather than on a holistic approach to rehabilitation (systematic review – FLANZER2005).

Families found the ecological systems approach to understanding and resolving difficulties very helpful because the focus was not solely on the young person, but on links with extended family and other professionals (TIGHE2012).

Families identified that extratherapeutic factors, such as the influence of other professionals and agencies (for example, school and youth offending services), and the role the criminal justice system played as a deterrent to future offending (TIGHE2012).

Those who struggled after the intervention had ended said they would have preferred a more tapered approach to ending, a 'weaning process' (TIGHE2012, p. 8).

**The way that services and systems work**

# APPENDIX 14:

# USER VOICE REPORT FOR THE NATIONAL

# COLLABORATING CENTRE FOR MENTAL HEALTH

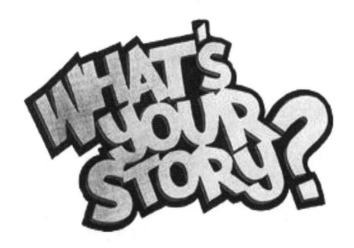

**SCOPING STUDY FOR THE DEVELOPMENT OF NICE GUIDELINES
ON ANTISOCIAL BEHAVIOUR AND CONDUCT DISORDERS IN
CHILDREN AND YOUNG PEOPLE: RECOGNITION, INTERVENTION
AND MANAGEMENT**

**A User Voice Report for the National Collaborating Centre for Mental Health**

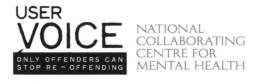

**Acknowledgements**

We would like to acknowledge the participation and contribution of all the young
people who took part in this study.

We would also like to thank the National Collaborating Centre for Mental Health
for recognising the importance of listening to the voice of young people.

**USER VOICE**

User Voice's work is led and delivered by ex-offenders who foster dialogue between users and providers of the criminal justice and related services. Our primary aim is to enable practitioners and policy makers to listen directly to service users, allowing unheard voices to make a difference.

The entrenched exclusion and complex needs of some of the people we work with can be a huge obstacle to service providers. While User Voice aims to be a powerful advocate on behalf of offenders, ex-offenders and others on the margins, it does this through robust but constructive engagement with those who have the power to design services and make decisions. Our aim is to act as a 'referee': ensuring that no one group's agenda dominates and that engagement benefits all.

We are well placed to gain the trust of people involved in crime. The involvement of ex-offenders has many benefits, not least of which is the narrative of success. Working with ex-offenders can be a powerful way of motivating people who have little self-belief that they can overcome the barriers they face. We recruit qualified and talented ex-offenders. This has a profound impact on employees' self-confidence and transforms their long-term employment prospects. User Voice demonstrates the hugely positive role ex-offenders can play given the right chance.

**History**

User Voice was founded by Mark Johnson, an ex-offender and former drug abuser, best-selling author of *Wasted* and social commentator. Mark's experiences of prison, and later as an employer of ex-offenders and consultant within the criminal justice system and voluntary sector, convinced him of the need to create a model of engagement that is fair and incentive led. His aim was to foster dialogue between service providers and users, which results in better and more cost-effective services.

**What do we do?**

User Voice empowers service users by focusing on their role in making change happen and providing them with a chance to develop their own proposals for change and innovation. The past experiences of User Voice's staff gives them a special understanding and rapport with people involved with the criminal justice system, which encourages participants to talk openly, often for the first time, about their feelings and experiences. Every project is different but falls into one of three main categories.

- *Raising awareness* through speeches and opinion, we present the models, practices and business case behind User Voice in order to inspire and influence. We create opportunities for the people we work with to meet and speak to those in power.
- *Bespoke consultations* like this one, where we work with clients to design projects aimed at accessing, hearing and acting upon the insights of service users. These

projects can include staff and user consultations, qualitative and quantitative work, and primary and secondary research.

- *User Voice Councils* developed for use within prisons or in the community for probation, youth offending teams and related services. In whatever context it occurs, the User Voice Council approach is underpinned by democratic models, which seek to engage participants in collective decision making within the confines of the particular service at hand.

Councils are designed to build people's skills in listening and communication, negotiation and problem solving and to provide a space where service users and staff can address problems and design solutions on a more equal footing. Their aim is to achieve wider goals such as increasing responsibility and active citizenship with consequent benefits in reducing reoffending, and improving chances of resettlement and employment.

## INTRODUCTION

This report outlines the key findings of a focus group facilitated by User Voice on behalf of the National Collaborating Centre for Mental Health (NCCMH). User Voice were approached by the NCCMH to assist them to incorporate the views of young people in the development of National Institute for Health and Care Excellence (NICE) guidelines on antisocial behaviour and conduct disorders in children and young people. The principle of incorporating the views of children and young people in the services designed to help them has been emphasised in previous, related, NICE guidance.

> *Put the voices of children, young people and their families at the heart of service design and delivery.*[121]

User Voice therefore considered this an exciting opportunity to incorporate the voices of young people who have had involvement with youth justice services into the development of further NICE guidelines. This group of young people tend to be neglected by health professionals and are often the most difficult to reach, both in terms of service delivery and for the purposes of service evaluation and research. This is largely due to their previously negative experiences of professionals and public services and their sense of alienation from and mistrust of those in positions of authority and control over them. User Voice has considerable experience of engaging with and representing the views of these young people. They are therefore uniquely placed to assist the NCCMH in their scoping study for the development of these guidelines.

---

[121]NICE (2010) *Promoting the Quality of Life of Looked-After Children and Young People*. NICE public health guidance 28. London: NICE. Available from: www.nice.org.uk/PH28

**Methodology**

A group of seven young people who had previously had involvement with User Voice youth activity volunteered to take part in the focus group: two young women and five young men, aged between 15 and 18 years old. In terms of ethnicity three were of black ethnic origin, three were mixed heritage and one was of white ethnic origin. Some group members had met before, others had not. Some had taken part in previous User Voice focus groups and others hadn't. All the young people had significant experience of the criminal justice system including time spent with associated agencies such as youth offending services, social services, police and youth services. Some had spent time in young offenders institutions, secure training centres and secure children's homes. All had been identified as having behaviour/conduct problems at school, with most spending time out of the mainstream classroom with behaviour support workers or in specialist behaviour units. Some had identified previous conflict issues at home with parents or family members and some had experienced periods of separation from their families when looked after by local authority social services departments. Some, but not all, had experience of CAMHS and of counselling services provided by other agencies such as schools and youth offending teams. Some had been diagnosed at various times in their childhood with disorders such as depression, anxiety and ADHD. For some it had been 'alluded to' that their diagnosed mental health disorders may have been a contributing factor to their antisocial behaviour. Some also had family members identified as having or requiring support from mental health services.

The life histories of the participants, therefore, shared characteristics commonly associated with offending. To this extent the young people were a small but representative sample of those young people considered at significant risk of developing a conduct disorder.

> *There are a number of risk factors that can predispose children to conduct disorders. These factors can be environmental or associated with the family or the children themselves. Environmental risk factors include social disadvantage, homelessness, low socioeconomic status, poverty, overcrowding and social isolation. Family risk factors include marital discord, substance misuse or criminal activities, and abusive and injurious parenting practices. Children with a 'difficult' temperament, brain damage, epilepsy, chronic illness or cognitive deficits are also more prone to conduct disorders.*[122]

The focus group took place at User Voice premises, in Kennington, London, with five participants travelling from London, one from Birmingham and one from the

---

[122]NICE (2007). *Parent-Training/Education Programmes in the Management of Children with Conduct Disorders.* NICE technology appraisal guidance 102. London: NICE. Available from: www.nice.org.uk/TA102

North West of England to attend. The day began with a morning presentation by Professor Stephen Scott, Professor of Child Health and Behaviour, and Professor Stephen Pilling, Director, NCCMH.

User Voice worked closely with the NCCMH in preparing the presentation to ensure that it was 'user friendly' in terms of its format and the language used to explain the consultation. The presentation introduced the young people to the scope of the project and they were also shown information on previously published NICE guidance.

For illustrative purposes a case study has been incorporated into this report to bring to life the narrative of one of the focus group participants. This young person volunteered to use her life story to offer additional insight into her experiences of access to care, interventions and delivery of care. The young person was assisted by a User Voice worker to write her story but the story is her own. Parts of her story are interwoven throughout the data analysis section of the report where relevant and her name has been changed to protect the young person's identity. The full case study is at the end of this report.


## THE YOUNG PEOPLE'S VIEWS

### Access to care

The focus group facilitators encouraged the young people to think about: how they had attempted to get help when they had needed this in the past; how they had decided who to approach for help and what type of help they might need; what had been helpful or unhelpful in this process; and their suggestions for what might make it easier for them or other young people to get help with any problems they may have in the future.

The young people were able to describe situations that either they or other young people they knew had encountered when they had needed help in the past. They indicated that who they would approach for help would be influenced, to an extent, by the nature of the problem and how serious it was. Broadly speaking most young people cited family and friends as the people they would be most likely to turn to if they needed help.

> *I've got a good relationship with my mum. I would go to my mum. She has lived with me for 17 years and she knows all about me. (male)*

> *I would go to a family member who would probably understand me the most. Basically I have got an older uncle... (male)*

> *I would go to my mum. (female)*

> *Mum always understands. (male)*

Some of the other young people in the group identified that they did not have a close family member they could approach for help.

> *That is where you are lucky. You have got a dad. Some of us have to be our own dads. (male)*

In these circumstances some of the young people identified that they, or others, would choose to approach friends for help.

> *They would probably just go to someone that they trust. You might have to go to someone that you trust, even if it is your friend. (male)*

> *Yes my friend is in that situation. She is in care. Her mum put her in care when she was a baby and her sister. If she wants anyone to speak to she always comes to me and tells me everything. She told me that she was getting videoed by her boyfriend, so I did some research and got a number for her to speak to. (female)*

Most of the young people identified the internet as a safe and trusted source of information to help them when they or people they knew had problems. For some young people this was most often their first port of call when seeking help.

> *Any problem, anything at all from A to Z, I would just go to Google. (male)*

This young person later clarified that he would prefer to seek help through the internet than approach professionals for help.

> *I feel that I could use the information myself and put that into effect.*

He was able to describe how he would check the reliability and accuracy of the information he had found.

> *Well I will scan the lot (websites) and just see the difference between each one and see what the most popular conclusion is. And work on it from there.*

Other young people agreed.

> *Google is a search engine so it would bring it up. The best place to resort to, to find internet websites that can help you. (male)*

Some of the young people indicated they would not trust public service websites such as the youth offending service website.

> *With them, like, they are all connected to the government which is different. So basically they all say the same thing but you don't really want to go there. (male)*

405

One young person identified Boots the chemist as a source of help with health-related problems.

> *I would go to Boots in town. They have a walk in doctor thing in Boots in town in Birmingham that you can go in, like my sister went in there yesterday and you can go there and they will give you paracetamol and tell you what is wrong with you. Just like a GP but it is anonymous. (female)*

Some young people did identify professionals they would approach if they needed help.

> *I would go to my YOT worker. Yes most people don't get along with their YOT worker but me and my YOT worker has got a good relationship. (female)*

Trust was often cited as a key consideration for the young people when considering who to approach for help. Mistrust of professionals based on previously negative experiences of public services was often cited as a barrier to young people seeking out or engaging with professional help.

---

Sophie had a mentor at primary school, 'L', who would take her out of class and talk about feelings and about her anger issues. Sophie enjoyed getting to know this mentor and built up trust and did share her feelings. However, Sophie remembers a time at school when they (teachers and mentor) asked why she didn't eat breakfast (Sophie states she never wanted to eat breakfast but there was always breakfast provided at home). Sophie states that she felt the things she told the mentor and their concerns over not eating breakfast were told to social services without her knowledge. Social workers came and visited Mum at their home, they saw there was lots of food in and didn't come again. From that point on, Sophie states she lost trust with mentor and any professional agencies working with the family and that this also had a huge impact upon her relationship with her Mum who felt betrayed that Sophie had spoken to outside agencies about the family, and Sophie felt bad that she had lost her Mum's trust.

---

> *It just takes one bad experience with like a person, like someone who is professional, like one bad experience with the police, to think that I am never talking to the police again. (female)*

> *I would go to no social worker. (male)*

Concerns about confidentiality were frequently cited when the issue of professional mistrust was being discussed.

Sophie thinks that now, looking back, the whole mistrust of professionals by her and her family stems from this early experience of trust being broken with her primary school mentor telling other agencies things without her knowing. Sophie states that when you tell one professional something about your feelings, they always go behind her back and tell someone else. She has never felt informed about her care and believes that it wouldn't have been as bad if someone had told her what was happening, what plans were being made or who they were going to tell, even when she was at primary school age.

*...but this is where you trust no one in this world, because you can't really trust anyone. That confidentiality is between you and that person. They could go handing it to someone else. (female)*

*...no information is safe anywhere today. (male)*

*But they are not allowed to give out your information. (male)*

*Yes they are. They are sometimes. (female)*

*They are all part of one big legal gang. (male)*

*Most young people now don't speak to the police. So come to the police, come to all those things with your GP and things like that because say you are under the age of 16, you get found in hospital...if you have taken an overdose they call the police because it is child security and then when the police come the police are the ones that put you on these things. Like they will put you in these homes and stuff like that. I have seen it happen. (female)*

*With these people in power you just can't win innit. You just feel that you can't win, probation and youth offending. Basically anything they say goes. If they say they will breach you, they will breach you, even if you didn't breach. (male)*

*....well I suppose counsellors are good for some people but personally I would not trust a counsellor because I had one and obviously if you are in danger they have got to say something. But ....unless you want that to be said ....I told my old counsellor something that I wish I didn't, you know what I mean, and that ....and it just – and now I regret. You have got to watch what you say. (female)*

This young woman clarified that concerns about confidentiality made her less likely to approach professionals for help.

*...because you don't want everyone to know your business. And most people now, like counsellors...and stuff they work like, youth offending and things like that, like*

407

*if you tell them something and if it is bad then, like even if you don't mean to say it, they are going to be telling the youth offending and the youth offending is going to write it down and you are going to have police knocking at your door asking you why you are making these accusations or why you are thinking these things whereas you want to just talk to and get help with your problems without thinking it is a big massive dilemma. It is not like you are admitting to murder, you are just saying how you feel about certain people but they take it as if you are making threats, but if you were going to [make] threats you would have done that in the first place.*

She described how her experience of confidentiality being breached by a counsellor she had seen at a CAMHS service had led to her withdrawing from this service.

*Cos I said something to my counsellor, and she has told, and like the next week my youth offending worker has told me, and I am thinking what the hell you are not supposed to, and I did actually say to the woman I don't want my youth worker to know. And she actually betrayed me which was like...and told her, and I would not go back there again after that.*

One young person explained why she would be reluctant to seek help from her doctor.

*Like if anything my doctor isn't going to find out because I know my doctor finds out something bad he will say something and my mum will find out and I don't want to tell her. And doctors have a thing about, even when they have perfectly competent children, doctors have got a thing about telling your parents things. (female)*

This generated a lot of discussion amongst the young people in the focus group.

*That is taking the piss don't you think? The doctor telling your mum and dad your personal business. You might not want them to know. That could cause havoc in the home you know. (male)*

*There are certain things you don't tell your mum and dad. There are certain things you can tell them but there are certain things you can't. That is how real it is. (male)*

*It's not you can't – you won't tell them. You just wouldn't want to. (male)*

*When they find out I know what it is like. (male)*

Interestingly, a coordinated, multi-agency approach to service provision often appeared to be a disincentive to use these services from the perspective of the young people.

*I think they work together to be honest. (male)*

*Hospitals, youth offending, police, probation, they all work together. (female)*

*…they are just working together to make you feel worse than what you already are. (female)*

Two young people, whilst acknowledging the need for multi-agency working, emphasised the importance of how information was shared between the different agencies and the need for transparency when doing so.

*In most situations it is important that they work together because it stops so many things from happening but it is the way that they do it rather than what they are doing. If they did it in a like a calm way, and said to the people, yes I have got to say things and say that because it is a risk Then I am sure young people would understand because it is risk. They could say I didn't mean it like that they could explain why they said it rather than not having to say something and then the probation worker is saying that she has put in a report and she would not have said these… (female)*

*Yes but I would understand sometimes if I was in that position and someone young was telling me that this is how they are feeling and that, I couldn't just – because of the way I am with kids – sit there and be like Oh my God – OK see you next week. I would have to do something about it. But I think it is just like the way that they are saying it, the way that they are putting it across. Like she put it across as if to say I said I was going to kill someone but I didn't I just said I felt like killing her because of the way she was going on. But the person I was talking about was my little sister but she did not understand, she thought I was actually going to kill my little sister but no I just felt like it because of the way she was going on. They just blow things out of proportion really. If she would have said to me, when I said to her don't tell anyone, if she would have said to me "I have got to tell this person because it is a risk....." Then I would have understood. Do you get me? But she didn't even tell me. She said, "OK". Basically saying that she is not going to say anything to them and I find out that she did. Anyone else and it would just have been arguments but because it is a counsellor you can't really argue with them. (female)*

These views were reflected by other young people who indicated that not knowing what information would be shared with which professional or agency in which circumstances led to them being reluctant to talk to professionals about their problems.

*It's like playing chess without knowing the rules. (male)*

*It's the without knowing the rules. That's the bit for me. That is the bit where it is not OK if it is your care. In my view, that is my personal opinion. (female)*

*Location of services*

The young people were asked if the location of services that were offered to them would have an influence on their willingness or ability to access these services. This appeared a less significant or important consideration for the young people compared to issues of professional mistrust, and misuse of authority. Most of the young people indicated that their preference for location would be dependent on the nature of the problem they were seeking help with.

> *I would say it all depends really. Some people would not want you going into their houses because their parents, they might find them intimidating. They can't say things because their parents are there. They would rather do it somewhere that is not at home like a community centre. (female)*

> *Yes. Community centre. Or like meet at a café or something. (female)*

> *Its more private isn't it. Relaxing, get a brew and sit down and chat. (female)*

> *School. Maybe certain lessons that you are going to see this particular kid that are always getting into trouble in that one lesson. Obviously there should be someone there so when you take them out of that lesson, talk to them, ask – like a mentor. (male)*

## Intervention

When discussing the services the young people had experienced in the past, the importance of establishing a relationship of trust with the professional involved in providing the service appeared to be the most significant consideration from the young people's perspective. Trust was often linked to the concerns about confidentiality highlighted previously. When describing experiences of positive and helpful relationships with professionals common themes that emerged included: the importance of consistency in professional involvement with the young person over time, the young person developing a sense that the professional concerned genuinely cared for them (most often demonstrated by the professional maintaining informal contact beyond the remit of their professional role) and the interpersonal style of the professional which helped the young person to engage with them therapeutically.

Some of the young people described how important it was for them to have an identified professional or worker who remained consistent in their lives over time.

> *What are social workers for? I am not being funny. Why? All they are there for is to put you into care. They don't give a shit because I had about like eight social workers from last year. They come and go. They come and expect me to tell my business to them or read my file, my personal business, and then leave without telling me that they are going to go off. Then another one comes. (female)*

*One worker, cos you can't get through to them all on an inter-personal level. (male)*

*So I had the same YOT worker throughout .... she got to know my personality innit. So like she could be more on a level with me like. Because to me having another YOT worker, or being introduced to one on one professionals, that you have got to create boundaries again. Not boundaries barriers. (male)*

*When I went in there (prison) I thought I ain't speaking to none of these screws but there was this one woman, she was my support officer and she was all right. I still speak to her now. She was all right like, she understood like my problems and that and she wanted – she helped me get bail – she helped me get my social worker and she even supports me now that I am not in prison. She will come down to Birmingham and she will come and check everything is fine and that. She doesn't have to you know. When I left prison she could have just said that's it she is not my problem no more. But she still makes time, she will still phone my probation to ..., she still makes time to try and find and make sure everything is OK. She says she doesn't want me reoffending again cos she cares. You know what, it makes me feel happy to know that there is someone who is not my family and is a professional that does care. Yes I don't want to let her down because she has got faith in me. So that's why when I am thinking about doing... I think no forget it. I am not having it like that now am I? But if you think about it I left prison in 2010, the last time I heard from her was 2 days ago. That is 2 years ago and she is still checking up on me. (female)*

*The only person that really helped me was that Trailblazers thing. You work for 6 months before and you stay 6 months now and that was a woman that is work-ing with me still and she was cool. Even though she is a woman she could relate to my problems. She used to tell me stories of her family and her past and even if it is not my day for her to come and see me if she is on the wing she will walk past, walk in my flat, how am I doing? Get my door pass for 5 minutes and obvi-ously just to talk – obviously with boys it is different you don't really want to show that much emotion but you go back to your cell thinking she is all right. I can see myself going back to her. Because there are some people that come to you and ask you questions like how your parents have been to you. I want to talk about me. I don't want to talk about my family. It is just the way they go about things. There is not really that much support for you. Obviously the guards are out there for support but they are just there to bend you up and throw you on the floor. (male)*

The interpersonal style of the worker was also cited as important by many of the young people. This included the worker's capacity to demonstrate an understanding of the young person's world and to enable the young person to feel at ease and able to talk about themselves and their problems or concerns.

*I think basically the YOT workers should be like more people who understand your situation more and have been there themselves. And can connect with you on a certain level. But if it is like more – but if there are people who are like stuck up and that you are just annoyed and it does not help the situation. It needs to be people who are like more.... (female)*

The style of clothing adopted by the worker was cited by most of the young people as a significant factor in whether they felt able to relate to them and feel comfortable talking to them. More specifically 'suits' were often identified as 'uniforms' that symbolised authority, control and professional detachment, in a negative way, for the young people.

*Even small things like the way someone dresses, that the way a YOT worker would dress that would just – it is much easier to break the tension between a young person and an adult if they have got the same mind frame. (male)*

*....when they (YOT workers) are at home you know if they didn't have the meeting they would not be wearing clothes like that. Obviously if they was lawyers or solicitors wearing a suit but why are you wearing a suit to work in a YOT office? (female)*

When asked if she felt the same about doctors this young woman confirmed that she did.

*Yes they should look like normal because I think it intimidates them – like police – police intimidate little kids as well. My little sister is shit scared of police because of the uniform. She is scared of them but if she saw a police officer like the police officer that came to college, my little sister was there and she was talking to him fine, and then obviously she found out he was a police officer – she said I didn't know he was because he wasn't wearing that funny uniform. So it is different. It is different perceptions because obviously people look at what they see, more than what they hear and what they know. (female)*

*It creates a whole different atmosphere. Definitely. (male)*

*It doesn't really matter how old they are, it doesn't really matter if they were a man or a woman, it is the way their personality is, the way they approach you and their body language. And it matters about their dress sense as well because I would not want to sit in a room with you and C if you was in a suit and he was in a suit looking all professional. (female)*

*It don't matter (if a worker is male or female) as long as they have come to show interest. As long as they show interest in – as long as you can genuinely know that they want to help you and want to make sure you are doing good then there should be no problems. They should just need that brief. There is nothing wrong about it as long as they want to help you and they are genuine about helping you and they focus on...(male)*

*Parenting programmes and family-based support services*
Most young people had either direct or indirect experience of these services. They expressed a range of views about their efficacy and made several suggestions about what might work better.

Some young people expressed concerns about their parents feeling judged or undermined by parenting programmes.

> *It could go two ways either it could make a positive effect of the outcome or it could be quite offensive towards the parents for someone else to come in and try to tell them how to raise their child. Because if someone was to come and tell me how to raise my kid and in my eyes I think I am doing it right and someone is coming to tell me I am doing it wrong. (male)*

> *I don't think my mum would like someone trying to tell her what to do cos to her that is like it is up to her to do and she brought me on this earth so it is up to her to do what she wants. Like if she wants to tell me off without reason ... that is what she is going to do. (male)*

> *...this person here could not come to my house and tell my mum what to do. She would just – she would look at him and tell him to walk out the door. (male)*

Others felt that this approach could work.

> *I think that can work though cos it just comes down to your parents and obviously the young person has to be open minded. You have to see eye to eye. On this thing here you have to not forget that it is your child, you have to forget that in a way that you are not telling them off. You need to see some sort of eye to eye level like we are not going look and shout – we are not going to interrupt I am going see where you are coming from, see why you are upset, why they are giving me trouble. If that is the case and obviously the young person is going to have to listen to them. (male)*

The young people made some useful suggestions about how parenting and family-based interventions could be more helpful:

1. The worker acting as a mediator between child and parent

> *...so rather than be feeling like it is a lecture, like people are coming in to lecture your parents and stuff it is more of a mediation kind of thing. You know we have not come here to lecture you, we are not trying to tell you how you are doing your job wrong as a parent. (male)*

2. Offering one to one work with the young person in the first instance to engage the parent in the process by noticing successful change

*Just sit down with the child, one on one, and then when the parents last see him the change, where did this change come from? And then obviously they arrive this is what I have been doing, this is what I have been seeing and then maybe that is where they will want to come and look at it because they see all right, this has helped my child. I have seen a change at home now he is tidying up and now he is coming in when I tell him. Why is it and then they will find out. (male)*

3. Videoing the individual session with the young person and showing this to the parent

*I reckon, how can I put it, a good tactic would be to – if you got the child on a one to one level without the parent around and you get down to the root of the problems if you get that videoed and show that back to the parent that could have a more positive effect because then she can't argue with the video. (male)*

*When you open your mouth you are not hearing what people are saying about your kids you are hearing your kids say it but they are not saying it to you but they are saying it to someone and then you are hearing. (female)*

One young person talked of how he would prefer his parents to be shown a video of his discussions with a worker than talk in his parents' presence about his feelings.

*No you don't want to show emotions to too many people. And you obviously don't want to show emotion to your parents sometimes cos you feel like you don't want your mum to see you like down in that. And then the parents are going to watch that and actually look at him and look at him and think that is how he feels. (male)*

Another young person expressed a preference for writing a letter to his parents rather than talking about his feelings on a video they would later be shown. He indicated this would feel unsafe for him given the nature of his relationship with his mother.

*Maybe a written letter. Post the letter and your mum picks it up and reads it – even so my mum the way she is – I wouldn't go on camera and talk about it because I know she might when I get home still go into a … Yes… talking my business on the camera. So there is a fine line between… you have got to know your parents. Because if you know what your parents are like then there is no point in going on video because then it is pointless. I would never go on video cos I know that would just be game over – she would just – even though you say to her but I feel like I can't tell you. But that is not the point. (male)*

Two young people described how a goal-focused approach could be helpful.

*Basically you just find out what is going on within the house. What the person is doing, how they feel about what they are doing, like if they are doing anything*

*positive in their life like working, going to college or whatever, and just basically knowing that there is progress and just talking to them about. (male)*

*The first time you meet them obviously you have like – not a target sheet but a …so how are things in your house now? And they will tell you. Obviously that is the first time you have met them. You would probably do an evaluation about once every 3 months or something. So in the next 3 months now you look at it again. So how are things and they are going to forget from the first – so you say how are things again and you just compare it from there to there so you know and say, All right. You decide if they are telling you the same sort of thing or are they now saying things are better at home and then you will know if there is progress and you are doing something right and if not then you have got to switch it up back to the drawing board and start it again. (male)*

*Education and school-based interventions*
Most of the young people in the group described difficulties they had encountered at school. They were able to describe both negative and positive experiences of teaching staff and behaviour support/intervention services they had received. Many indicated that getting a good education had been important to them and expressed a sense of disappointment that their potential had not been recognised or supported by teaching staff. They gave some useful examples of what had worked and what hadn't worked in helping them to learn and engage with the education system.

The young people frequently referred to feeling they had been labelled as difficult or problematic children from an early age and that this label had stuck throughout their time in the education system.

*…if you start getting into trouble in Year 7, that is the first year of secondary school, if you get in trouble within that first year, you are labelled as one to watch and then that is it from then. It happened to me and they kicked me out in Year 11 though. Why didn't you kick me out in Year 9 not 11 and go to a new school and start afresh then? Kick me out in Year 11 during mock exams. (male)*

*But most of these kids that teachers claim that are being a problem, most of them are mighty smart. I was so smart, not I was, I am smart, in school. I was smart but the teachers they used to just violate me and obviously because of the way I am… and I have got that intellectual side and when a teacher pisses me off I am going to switch and then I will get kicked out. (male)*

*It's like they heed that you are smart but you are not the perfect role model for them to brag about they don't want you in their class so they would rather give you the fling to someone else. Even though you are the one asking the questions, you are the one doing the work. (male)*

Some young people described how they had felt their work had not been valued by teachers in view of the negative view the teachers had formed of them.

*I get written off…but when Ofsted come they want to show them my work. (male)*

*They always put my work to the front like, they come round to see me first open at my best page in the book but any other day I am not worth nothing to them but when Ofsted want to come they want to show how good their school is – so I remember one time they come along I told them how shit the school was… (male)*

*They don't really care about our education. (male)*

*Yes they just don't understand young children, that's what it is. Teachers don't understand young children. (male)*

Some young people were also able to describe positive experiences of teachers and school-based behaviour intervention programmes. This led to a general discussion of what had been different about teachers who had been helpful.

*When I went to my secondary school it was like we had people that were behaviour officers. They understood us. They understood us completely. (male)*

*The behaviour officers like, you would think all of them were just like……they used to joke around with us, understand…well even cuss some of the teachers as well cos they understand and we would go to them like. There would always be kids in our school that would get into trouble just to go and talk to them about something. (male)*

*…but there was like this one teacher called Miss Smith and like she used to let us listen to music, we do like half an hour of work and half an hour on the computer, but like in her lesson like all the teachers noticed there were no problems with one student because, if you think about it, if everyone is listening to their music they are not going to be tempted to talk either. (female)*

*They are concentrating. (male)*

Most of the young people were in agreement that being allowed to listen to music (on their headphones) had improved, or would be likely to improve, their concentration within the classroom.

*So obviously you are not going to have no problems because no one is going to be shouting over the class or getting hyped or distracting other people cos they are doing their work. (female)*

*And also when you have got a short attention span you have to break the silence sometimes, like you can't just sit there in that quiet atmosphere like an exam. And in exam time, you get me? All the work you want me to do definitely. (male)*

*It is more relaxing, like I feel more comfortable. (male)*

*It's like I can't hear nothing around I can still think and rap at the same time. No distractions. (male)*

*Or even let us listen to a little bit of music and just do our work and concentrate. (male)*

*I would have my headphones in and I would do my work. (male)*

*If I could have my music I would be an A\* student. (male)*

*Just put your headphones in to get on with your work. (male)*

The young people also described how teachers who had been helpful had been effective in creating a more relaxed atmosphere within the classroom.

*I mean basically as long as the teachers understand that students need to learn and that students just need a little bit of freedom to learn and that everything is just controlled but a bit of freedom as well and encouragement. (male)*

*The teacher is much more relaxed like. If they let us talk but as long as we do the work then... (male)*

*It is usually the nice teachers that are not really taken for mugs but are more respected. (male)*

One young person identified that having a mentor or counsellor, someone like a User Voice focus group facilitator who had encountered similar problems, would be helpful.

*I reckon that you (User Voice) working in a school would understand and to the students would be very helpful. (male)*

When asked to elaborate on this he responded:

*...he has been through the same thing. He can tell me how I can stop and just learn. Don't mind the teachers. Just get your education. Do your mocks, do your exams, leave. Do what you are doing afterwards. (male)*

Teachers who were inflexible and uncompromising were seen as being less helpful. Exclusions from class were often felt to be unjustified, particularly when the young person felt the teacher had been unable or unwilling to give them the help they had needed to learn. This was attributed by one young person to an inadequate teacher-to-pupil ratio and excessive class sizes.

> *And they say they are doing it to make you better but it is not helping – you kicking me out of my lesson. Where am I going to learn? And sending me into isolation for the next four days helping me – sitting with them people in there – who all they want to say to me is 'Oh C you should be good in school'. It is not my fault the teacher wants to kick me out just because I don't understand the work. There are teachers like...I think there need to be more than one teacher in a class cos when there is only teacher in the class it does not work you know because not everyone is getting the attention so the boys over there are getting upset because they don't know what they are doing and yet the teacher is saying the work has got to be in ten minutes. But they do not know what they are doing because there is one teacher and she is standing over there. (female)*

> *Yes they have got to teach properly if they expect you to do the work. See in an English class I didn't do work because I was not taught properly because she was just nagging at the whole class that refused to work. You could get told off by the head of English for that. That is not my problem. She should have just carried on with the lesson. (male)*

**Delivery of care**

The young people were asked to think about what had been most useful about the services they had received in the past and what could be changed to make them more likely to use these services if they needed help in the future.

The themes of professional mistrust, concerns about confidentiality and the significance of forming trusting relationships with those who are trying to help them reemerged during this part of the focus group discussion. Other themes that emerged included: negative experiences of assessments, the significance of help being offered at periods of crisis and change for the young person; the importance of feeling listened to and understood by those trying to help them (the significance of mentoring); and having choice about who they see and when (self-referrals being seen as more helpful than professional/agency referrals).

Some young people described how they had found professional assessments unhelpful and intrusive. This appeared to be linked to: concerns about confidentiality; previously negative experiences of professional assessments when they felt their behaviour, or what they had told professionals, had been misunderstood or misinterpreted; and their experience of lack of continuity of care, having encountered frequent changes of professional or multiprofessional involvement in their lives. In this context assessments were experienced as being asked the same questions by a number of professionals who they had not yet formed a trusting relationship with, and where there was no obvious benefit to the young person in engaging in the assessment process.

> *...but you know sometimes it gets too much like when – it is like you being a social worker and you be the counsellor. You have asked me this question about what is going on in my life – I have told you but you two are still working together, but you are asking the same questions but you were already in the room listening to what I said and they just ask you to repeat it and repeat it, and they are just writing notes, but they are not telling you what they are writing, they are just looking at you and writing notes and you don't get to see the notes you know. They are taking the notes away for whatever and they could have been writing that I am a bitch or this that this and I would not know. (female)*

This young person went on to describe how an interview with a counsellor was similar to a police interview. She emphasised how an open-recording policy would have helped her feel more able to engage with the counselling process.

> *I would be better if you could see the notes they were writing so you could approve it before they take it in writing because I know counsellors need to write up what they have been doing but it would be better if we could say, no, no, no I don't like this and they took it off and then publish it afterwards and took it away. Because I wouldn't mind my GP seeing something like that but when it is them writing every single word, even if I just said crap, x said 'crap'. Things like that it is like a police interview. (female)*

A mistrust of professional assessments often appeared to be linked to previously negative experiences of professional assessments, particularly for those young people who had been the subjects of child safeguarding procedures or had been looked after by local authority social services departments.

When asked what would make her more likely to engage with professional help this young woman gave the following response.

> *It all depends how nosey they were because people now, like people who are professional that are nosey you know – even – because they think we are young – they think we don't clock what they are doing but they come up with their snide remarks like – when I was in school 'What did you have to eat this morning?' I don't eat breakfast but when I was young – when I went to my mum they started giving me toast at school and I am thinking 'What?' and the teacher would go to my mum and tell, and then bam – they tried to take me off my mum – why? – because C don't eat breakfast. I told them I don't like to eat breakfast. They have gone to my house, they have seen there is a million breakfast cereals in the kitchen cupboard because my brothers and sisters like them but I personally don't eat breakfast, but their story is Oh she is being neglected. They don't look into it properly like – I know they need to do that just in case I was being neglected but sometimes it is too much like they need to find out the full facts before taking*

*action. It's just like me saying Ah that door is cream but maybe it could have been a different colour before but I am not finding out the full facts. (female)*

When asked if it would have helped for professionals to have explained what was happening she responded:

*Yes. Like now they are sneaky man. They are not going to explain it to you because they want to try to catch people out. (female)*

Feeling listened to and understood by professionals frequently emerged as a theme during the focus group discussions.

---

Sophie remembers that she had two bereavement counselling sessions at school in Year 8 after her step-dad died. She only went to two sessions and then stopped because she felt the counsellor was bringing up questions about the death of her step-dad very directly and in a way that made her feel uncomfortable. Sophie states she felt pushed into talking about her feelings too soon before she had a relationship with the counsellor. She reflects that it could have been better if they had taken time to get to know her, who she was before; she would feel able to talk openly about her feelings.

---

The importance of professionals taking the time and interest to establish the reasons for the young person's difficulties or problematic behaviour were illustrated by the following young person.

*To be honest – schools could have helped. At them ages I was just – my dad just died and I weren't going to school and it would have helped if the school was understanding about it instead of sending my mum cruel letters about parenting and that. If they would have just understood because obviously my mum is not the type of person to tell people everything so my school did not know my dad died. Do you get me? The school did not know until I was leaving school. So it was just like...because obviously...it just got blurted out then.....but if they took the time to understand the reason why....because nowadays if my little cousin misses a day of school they are phoning, they are sending letters out to my auntie's address for one day. They are phoning auntie like if you don't show us proof... you going to court like. (female)*

---

Sophie remembers that in Year 8 there was an incident when her Mum was called to school by the head teacher stating they thought that she may have autism and ADHD. Her mum did not agree with this diagnosis and had a fight with the head teacher. This was never raised again and Sophie does not remember ever being

---

assessed about it and states that her mum didn't agree to the assessments about autism or ADHD. Sophie's perspective is that she got angry about the teacher and the type of lessons and that led to her disruptive behaviour and in her view was not to do with autism or ADHD, but that the work at school wasn't matched to her ability; she found the work too easy so became disruptive. From then she remembers being in isolation most of the time, but mixed with friends at lunchtime and started smoking cannabis and cigarettes at school.

Linked to issues of power and control, the young people also talked of the importance of being given choices about the support offered to them. Broadly speaking interventions that were considered mandatory rather than voluntary were seen as less helpful and interventions where young people were given choices about the worker they were referred to and felt involved in identifying the goals of the intervention were considered most helpful. Many of the young people also talked of the importance of feeling they could have choices about the help offered to them in terms of who they saw and when, and how this was a significant factor in whether they were prepared to meaningfully engage and benefit from the help offered.

> *I just turned round and said I don't want another social worker but they still come. This one turned around and said, 'I'll just come for a chat and see how it goes'. And I just think to myself, 'No, go away'. (female)*

> *I think it would be good you know when you get to that age of 14, 15, 16 – I know that like when you get to the age of 16 if you have got a social worker – like if your social workers thinks they can close the case she wants to close the case, but I think it should be a thing where, say if you have had a social worker since you were 10 and you get to that age of 14 and you don't need it no more you could say, 'I don't want a social worker no more'. Not make you have one till you are 16. (female)*

> *But it's not fair you can't turn round and say I don't want one no more. (female)*

> *And it is your life they have control over. (female)*

One young woman described how she hadn't trusted school-based counsellors as they were only accessible through teacher referrals and hence issues of trust and confidentiality came to the fore again.

> *Like in my school we have got school counsellors any time. But they don't like …the counsellors are only there when the head teacher sends you to the counsellor and like they speak to you like you are an idiot like. So they will be speaking on their phone? And then they will say so, why did you do this today? And I am*

*thinking it is just – why do you speak to me like that? Why can't you just speak normal? And like sometimes it's – them counsellors are still telling your teachers everything you are saying. And the teachers as well, the teachers are . . . . because teachers will wind you up. I was always the bad one in class. My teacher used to wind me up 24/7 just so she could kick me out the class because she knew I didn't like her ... from when – she told me my maths was wrong and she was wrong you know and I was right and she kicked me out because of that and since then I didn't like her. I never forgot. I see her now and she just runs away from me. (female)*

The importance of engaging with workers who the young people felt had some understanding of their situation also reemerged during this session of the focus group, such as the use of mentors who may have previously experienced similar problems in the past. One young woman described how she considered this was particularly needed for young males, like her younger brother, who would find it difficult to talk to their families or to professionals they were unable to trust.

*He is just stubborn. If he wanted help he could get help, but he wants help to come to him. He doesn't know about the help you get. If there was something or some-one that was telling young boys about the help they could get and it was all confi-dential, all anonymous and they could just speak to someone like you (User Voice facilitator), you know what I mean, I go to them because we have things to relate to but they have no one to relate to – because not everyone is on this programme.*

*So it is hard for them because they are going to think I don't want to talk to my mum about...I can't talk to my mum because I am shouting...or I can't talk to my mum because I am doing this, because my mum is going to go mad. . . . Sometimes their dad is not even there and the dad is the worst one to go to. So they just need someone outside that is not going to police, who can just talk to them because they have been through it themselves. So this is not very good because of this and this and this – not you are wrong. (female)*

Some of the young people described how they had been most receptive to help at times of significant change and crisis in their lives.

*You know what the most helpful thing for me was going to prison. Like being, like all the young girls in there, obviously I still know the boys round my area and that going into prison. . ... but there are not many girls go to a prison and see it is full of women and find out what most of the girls were in for – like it is heart breaking you know. Cos most of the girls are in there because of something that has happened to them and something that is not their fault. And for them not to be understood because it is not their fault and end up in prison for it. But then it was good like, it was life changing because it made me realise what to do. Like I was far away from everyone. It was a good little break to be honest. It made me clear my head and think when I get back there is no way I am coming back here. (female)*

*I got loads of support when I was in there but I had like a drugs counsellor in there and it is not where you have to do it because you have been on drugs it's all mandatory like if you do not want to go to education, the only thing that would happen is that you have to be in your room all day. They have got everything in there. They have got church in there, anything you want to do they will help you do it. I was doing catering in there, hairdressing, and if you can't do it in that prison they will transport you to a different prison to do it. And it is good in there.... it is supportive because you have got your own personal officer to speak to and there are various people that come in that are nothing to do with the police, like mentors, that will help you through it in there. (female)*

*Prison, it changed me. It changed my way of thinking. Just sitting in there knowing that I can't even open my door to go to the shop. Can't even use my phone and say 'Hi what is going on'. I can't do nothing. (male)*

*So what helped me get out of trouble? This sounds mean but I think the best thing that helped me was falling out with my mum, because I ended up living nowhere. Like crashing at my mates house or just staying out all night and then the police called my social services and then I thought 'What am I doing. I have lost my family.' And I only had my best mate. And I realised that I was going to end up being put into care if I didn't go back. So that's what I did. (female)*

## CONCLUSIONS

The young people who took part in this focus group formed a small but representative group of those young people considered most likely to develop difficult or problematic behaviour. Remarkably, given their often previously negative experiences of professionals and public service intervention into the lives of themselves and their families, they were able to speak freely about those experiences and in so doing demonstrated valuable insights into how these services can be improved.

The young people demonstrated considerable resilience and resourcefulness in managing the problems they had encountered throughout their childhoods. They had sought help from trusted family members and friends and had used websites available on the internet in an attempt to resolve their problems. They had also been a resource to others experiencing difficulties, such as friends and family members, and demonstrated considerable insight into their own needs and the needs of others.

### Access to care

Unsurprisingly, these young people indicated that they had been cautious about seeking out or engaging with professional help offered by public services. This caution was largely due to their previously negative experiences of professional involvement and concerns in particular about confidentiality. This is a particularly salient issue for young people who have had involvement with the criminal justice system when professional assessments and information collated about them can have a significant impact on their liberty and freedom. For these young people professionals often represent figures of power and authority over their lives and are therefore not to be trusted. These young people do not necessarily differentiate between professionals with statutory powers over them, for example police and social workers, and those without statutory powers, for example counsellors and other related health professionals. Indeed the young people are only too aware that these professionals talk to each other and therefore they are cautious about what they say to any professional.

Most of the young people were able to acknowledge the need for information about them to be shared amongst professionals in certain circumstances. Their concern, often based on previous experience, was the process in which this information would be shared. Transparency about what information would be shared with whom and in what circumstances was considered very important by the young people in establishing a relationship of trust with professionals trying to help them.

Consistency of care and the interpersonal style of the professional or worker was also considered important. Many of the young people had encountered disrupted family relationships throughout their childhoods which had to an extent been compounded by frequent changes in professionals they had encountered during this time. This was often experienced as lack of care and interest on the part of the professionals and therefore the young person felt less investment or confidence in the professional relationship. Trusted professionals were those who demonstrated a commitment to the young person over time, often beyond the remit of their professional role. They were also professionals who had good interpersonal skills that enabled the young person to feel at ease when talking to them.

Many of the young people identified that talking to someone who had encountered similar problems to their own, that they could relate to on a personal level, such as a mentor, would be helpful, particularly in 'brokering' relationships with, and assisting them to engage, in wider professional networks and support services.

**Intervention**

The young people were able to describe positive examples of professionals who had helped them and made some specific suggestions of how professionals could work constructively with them and their families. This was particularly the case for professionals involved in parenting and family support programmes and for teachers working with young people who are finding it difficult to learn at school.

Some of the young people described how attempts made by professionals to engage their parents in parenting programmes had resulted in their parents becoming angry and defensive, which had resulted in the young people feeling unsafe and less willing to engage in these programmes in the future. In this context the provision of this service had more potential harm than benefit for the young person.

Many of the young people gave suggestions of more indirect ways of engaging their parents in support services designed to improve family relationships. These included individual sessions with the young person that could be used to explore safe ways of them communicating their needs and wishes to the parent (through video recordings or letter writing) and to attempt to engage the parent in the process by demonstrating that they (the young person) were willing and able to change their behaviour.

The young people were also able to describe positive experiences of teachers and education-based behaviour support workers who had helped them to learn whilst at school. Teachers who were able to demonstrate that they cared about the young person's education and who created a class-room ethos of 'flexible control', whereby the young person was given some freedom to choose the best way of learning for them, were most respected and valued. Being allowed to listen to music through headphones within a classroom setting was frequently cited as an example of what had helped them to learn in the past.

The young people particularly valued professionals who had taken time to get to know them and who had demonstrated they cared and who had given them choices and control over the help they were offered.

## Delivery of care

The location of services appeared to be a less significant issue for the young people than the issues of trust and confidentiality outlined above. A key consideration was the ability to establish a relationship with someone they could trust, who enabled them to feel relaxed and at ease about talking about their problems or concerns. A location that assisted in this process was, to this extent considered important. For example some young people described how meeting in cafes and community centres would help them to have a more relaxed conversation with their worker. Such relationships had, however, also been established within prison. Workers who could be flexible and responsive to the preferences of the young people, within the limits of the service being offered, were most valued.

Professional assessments were often described as intrusive and unhelpful by the young people. This appeared linked to concerns about confidentiality, previous experiences of multiple professional and multi-agency involvement in their lives and frequent changes in the workers responsible for their care. This was often experienced by the young people as being asked the same questions by several different professionals they had not yet formed a trusting relationship with, and where there appeared to be no tangible benefits or incentive for the young person to engage in the assessment. Assessments that involved more than one professional, and where professionals openly took notes throughout the assessment interview, were described as particularly unhelpful. Transparency about confidentiality issues, open recording policies and the importance of involving the young person in any changes and transfers in professionals working with them were all suggested as helpful ways forward in helping the young people develop more confidence in the services being offered to them.

The importance of self-referrals and of being offered choice and an element of control about who they approached for help, were also common themes that emerged during the focus group discussions. Having easy access to workers who they could approach when they needed help, and which didn't require them to be referred by other professionals was often considered most helpful. The use of mentors, or workers they felt they could relate to in a more informal and relaxed manner, and who could act as mediators or advocates to assist the young person to get appropriate help from more formal statutory and public services, was seen as particularly valuable.

Some young people described how they had been helped most during periods of crisis and significant change in their lives, such as imprisonment or family breakdown. This may indicate that services that are offered to young people at such points in their life are likely to be more effective.

Generally there appeared to be little difference in the experiences or views expressed between the young women and young men within the group and therefore gender did not appear to be a significant factor, in terms of access to care, intervention, or service delivery for this particular group of young people.

## PROPOSALS FOR RECOMMENDATIONS

### Access to care

1. The largest barrier to these young people accessing services was their mistrust of professionals linked to concerns about confidentiality and previously negative experiences of professional involvement in their lives. Services attempting to engage these young people therefore need to develop clear policies on confidentiality that encourage openness and transparency with the young person about what information will be shared with other agencies and in what circumstances.

### Intervention

2. Being able to develop a trusting relationship with professionals trying to help them was the most important consideration for the young people when describing positive experiences of services they had received. This finding supports recommendations made by previous related NICE Guidance:

   *'Build a trusting relationship, work in an open, engaging and non-judgemental manner, and be consistent and reliable.'*[123]

3. Family-based behaviour support programmes should only be offered when it has been established the young person feels safe and supported enough to work openly with their parents about changes that need to be made to help them improve their behaviour. The young person needs to be central to this process and their ideas about how to engage parents utilised.

---

[123]*Antisocial Personality Disorder* (NICE clinical guideline 77).

4. School-based behaviour intervention programmes need to offer young people flexibility and choice about methods and techniques that help them to learn the most.

**Delivery of care**

5. Professional assessments need to be undertaken over time, enabling the young person to establish a relationship of trust with the professional undertaking the assessment. Open note taking during formal assessments and the involvement of more than one professional during assessment interviews should be avoided. Offering young people choice about the location of the assessment interview and who they might like to be there to help them in this process (for example, a mentor or advocate) is more likely to engage the young person in the assessment process.

6. These young people valued being offered an element of autonomy and choice in the services made available to them. This finding also supports previous, related NICE guidance:

> *Work in partnership with people with antisocial personality disorder to develop their autonomy and promote choice by: ensuring that they remain actively involved in finding solutions to their problems, including during crises; encouraging them to consider the different treatment options life choices available to them and the consequences of the choices they make.'*[124]

7. Offering services to young people at a time when they are encountering crises and periods of significant change in their life, and therefore more receptive to support services offered to them may be a more effective means of engaging these young people in meaningful change.

**CASE STUDY**

Sophie is 18 years old; she has three older sisters and one older brother, and two younger sisters and one younger brother. Her sister died in January of this year at 19 years of age. Her step-father died 6 years ago. At the age of 6 Sophie suffered sexual abuse from a neighbour who was in a position of trust in the family and used to look after the children at times. After this, Sophie states her mum struggled to cope with what had happened and that her mum's mental health deteriorated from there. This meant that there were problems in trusting people with Sophie's care, and this impacted negatively on the relationship between her mum and dad, often meaning that her dad wasn't allowed to see Sophie without her mum being there. Sophie states she doesn't remember being offered any therapeutic help

---

[124]NICE. 2009. *Antisocial Personality Disorder: Treatment, Management and Prevention*. NICE clinical guideline 77. London: NICE. Available from: www.nice.org.uk/guidance/CG77

and talked about how hard it was knowing her mum could hear her giving video evidence to the police (even though she was behind a screen and not in the room). She remembers feeling worried about how much her telling things to the police might be hurting her mum. Sophie states her mum smoked more after this and struggled to cope so Sophie went to stay at her Nan's a lot.

At around age 10 Sophie started self-harming and was cutting at home and at school. She remembers that at school the health nurses and teachers would see her arms and ask about it as there was blood on her school shirt; Sophie said she would tell them her cat scratched her and nothing further happened.

Sophie remembers how her step mum taught her how to hurt herself and burn herself and how doing it can help you cope with anger. After her step dad died at around age 12/13, Sophie stayed at her step mum's house for a few weeks and was given a knife to cut herself with by her step mum and told this was a good way to cope instead of crying. Sophie remembers that her mum found glass in her pencil case when she was aged 13, which led to a big fight between them. Her mum threatened to cut herself too and suggested to Sophie that maybe 'they should die together'. Sophie was shocked by this and states she never cut herself again.

At 16, Sophie's mum suffered a stroke and now has impaired mobility. Sophie states around this time she started to hang round with girls who were offending which led to her spending time on remand for a month and a half in prison. This is where she states she finally got help and that she knows this means something because the woman is still in touch with her now and rings for a chat and to meet up to see how she is doing. Sophie says she knows this woman genuinely cared because she keeps in touch now even though she isn't paid to do so. Sophie says it makes her feel like someone has faith in her, she trusts her and doesn't want to let her down by getting into trouble.

Sophie talks about her 7 year old sister who hasn't had any counselling about the bereavements (step-dad and recently 19 year old sister) in the family. Sophie says her sister tells her she wants to kill herself, and her little brother is naughty too. Her mum struggles to cope with the younger children due to her stroke. Carers go to the house three times a day to help with her mum's care and Sophie goes there every other day and cares for her two younger siblings to help her mum. Sophie describes how her little sister is trying to care for their mum too.

Sophie is currently living in a hostel and is hoping to get a flat soon so she can have her two younger siblings there some of the time to help her mum out with their care and allow her time to rest.

For more information please contact:
User Voice
20 Newburn Street
London SE11 5PJ
Tel: 020 3137 7471
Email: info@uservoice.org
Website: www.uservoice.org

# 11   REFERENCES

Achenbach TM. Manual for the Child Behavior Checklist and 1991 Profile. Burlington, VT: University of Vermont, Department of Psychiatry; 1991.

Achenbach TM. Diagnosis, assessment, taxonomy, and case formulations. In: Ollendick TH, Hersen M, eds. Handbook of Child Psychopathology. 3rd edn. New York, NY: Plenum Press; 1998. p. 63–87.

Achenbach TM, Rescorla LA. Manual for the ASEBA Preschool Forms and Profiles. Burlington, VT: University of Vermont, Research Center for Children, Youth, & Families; 2001.

Achenbach TM, McConaughy SH, Howell CT. Child/adolescent behavioral and emotional problems: implications of cross-informant correlations for situational specificity. Psychological Bulletin. 1987;101:213–32.

Adams JF. Impact of parent training on family functioning. Child and Family Behavior Therapy. 2001;23:29–42.

Adamshick PZ. The lived experience of girl-to-girl aggression in marginalized girls. Qualitative Health Research. 2010;20:541–55.

Adelman HS, Taylor L. On Understanding Intervention in Psychology and Education. Westport, CT: Praeger; 1994.

AGREE Collaboration. Development and validation of an international appraisal instrument for assessing the quality of clinical practice guidelines: the AGREE project. Quality and Safety in Health Care. 2003;12:18–23.

Aldgate J, Rose W, McIntosh M. Changing Directions for Children with Challenging Behaviour and their Families: Evaluation of CHILDREN 1st's Directions Projects. Glasgow: The Open University; 2007.

Alexander JF. Short-term behavioral intervention with delinquent families: impact on family process and recidivism. Journal of Abnormal Psychology. 1973;81:219–25.

Alexander JF, Robbins MS. Functional family therapy: a phase-based and multi-component approach to change. In: Murrihy RC, Ollendick TH, Kidman AD, eds. Clinical Handbook of Assessing and Treating Conduct Problems in Youth. 1st edn. New York, NY: Springer-Verlag; 2010. p. 245–71.

Allen G. Early intervention: the next steps (an independent report to Her Majesty's Government). London: HM Government Cabinet Office; 2011.

Altman DG, Bland JM. Diagnostic tests 1: sensitivity and specificity. BMJ. 1994a;308:1552.

Altman DG, Bland JM. Diagnostic tests 2: predictive values. BMJ. 1994b;309:102.

Aman MG, De Smedt G, Derivan A, Lyons B, Findling RL, Risperidone Disruptive Behavior Study Group. Double-blind, placebo-controlled study of risperidone for the treatment of disruptive behaviors in children with subaverage intelligence. American Journal of Psychiatry. 2002;159:1337–46.

*References*

American Psychiatric Association. Diagnostic and Statistical Manual of Mental Disorders (DSM-IV). 4th edn. Washington, DC: American Psychiatric Association; 1994.

American Psychiatric Association. Diagnostic and Statistical Manual of Mental Disorders: Text Revision (DSM-IV-TR). Washington, DC: American Psychiatric Association; 2000.

Arbuthnot J, Gordon DA. Behavioral and cognitive effects of a moral reasoning development intervention for high-risk behavior-disordered adolescents. Journal of Consulting and Clinical Psychology. 1986;54:208–16.

Ashkar PJ, Kenny DT. Views from the inside: young offenders' subjective experiences of incarceration. International Journal of Offender Therapy and Comparative Criminology. 2008;52:584–97.

Augimeri LK, Farrington DP, Koegl DP, Day DM. The SNAPTM Under 12 Outreach Project: effects of a community based program for children with conduct problems. Journal of Child and Family Studies. 2007;16:799–807.

August GJ, Realmuto GM, Hektner JM, Bloomquist ML. An integrated components preventive intervention for aggressive elementary school children: the Early Risers program. Journal of Consulting and Clinical Psychology. 2001;69:614–26.

August GJ, Lee SS, Bloomquist ML, Realmuto GM, Hektner JM. Dissemination of an evidence-based prevention innovation for aggressive children living in culturally diverse, urban neighborhoods: the Early Risers effectiveness study. Prevention Science. 2003;4:271–86.

August GJ, Bloomquist ML, Lee SS, Realmuto GM, Hektner JM. Can evidence-based prevention programs be sustained in community practice settings? The Early Risers' Advanced-Stage Effectiveness Trial. Prevention Science. 2006;7:151–65.

Axberg U, Hanse JJ, Broberg AG. Parents' description of conduct problems in their children: a test of the Eyberg Child Behavior Inventory (ECBI) in a Swedish sample aged 3–10. Scandinavian Journal of Psychology. 2008;49:497–505.

Azrin NH, Donahue B, Teichner G, Crum T, Howell J, DeCato L. A controlled evaluation and description of individual-cognitive problem solving and family-behavioral therapies in conduct-disordered and substance-dependent youth. Journal of Child and Adolescent Substance Abuse. 2001;11:1–43.

Baker-Henningham H, Walker SP, Powell C, Gardner JM. Preventing behaviour problems through a universal intervention in Jamaican basic schools: a pilot study. West Indian Medical Journal. 2009;58:460–64.

Baker-Henningham H, Scott S, Jones K, Walker S. Reducing child conduct problems and promoting social skills in a middle-income country: cluster randomised controlled trial. British Journal of Psychiatry. 2012;201:1–8.

Bangs ME, Hazell P, Danckaerts M, Hoare P, Coghill DR, Wehmeier PM, et al. Atomoxetine for the treatment of attention-deficit/hyperactivity disorder and oppositional defiant disorder. Pediatrics. 2008;121:e314–20.

Bank L, Marlowe JH, Reid JB, Patterson GR, Weinrott MR. A comparative evaluation of parent-training interventions for families of chronic delinquents. Journal of Abnormal Child Psychology. 1991;19:15–33.

Banks R, Hogue A, Timberlake T, Liddle H. An Afrocentric approach to group social skills training with inner-city African American adolescents. Journal of Negro Education. 1996;65:414–23.

Barber AJ, Tischler VA, Healy E. Consumer satisfaction and child behaviour problems in child and adolescent mental health services. Journal of Child Health Care. 2006;10:9–21.

Barnes J, Ball M, Meadows P, McLeish J, Belsky J, FNP Implementation Research Team. Nurse-Family Partnership Programme: First Year Pilot Sites Implementation in England: Pregnancy and the Post-partum Period. Research Report DCSF-RW051. London: Department for Children Schools and Families; 2008.

Barnoski R. Outcome Evaluation of Washington State's Research-based Programs for Juvenile Offenders. Document No. 04–01-1201. Olympia, WA: Washington State Institute for Public Policy; 2004.

Barrett B, Byford S, Chitsabesan P, Kenning C, Barrett B, Byford S, et al. Mental health provision for young offenders: service use and cost. British Journal of Psychiatry. 2006;188:541–46.

Barrett PM, Turner CM, Rombouts S, Duffy AL. Reciprocal skills training in the treatment of externalising behaviour disorders in childhood: a preliminary investigation. Behaviour Change. 2000;17:221–34.

Barzman DH, DelBello MP, Adler CM, Stanford KE, Strakowski SM. The efficacy and tolerability of quetiapine versus divalproex for the treatment of impulsivity and reactive aggression in adolescents with co-occurring bipolar disorder and disruptive behavior disorder(s). Journal of Child and Adolescent Psychopharmacology. 2006;16:665–70.

Bauer SR, Sapp M, Johnson D. Group counseling strategies for rural at-risk high school students. The High School Journal. 2000;83:41–50.

Beauchaine TP, Hong J, Marsh P. Sex differences in autonomic correlates of conduct problems and aggression. Journal of the American Academy of Child and Adolescent Psychiatry. 2008;47:788–96.

Begg CB, Mazumdar M. Operating characteristics of a rank correlation test for publication bias. Biometrics. 1994;50:1088–101.

Behan J, Fitzpatrick C, Sharry J, Carr A, Waldron B. Evaluation of the Parenting Plus Programme. Irish Journal of Psychology. 2001;22:238–56.

Belsky J, Melhuish E, Barnes J, Leyland AH, Romaniuk H. Effects of Sure Start local programmes on children and families: early findings from a quasi-experimental, cross sectional study. BMJ. 2006;332:1476.

Berlin JA. Does blinding of readers affect the results of meta-analyses? University of Pennsylvania Meta-analysis Blinding Study Group. Lancet. 1997;350:185–86.

Bernal ME, Klinnert MD, Schultz LA. Outcome evaluation of behavioral parent training and client-centered parent counseling for children with conduct problems. Journal of Applied Behavior Analysis. 1980;13:677–91.

Blader JC, Schooler NR, Jensen PS, Pliszka SR, Kafantaris V. Adjunctive divalproex versus placebo for children with ADHD and aggression refractory to stimulant monotherapy. American Journal of Psychiatry. 2009;166:1392–401.

Blair RJR, Mitchell D, Blair K. The Psychopath: Emotion and the Brain. London: Blackwell Publishing; 2005.

## References

Bodenmann GC. The efficacy of the Triple P-Positive Parenting Program in improving parenting and child behavior: A comparison with two other treatment conditions. Behaviour Research and Therapy. 2008;46:411–27.

Bonin EM, Stevens M, Beecham J, Byford S, Parsonage M. Costs and longer-term savings of parenting programmes for the prevention of persistent conduct disorder: a modelling study. BMC Public Health. 2011;11:803.

Borduin CM, Mann BJ, Cone LT, Henggeler SW, Fucci BR, Blaske DM, et al. Multisystemic treatment of serious juvenile offenders: long-term prevention of criminality and violence. Journal of Consulting and Clinical Psychology. 1995;63:569–78.

Borduin CM, Schaeffer CM. Multisystemic treatment of juvenile sexual offenders: a progress report. Journal of Psychology and Human Sexuality. 2002;13:25–42.

Borenstein M, Hedges L, Higgins J, Rothstein H. Comprehensive Meta-analysis [Computer program]. Version 2. Englewood, NJ: Biostat; 2005.

Botvin GJ, Griffin KW, Nichols TD. Preventing youth violence and delinquency through a universal school-based prevention approach. Prevention Science. 2006;7:403–08.

Bradley SJ, Jadaa DA, Brody J, Landy S, Tallett SE, Watson W, et al. Brief psychoeducational parenting program: an evaluation and 1-year follow-up. Journal of the American Academy of Child and Adolescent Psychiatry. 2003;42:1171–78.

Braet C, Meerschaert T, Merlevede E, Bosmans G, Van Leeuwen K, De Mey W. Prevention of antisocial behaviour: evaluation of an early intervention programme. European Journal of Developmental Psychology. 2009;6:223–40.

Braswell L, August GJ, Bloomquist ML, Realmuto GM, Skare SS, Crosby RD. School-based secondary prevention for children with disruptive behavior: initial outcomes. Journal of Abnormal Child Psychology. 1997;25:197–208.

Brennan PA, Grekin ER, Mednick SA. Prenatal and perinatal influences on conduct disorder and serious delinquency. In: Lahey BL, Moffitt TE, Caspi A, eds. Causes of Conduct Disorder and Juvenile Delinquency. New York, NY: Guilford Press; 2003. p. 319–44.

Brody GH, Kogan SM, Chen YF, McBride Murry V. Long-term effects of the Strong African American Families program on youths' conduct problems. Journal of Adolescent Health. 2008;43:474–81.

Brody GH, Chen YF, Kogan SM, Yu T, Molgaard VK, DeClemente RJ, et al. Family-centered program deters substance use, conduct problems, and depressive symptoms in black adolescents. Pediatrics. 2012;129:108–15.

Brookman-Frazee L, Garland AF, Taylor R, Zoffness R. Therapists' attitudes towards psychotherapeutic strategies in community-based psychotherapy with children with disruptive behavior problems. Administration and Policy in Mental Health. 2009;36:1–12.

Brotman LM, Klein RG, Kamboukos D, Brown EJ, Coard SI, Sosinsky LS. Preventive intervention for urban, low-income preschoolers at familial risk for conduct problems: a randomized pilot study. Journal of Clinical Child and Adolescent Psychology. 2003;32:246–57.

Brotman LM, Gouley KK, Chesir-Teran D, Dennis T, Klein RG, Shrout P. Prevention for preschoolers at high risk for conduct problems: immediate outcomes on parenting practices and child social competence. Journal of Clinical Child and Adolescent Psychology. 2005;34:724–34.

Brunk M, Henggeler SW, Whelan JP. Comparison of multisystemic therapy and parent training in the brief treatment of child abuse and neglect. Journal of Consulting and Clinical Psychology. 1987;55:171–78.

Budd T, Sharp C, Mayhew P. Offending in England and Wales: first results from the 2003 Crime and Justice Survey Home Office. London: Home Office Research Development and Statistics Directorate; 2005.

Buitelaar JK, Van der Gaag RJ, Cohen-Kettenis P, Melman CT. A randomized controlled trial of risperidone in the treatment of aggression in hospitalized adolescents with subaverage cognitive abilities. Journal of Clinical Psychiatry. 2001;62:239–48.

Burke JD, Loeber R, Lahey BB, Rathouz PJ. Developmental transitions among affective and behavioral disorders in adolescent boys. Journal of Child Psychology and Psychiatry. 2005;46:1200–10.

Burns GL, Owen SM. Disruptive behaviors in the classroom: initial standardization data on a new teacher rating scale. Journal of Abnormal Child Psychology. 1990;18:515–25.

Burns GL, Patterson DR. Factor structure of the Eyberg Child Behavior Inventory: unidimensional or multidimensional measure of disruptive behavior? Journal of Clinical Child Psychology. 1991;20:439–44.

Burns GL, Patterson DR. Factor structure of the Eyberg Child Behavior Inventory: a parent rating scale of oppositional defiant behavior toward adults, inattentive behavior, and conduct problem behavior. Journal of Clinical Child Psychology. 2000;29:569–77.

Bushman BB, Peacock GG. Does teaching problem-solving skills matter? An evaluation of problem-solving skills training for the treatment of social and behavioral problems in children. Child and Family Behavior Therapy. 2010;32:103–24.

Butler S, Baruch G, Hickey N, Fonagy P. A randomized controlled trial of multisystemic therapy and a statutory therapeutic intervention for young offenders. Journal of the American Academy of Child and Adolescent Psychiatry. 2011;50:1220–35.

Butz AM, Pulsifer M, Marano N, Belcher H, Lears MK, Royall R. Effectiveness of a home intervention for perceived child behavioral problems and parenting stress in children with in utero drug exposure. Archives of Pediatrics and Adolescent Medicine. 2001;155:1029–37.

Bywater T, Hutchings J, Linck P, Whitaker C, Daley D, Yeo ST, et al. Incredible Years parent training support for foster carers in Wales: a multi-centre feasibility study. Child: Care, Health and Development. 2011;37:233–43.

Caldwell MF, Vitacco M, Rybroek GJ. Are violent delinquents worth treating? A cost-benefit analysis. Journal of Research in Crime and Delinquency 2006;43:148–68.

Callaghan J, Young B, Pace F, Vostanis P. Evaluation of a new mental health service for looked after children. Clinical Child Psychology and Psychiatry. 2004;9:130–48.

Campbell SB, Ewing LJ. Follow-up of hard-to-manage preschoolers: adjustment at age 9 and predictors of continuing symptoms. Journal of Child Psychology and Psychiatry. 1990;31:871–89.

Campbell M, Small AM, Green WH. Lithium and haloperidol in hospitalized aggressive children. Psychopharmacology Bulletin. 1982;18:126–30.

Campbell M, Adams PB, Small AM, Kafantaris V, Silva RR, Shell J, et al. Lithium in hospitalized aggressive children with conduct disorder: a double-blind and placebo-controlled study. Journal of the American Academy of Child and Adolescent Psychiatry. 1995;34:445–53. Erratum in: 1995;34:694.

Campbell SB, Spieker S, Burchinal M, Poe MD, Network NECCR. Trajectories of aggression from toddlerhood to age 9 predict academic and social functioning through age 12. Journal of Child Psychology and Psychiatry. 2006;47:791–800.

Carnes-Holt K. Child-parent relationship therapy (CPRT) with adoptive families: effects on child behavior, parent-child relationship stress, and parental empathy [dissertation]. Denton, TX: University of North Texas; 2010.

Cavell TA, Hughes JN. Secondary prevention as context for assessing change processes in aggressive children. Journal of School Psychology. 2000;38:199–235.

Ceballos PL, Bratton SC. Empowering Latino families: effects of a culturally responsive intervention for low-income immigrant Latino parents on children's behaviors and parental stress. Psychology in the Schools. 2010;47:761–75.

Cefai C, Cooper P. Students without voices: the unheard accounts of secondary school students with social, emotional and behaviour difficulties. European Journal of Special Needs Education. 2010;25:183–98.

Centre for Criminal Justice. Mainstreaming Methodology for Estimating Costs of Crime: Costing Principles and Methodology. York: University of York; 2008.

Centre for Reviews and Dissemination. NHS Economic Evaluation Database Handbook. Available from: www.york.ac.uk/inst/crd/pdf/nhseed-handbook2007.pdf. York: Centre for Reviews and Dissemination, University of York; 2007.

Chamberlain P, Reid JB. Comparison of two community alternatives to incarceration for chronic juvenile offenders. Journal of Consulting and Clinical Psychology. 1998;66:624–33.

Chamberlain P, Leve LD, Degarmo DS. Multidimensional treatment foster care for girls in the juvenile justice system: 2-year follow-up of a randomized clinical trial. Journal of Consulting and Clinical Psychology. 2007;75:187–93.

Chamberlain P, Price J, Leve L, Laurent H, Landsverk J, Reid JB. Prevention of behavior problems for children in foster care: outcomes and mediation effects. Prevention Science. 2008;9:17–27.

Champion LA, Goodall G, Rutter M. Behavioural problems in childhood and stressors in early adult life: 1. A 20 year follow-up of London school children. Psychological Medicine 1995;25:231–46.

Chao P-C, Bryan T, Burstein K, Ergul C. Family-centered intervention for young children at risk for language and behavior problems. Early Childhood Education Journal. 2006;34:147–53.

Cheney DA, Stage SA, Hawken LS, Lynass L, Mielenz C, Waugh M. A 2-year outcome study of the check, connect, and expect intervention for students at risk for severe behavior problems. Journal of Emotional and Behavioral Disorders. 2009;17:226–43.

Cheng TL, Haynie D, Brenner R, Wright JL, Chung SE, Simons-Morton B. Effectiveness of a mentor-implemented, violence prevention intervention for assault-injured youths presenting to the emergency department: results of a randomized trial. Pediatrics. 2008;122:938–46.

Choi AN, Lee MS, Lee J-S. Group music intervention reduces aggression and improves self-esteem in children with highly aggressive behavior: a pilot controlled trial. Evidence-based Complementary and Alternative Medicine. 2010;7:213–17.

Clark HB, Prange ME, Lee B, Boyd LA, McDonald BA, Stewart ES. Improving adjustment outcomes for foster children with emotional and behavioral disorders: early findings from a controlled study on individualized services. Journal of Emotional and Behavioral Disorders. 1994;2:207.

Coatsworth JD, Santisteban DA, McBride CK, Szapocznik J. Brief strategic family therapy versus community control: engagement, retention, and an exploration of the moderating role of adolescent symptom severity. Family Process. 2001;40:313–32.

Cochrane Collaboration, The. Review Manager (RevMan) [Computer programme]. Version 5.1. Copenhagen: The Nordic Cochrane Centre, The Cochrane Collaboration; 2011.

Cohen MA. The monetary value of saving a high-risk youth. Journal of Quantitative Criminology. 1998;14:5–33.

Cohen MA, Miller TR. Cost of mental health care for victims of crime. Journal of Interpersonal Violence. 1998;13:93–110.

Cohen MA, Piquero AP. New evidence on the monetary value of saving a high risk youth. Journal of Quantitative Criminology. 2009;25:25–49.

Cohen P, Cohen J, Brook J. An epidemiological study of disorders in late childhood and adolescence: II. Persistence of disorders. Journal of Child Psychology and Psychiatry. 1993;34:869–77.

Coie JD. The impact of negative social experiences on the development of antisocial behavior. In: Kupersmidt JB, Dodge KA, eds. Children's Peer Relations: From Development to Intervention. Washington, DC: American Psychological Association; 2004. p. 243–67.

Collishaw S, Maughan B, Goodman R, Pickles A. Time trends in adolescent mental health. Journal of Child Psychology and Psychiatry. 2004;45:1350–62.

Colvin A, Eyberg SM, Adams C. Standardization of the Eyberg Child Behavior Inventory with Chronically Ill Children. Available from: www.pcit.org. Gainesville, FL: University of Florida, Child Study Laboratory; 1999.

Commission for Health Improvement. The Experience of Service Questionnaire Handbook. London: Department of Health; 2002.

Conduct Problems Prevention Research Group. A developmental and clinical model for the prevention of conduct disorders: the FAST Track program. Development and Psychopathology. 1992;4:509–27.

Conduct Problems Prevention Research Group. Initial impact of the Fast Track prevention trial for conduct problems: II. Classroom effects. Conduct Problems Prevention Research Group. Journal of Consulting and Clinical Psychology. 1999;67:648–57.

*References*

Conduct Problems Prevention Research Group. The effects of the Fast Track preventive intervention on the development of conduct disorder across childhood. Child Development. 2011;82:331–45.

Connell S, Sanders MR, Markie-Dadds C. Self-directed behavioral family intervention for parents of oppositional children in rural and remote areas. Behavior Modification. 1997;21:379–408.

Conners CK, Eisenberg L. The effects of methylphendiate on symptomatology and learning in disturbed children. American Journal of Psychiatry. 1963;120:458–64.

Conners CK, Kramer R, Rothschild GH, Schwartz L, Stone A. Treatment of young delinquent boys with diphenylhydantoin sodium and methyphenidate. A controlled comparison. Archives of General Psychiatry. 1971;24:156–60.

Conners CK, Wells KC, Parker JD, Sitarenios G, Diamond JM, Powell JW. A new self-report scale for assessment of adolescent psychopathology: factor structure, reliability, validity, and diagnostic sensitivity. Journal of Abnormal Child Psychology. 1997;25:487–97.

Connor DF, McLaughlin TJ, Jeffers-Terry M. Randomized controlled pilot study of quetiapine in the treatment of adolescent conduct disorder. Journal of Child and Adolescent Psychopharmacology. 2008;18:140–56.

Connor DF, Findling RL, Kollins SH, Sallee F, López FA, Lyne A, et al. Effects of guanfacine extended release on oppositional symptoms in children aged 6–12 years with attention-deficit hyperactivity disorder and oppositional symptoms: a randomized, double-blind, placebo-controlled trial. CNS Drugs. 2010;24:755–68.

Côté S, Tremblay RE, Nagin D, Zoccolillo M, Vitaro F. The development of impulsivity, fearfulness, and helpfulness during childhood: patterns of consistency and change in the trajectories of boys and girls. Journal of Child Psychology and Psychiatry. 2002;43:609–18.

Cowan PA, Cowan CP, Kline Pruett M, Pruett K, Wong JJ. Promoting fathers' engagement with children: preventive interventions for low-income families. Journal of Marriage and Family. 2009;71:663–79.

Cueva JE, Overall JE, Small AM, Armenteros JL, Perry R, Campbell M. Carbamazepine in aggressive children with conduct disorder: a double-blind and placebo-controlled study. Journal of the American Academy of Child and Adolescent Psychiatry. 1996;35:480–90.

Cummings EM, Davies PT. Effects of marital conflict on children: recent advances and emerging themes in process-oriented research. Journal of Child Psychology and Psychiatry. 2002;43:31–63.

Cummings JG, Wittenberg JV. Supportive expressive therapy–parent child version: an exploratory study. Psychotherapy (Chicago). 2008;45:148–64.

Cunningham CE, Bremner R, Boyle M. Large group community-based parenting programs for families of preschoolers at risk for disruptive behaviour disorders: utilization, cost effectiveness, and outcome. Journal of Child Psychology and Psychiatry. 1995;36:1141–59.

Curtis L. Unit Costs of Health and Social Care 2011. Canterbury: University of Kent; 2011.

Dadds MR, McHugh TA. Social support and treatment outcome in behavioral family therapy for child conduct problems. Journal of Consulting and Clinical Psychology. 1992;60:252–59.

Davies J, Wright J. Children's voices: a review of the literature pertinent to looked-after children's views of mental health services. Child and Adolescent Mental Health. 2008;13:26–31.

Deffenbacher JL, Lynch RS, Oetting ER, Kemper CC. Anger reduction in early adolescents. Journal of Counseling Psychology. 1996;43:149–57.

Dell'Agnello G, Maschietto D, Bravaccio C, Calamoneri F, Masi G, Curatolo P, et al. Atomoxetine hydrochloride in the treatment of children and adolescents with attention-deficit/hyperactivity disorder and comorbid oppositional defiant disorder: a placebo-controlled Italian study. European Neuropsychopharmacology. 2009;19:822–34.

Dembo R, Ramirez-Garnica G, Schmeidler J, Pacheco K. The impact of a family empowerment intervention on target youth recidivism: a one year follow-up. Program/project evaluations Contract No.: NCJ 171841. Bethesda, MD: National Institute of Health; 1997.

Dembo R, Ramirez-Garnica G, Rollie M, Schmeidler J, Livingston S, Hartsfield A. Youth recidivism twelve months after a family empowerment intervention: final report. Journal of Offender Rehabilitation. 2000;31:29–65.

Dembo R, Schmeidler J, Seeberger W, Shemwell M, Rollie M, Pacheco K, et al. Long-term impact of a family empowerment intervention on juvenile offender psychosocial functioning. Journal of Offender Rehabilitation. 2001;33:59–109.

Department of Health. A national service framework for mental health: modern standards and service models. Available at: http://www.dh.gov.uk/en/Publicationsandstatistics/Publications/PublicationsPolicyAndGuidance/DH_4009598. London: Department of Health; 1999.

DeRosier ME, Gilliom M. Effectiveness of a parent training program for improving children's social behavior. Journal of Child and Family Studies. 2007;16:660–70.

Desbiens N, Royer E. Peer groups and behaviour problems: a study of school-based intervention for children with EBD. Emotional and Behavioural Difficulties. 2003;8:120–39.

Dick DM, Aliev F, Krueger RF, Edwards A, Agrawal A, Lynskey M, et al. Genome-wide association study of conduct disorder symptomatology. Molecular Psychiatry. 2011;16:800–08.

Dionne R, Davis B, Sheeber L, Madrigal L. Initial evaluation of a cultural approach to implementation of evidence-based parenting interventions in American Indian communities. Journal of Community Psychology. 2009;37:911–21.

Dirks-Linhorst PA. An evaluation of a family court diversion program for delinquent youth with chronic mental health needs [dissertation]. St Louis, MO: University of Missouri; 2003.

Dishion TJ, Andrews DW. Preventing escalation in problem behaviors with high-risk young adolescents: immediate and 1-year outcomes. Journal of Consulting and Clinical Psychology. 1995;63:538–48.

*References*

Dishion TJ, Shaw D, Connell A, Gardner F, Weaver C, Wilson M. The family check-up with high-risk indigent families: preventing problem behavior by increasing parents' positive behavior support in early childhood. Child Development. 2008;79:1395–414.

Dittmann RW, Schacht A, Helsberg K, Schneider-Fresenius C, Lehmann M, Lehmkuhl MD, et al. Atomoxetine versus placebo in children and adolescents with attention-deficit/hyperactivity disorder and comorbid oppositional defiant disorder: A double-blind, randomized, multicenter trial in Germany. Journal of Child and Adolescent Psychopharmacology. 2011;21:97–110.

Dodge K, Rutter M, eds. Gene-environment Interactions in Developmental Psychopathology. New York, NY: Guildford Press; 2011.

Dodge KA. Translational science in action: hostile attributional style and the development of aggressive behavior problems. Development and Psychopathology. 2006;18:791–814.

Dodgen DW. Skills training for incarcerated juvenile delinquents [dissertation]. Houston, TX: University of Houston; 1995.

Domitrovich CE, Cortes RC, Greenberg MT. Improving young children's social and emotional competence: a randomized trial of the preschool 'PATHS' curriculum. The Journal of Primary Prevention. 2007;28:67–91.

Donovan SJ, Stewart JW, Nunes EV, Quitkin FM, Parides M, Daniel W, et al. Divalproex treatment for youth with explosive temper and mood lability: a double-blind, placebo-controlled crossover design. American Journal of Psychiatry. 2000;157:818–20. Erratum in: 2000;157:1192.

Dozier M, Peloso E, Lindhiem O, Gordon MK, Manni M, Sepulveda S, et al. Developing evidence-based interventions for foster children: an example of a randomized clinical trial with infants and toddlers. Journal of Social Issues. 2006;62:767–85.

Dretzke J, Frew E, Davenport C, Barlow J, Stewart-Brown S, Sandercock J, et al. The effectiveness and cost-effectiveness of parent training/education programmes for the treatment of conduct disorder, including oppositional defiant disorder, in children. Report No.: 50. Southampton: Health Technology Assessment; 2005.

Drugli MB, Larsson B. Children aged 4–8 years treated with parent training and child therapy because of conduct problems: generalisation effects to day-care and school settings. European Child and Adolescent Psychiatry. 2006;15:392–99.

Dubourg R, Hamed J, Thorns J. The economic and social costs of crime against individuals and households 2003/04. Home Office On-Line Report 30/05. Available at: webarchive.nationalarchives.gov.uk/20100413151441/crimereduction.homeoffice.gov.uk/statistics/statistics39.htm; 2005.

Dumas JE. Conduct disorder. In: Turner SM, Calhoun KS, Adams HE, eds. Handbook of Clinical Behavior Therapy. 2nd edn. New York, NY: Wiley; 1992. p. 285–316.

Dupper DR, Krishef CH. School-based social-cognitive skills training for middle school students with school behavior problems. Children and Youth Services Review. 1993;15:131–42.

DuRant RH, Treiber F, Getts A, McCloud K, Linder CW, Woods ER. Comparison of two violence prevention curricula for middle school adolescents. Journal of Adolescent Health. 1996;19:111–17.

Durlak JA, Weissberg RP, Dymnicki AB, Taylor RD, Schellinger KB. The impact of enhancing students' social and emotional learning: a meta-analysis of school-based universal interventions. Child Development. 2011;82:405–32.

Duval S, Tweedie R. A nonparametric 'trim and fill' method of accounting for publication bias in meta-analysis. Journal of the American Statistical Association. 2000;95:89–98.

Eccles M, Freemantle N, Mason J. North of England evidence based guideline development project: methods of developing guidelines for efficient drug use in primary care. BMJ. 1998;316:1232–35.

Edwards RT, Céilleachair A, Bywater T, Hughes DA, Hutchings J. Parenting programme for parents of children at risk of developing conduct disorder: cost effectiveness analysis. BMJ. 2007;334:682–85.

Elias LC, Marturano EM, Motta AM, Giurlani AG. Treating boys with low school achievement and behavior problems: comparison of two kinds of intervention. Psychological Reports. 2003;92:105–16.

Elrod HP, Minor KI. Second wave evaluation of a multi-faceted intervention for juvenile court probationers. International Journal of Offender Therapy and Comparative Criminology. 1992;36:247–62.

Emshoff JG, Blakely CH. The diversion of delinquent youth: family focused intervention. Children and Youth Services Review. 1983;5:343–56.

Eyberg S. Parent and teacher behavior inventories for the assessment of conduct problem behaviors in children. In: VandeCreek L, Knapp S, Jackson TL, eds. Innovations in Clinical Practice: A Source Book. Sarasota, FL: Professional Resource Exchange; 1992. p. 377–82.

Eyberg SM, Robinson EA. Conduct problem behavior: standardization of a behavioral rating. Journal of Clinical Child Psychology. 1983;12:347–54.

Eyberg SM, Pincus D. Eyberg Child Behavior Inventory and Sutter-Eyberg Student Behavior Inventory: Professional Manual. Odessa, FL: Psychological Assessment Resources; 1999.

Farmer EMZ, Burns BJ, Wagner HR, Murray M, Southerland DG. Enhancing 'usual practice' treatment foster care: findings from a randomized trial on improving youth outcomes. Psychiatric Services. 2010;61:555–61.

Farrell AD, Meyer AL, White KS. Evaluation of Responding in Peaceful and Positive Ways (RIPP): a school-based prevention program for reducing violence among urban adolescents. Journal of Clinical Child Psychology. 2001;30:451–63.

Farrell AD, Meyer AL, Sullivan TN, Kung EM. Evaluation of the Responding in Peaceful and Positive Ways (RIPP) seventh grade violence prevention curriculum. Journal of Child and Family Studies. 2003;12:101–20.

Farrington DP. Editorial. Criminal Behaviour and Mental Health. 1994;4:83–86.

Farrington DP. The importance of child and adolescent psychopathy. Journal of Abnormal Child Psychology. 2005;33:489–97.

Feindler EL, Marriott S, Iwata M. Group anger control training for junior high school delinquents. Cognitive Therapy and Research. 1984;8:299–311.

Feinfield KA, Baker BL. Empirical support for a treatment program for families of young children with externalizing problems. Journal of Clinical Child and Adolescent Psychology. 2004;33:182–95.

Fergusson DM, Horwood LJ, Lynskey MT. The stability of disruptive childhood behaviors. Journal of Abnormal Child Psychology. 1995;23:379–96.

Fergusson DM, Horwood LJ, Lynskey MT. Childhood sexual abuse and psychiatric disorder in young adulthood: II. Psychiatric outcomes of childhood sexual abuse. Journal of the American Academy of Child and Adolescent Psychiatry. 1996;35:1365–74.

Fergusson DM, Horwood LJ, Ridder EM. Show me a child at seven: consequences of conduct problems in childhood for psychosocial functioning in adulthood. Journal of Child Psychology and Psychiatry. 2005;46:837–49.

Field F. The foundation years: preventing poor children becoming poor adults. The report of the Independent Review on Poverty and Life Chances. London: Cabinet Office; 2010.

Findling RL, McNara NK, Branicky LA, Schluchter MD, Lemon E, Blumer JL. A double-blind pilot study of risperidone in the treatment of conduct disorder. Journal of the American Academy of Child and Adolescent Psychiatry. 2000;39:509–16.

Fischer JE, Bachmann LM, Jaeschke R. A readers' guide to the interpretation of diagnostic test properties: clinical example of sepsis. Intensive Care Medicine. 2003;29:1043–51.

Fisher PA, Kim HK. Intervention effects on foster preschoolers' attachment-related behaviors from a randomized trial. Prevention Science. 2007;8:161–70.

Flannery DJ, Vazsonyi AT, Liau AK, Guo S, Powell KE, Atha H, et al. Initial behavior outcomes for the peacebuilders universal school-based violence prevention program. Developmental Psychology. 2003;39:292–308.

Flanzer J. The status of health services research on adjudicated drug-abusing juveniles: selected findings and remaining questions. Substance Use and Misuse. 2005;40:887–911.

Flay BR, Graumlich S, Segawa E, Burns JL, Holliday MY. Effects of 2 prevention programs on high-risk behaviors among African American youth – a randomized trial. Archives of Pediatrics and Adolescent Medicine. 2004;158:377–84.

Fonagy P, Target M, Cottrell D, Phillips J, Kurtz Z. What Works for Whom? A Critical Review of Treatments for Children and Adolescents. New York, NY: Guilford Publications; 2002.

Fontaine N, Carbonneau R, Barker ED, Vitaro F, Hébert M, Côté SM, et al. Girls' hyperactivity and physical aggression during childhood and adjustment problems in early adulthood: a 15-year longitudinal study. Archives of General Psychiatry. 2008;65:320–28.

Foote R, Eyberg S, Schuhmann E. Parent-child interaction approaches to the treatment of child behavior problems. In: Ollendick TH, Prinz RJ, eds. Advances in Clinical Child Psychology. New York, NY: Plenum Press; 1998. p. 125–51.

Ford T, Goodman R, Meltzer H. Service use over 18 months among a nationally representative sample of British children with psychiatric disorder. Clinical Child Psychology and Psychiatry. 2003;8:37–51.

Forehand RL, Merchant MJ, Long N, Garai E. An examination of parenting the strong-willed child as bibliotherapy for parents. Behavior Modification. 2010;34:57–76.

Forehand RL, Merchant MJ, Parent J, Long N, Linnea K, Baer J. An examination of a Group Curriculum for parents of young children with disruptive behavior. Behavior Modification. 2011;35:235–51.

Forgatch MS, DeGarmo DS. Parenting through change: an effective prevention program for single mothers. Journal of Consulting and Clinical Psychology. 1999;67:711–24.

Foster EM, Jones DE, Conduct Problems Prevention Research Group. The high costs of aggression: public expenditures resulting from conduct disorder. American Journal of Public Health. 2005;95:1767–72.

Foster EM, Jones D, Conduct Problems Prevention Research Group. Can a costly intervention be cost-effective? An analysis of violence prevention. Archives of General Psychiatry. 2006;63:1284–91.

Foster EM, Olchowski AE, Webster-Stratton CH. Is stacking intervention components cost-effective? An analysis of the Incredible Years program. Journal of the American Academy of Child and Adolescent Psychiatry. 2007;46:1414–24.

Fowles TR. Preventing recidivism with cell-phones: telehealth aftercare for juvenile offenders [dissertation]. Salt Lake City, UT: University of Utah; 2009.

Frankham J, Edwards-Kerr D, Humphrey N, Roberts L. School exclusions: learning partnerships outside mainstream education. York: Joseph Rowntree Foundation; 2007.

Franz M, Weihrauch L, Schäfer R. PALME: A preventive parental training program for single mothers with preschool aged children. Journal of Public Health. 2011;19:305–19.

Fraser MW, Day SH, Galinsky MJ, Hodges VG, Smokowski PR. Conduct problems and peer rejection in childhood: a randomized trial of the making choices and strong families programs. Research on Social Work Practice. 2004;14:313–24.

Freiden J. GAME: a clinical intervention to reduce adolescent violence in schools [dissertation]. Memphis, TN: University of Memphis; 2006.

Funderburk BW, Eyberg S. Psychometric characteristics of the Sutter-Eyberg Student Behavior Inventory: a school behavior rating scale for use with preschool children. Behavioral Assessment. 1989;11:297–313.

Funderburk BW, Eyberg S, Behar L. Psychometric properties of the Sutter-Eyberg Student Behavior Inventory with high-SES Preschoolers. Annual meeting of the American Psychological Association; August 1989; New Orleans, LA.

Fung MT, Raine A, Loeber R, Lynam DR, Steinhauer SR, Venables PH, et al. Reduced electrodermal activity in psychopathy-prone adolescents. Journal of Abnormal Psychology. 2005;114:187–96.

Furlong M, McGilloway S, Bywater T, Hutchings J, Smith SM, Donnelly M. Behavioural and cognitive-behavioural group-based parenting programmes for early-onset conduct problems in children aged 3 to 12 years. Cochrane Database of Systematic Reviews. 2012;15:Art. No.: CD008225. DOI: 10.1002/14651858. CD008225.pub2.

*References*

Gallart SC, Matthey S. The effectiveness of Group Triple P and the impact of the four telephone contacts. Behaviour Change. 2005;22:71–80.

Gardner F, Burton J, Klimes I. Randomised controlled trial of a parenting intervention in the voluntary sector for reducing child conduct problems: outcomes and mechanisms of change. Journal of Child Psychology and Psychiatry and Allied Disciplines. 2006;47:1123–32.

Gardner F, Shaw D, Dishion T, Burton J, Supplee L. Randomized prevention trial for early conduct problems: effects on proactive parenting and links to toddler disruptive behavior. Journal of Family Psychology. 2007;21:398–406.

Garralda ME, Yates P, Higginson I. Child and adolescent mental health service use: HoNOSCA as an outcome measure. The British Journal of Psychiatry. 2000;177:52–58.

Garrison SR, Stolberg AL. Modification of anger in children by affective imagery training. Journal of Abnormal Child Psychology. 1983;11:115–29.

Garza Y. Effects of culturally responsive child-centered play therapy compared to curriculum-based small group counseling with elementary-age Hispanic children experiencing externalizing and internalizing behavior problems: a preliminary study [dissertation]. Denton, TX: University of North Texas; 2004.

General Medical Council. Good practice in prescribing and managing medicines and devices. London: General Medical Council; 2013.

Glisson C, Schoenwald SK, Hemmelgarn A, Green P, Dukes D, Armstrong KS, et al. Randomized trial of MST and ARC in a two-level evidence-based treatment implementation strategy. Journal of Consulting and Clinical Psychology. 2010;78:537–50.

Goodman A, Patel V, Leon DA. Why do British Indian children have an apparent mental health advantage? Journal of Child Psychology and Psychiatry. 2010;51:1171–83.

Goodman R. The Strengths and Difficulties Questionnaire: a research note. Journal of Child Psychology and Psychiatry. 1997;38:581–6.

Goodman R. The extended version of the Strengths and Difficulties Questionnaire as a guide to child psychiatric caseness and consequent burden. Journal of Child Psychology and Psychiatry, and Allied Disciplines. 1999;40:791–9.

Goodman R. Psychometric properties of the Strengths and Difficulties Questionnaire. Journal of the American Academy of Child and Adolescent Psychiatry. 2001;40:1337–45.

Goodman R, Scott S. Comparing the Strengths and Difficulties Questionnaire and the Child Behaviour Checklist: is small beautiful? Journal of Abnormal Child Psychology. 1999;27:17–24.

Goodman R, Meltzer H, Bailey V. The Strengths and Difficulties Questionnaire: a pilot study on the validity of the self-report version. European Child and Adolescent Psychiatry. 1998;7:125–30.

Goodman R, Ford T, Simmons H, Gatward R, Meltzer H. Using the Strengths and Difficulties Questionnaire (SDQ) to screen for child psychiatric disorders in a community sample. The British Journal of Psychiatry. 2000a;177:534–9.

Goodman R, Renfrew D, Mullick M. Predicting type of psychiatric disorder from Strengths and Difficulties Questionnaire (SDQ) scores in child mental health clinics in London and Dhaka. European Child and Adolescent Psychiatry. 2000b;9:129–34.

Goodman R, Ford T, Meltzer H. Mental health problems of children in the community: 18 month follow up. BMJ. 2002;324:1496–97.

Goodman R, Ford T, Corbin T, Meltzer H. Using the Strengths and Difficulties Questionnaire (SDQ) multi-informant algorithm to screen looked-after children for psychiatric disorders. European Child and Adolescent Psychiatry. 2004;13 (Suppl. 2):II25-II31.

Gordon RS, Jr. An operational classification of disease prevention. Public Health Reports. 1983;98:107–9.

Gottfredson D, Kumpfer K, Polizzi-Fox D, Wilson D, Puryear V, Beatty P, et al. The Strengthening Washington D.C. Families Project: a randomized effectiveness trial of family-based prevention. Prevention Science. 2006;7:57–74.

Gould N, Richardson J. Parent-training/education programmes in the management of children with conduct disorders: developing an integrated evidence-based perspective for health and social care. Journal of Children's Services. 2006;1:47–60.

Green H, McGinnity A, Meltzer H, Ford T, Goodman R. Mental health of children and young people in Great Britain, 2004: summary report. Newport: Office for National Statistics; 2005.

Greene RW, Biederman J, Zerwas S, Monuteaux MC, Goring JC, Faraone SV. Psychiatric comorbidity, family dysfunction, and social impairment in referred youth with oppositional defiant disorder. American Journal of Psychiatry. 2002;159:1214–24.

Greene RW, Ablon JS, Goring JC, Raezer-Blakely L, Markey J, Monuteaux MC, et al. Effectiveness of collaborative problem solving in affectively dysregulated children with oppositional-defiant disorder: initial findings. Journal of Consulting and Clinical Psychology. 2004;72:1157–64.

Gross D, Fogg L, Webster-Stratton C, Garvey C, Julion W, Grady J. Parent training of toddlers in day care in low-income urban communities. Journal of Consulting and Clinical Psychology. 2003;71:261–78.

Grossman JB, Tierney J. Does mentoring work? An impact study of the Big Brothers Big Sisters program. Evaluation Review. 1998;22:403–26.

Haas SM, Waschbusch DA, Pelham WE, Jr., King S, Andrade BF, Carrey NJ. Treatment response in CP/ADHD children with callous/unemotional traits. Journal of Abnormal Child Psychology. 2011;39:541–52.

Hanisch C, Freund-Braier I, Hautmann C, Jänen N, Plück J, Brix G, et al. Detecting effects of the indicated prevention Programme for Externalizing Problem behaviour (PEP) on child symptoms, parenting, and parental quality of life in a randomized controlled trial. Behavioural and Cognitive Psychotherapy. 2010;38:95–112.

Hannon C, Bazalgette L, Wood C. In Loco Parentis. Available from: www.demos.co.uk/publications/inlocoparentis. London: Demos; 2010.

Harwood MD. Early identification and intervention for disruptive behavior in primary care: a randomized controlled trial [dissertation]. Gainesville, FL: University of Florida; 2006.

*References*

Hawes DJ, Dadds MR. The treatment of conduct problems in children with callous-unemotional traits. Journal of Consulting and Clinical Psychology. 2005;73:737–41.

Hazell P, Zhang S, Wolanczyk T, Barton J, Johnson M, Zuddas A, et al. Comorbid oppositional defiant disorder and the risk of relapse during 9 months of atomoxetine treatment for attention-deficit/hyperactivity disorder. European Child and Adolescent Psychiatry. 2006;15:105–10.

Hazell PL, Stuart JE. A randomized controlled trial of clonidine added to psychostimulant medication for hyperactive and aggressive children. Journal of the American Academy of Child and Adolescent Psychiatry. 2003;42:886–94.

Henggeler SW, Melton GB, Smith LA. Family preservation using multisystemic therapy: an effective alternative to incarcerating serious juvenile offenders. Journal of Consulting and Clinical Psychology. 1992;60:953–61.

Henggeler SW, Melton GB, Brondino MJ, Scherer DG, Hanley JH. Multisystemic therapy with violent and chronic juvenile offenders and their families: the role of treatment fidelity in successful dissemination. Journal of Consulting and Clinical Psychology. 1997;65:821–33.

Henggeler S, Schoenwald S, Borduin C, Rowland M, Cunningham P. Multisystemic Treatment of Antisocial Behavior in Children and Adolescents: Treatment Manuals for Practitioners. New York, NY: Guilford Press; 1998.

Henggeler SW, Pickrel SG, Brondino MJ. Multisystemic treatment of substance-abusing and dependent delinquents: outcomes, treatment fidelity, and transportability. Mental Health Services Research. 1999;1:171–84.

Henggeler SW, Halliday-Boykins CA, Cunningham PB, Randall J, Shapiro SB, Chapman JE. Juvenile drug court: enhancing outcomes by integrating evidence-based treatments. Journal of Consulting and Clinical Psychology. 2006;74:42–54.

Herrmann DS, McWhirter JJ. Anger and aggression management in young adolescents: an experimental validation of the SCARE program. Education and Treatment of Children. 2003;26:273–302.

Heywood S, Stancombe J, Street E, Mittler H, Dunn C, Kroll L. A brief consultation and advisory approach for use in child and adolescent mental health services: a pilot study. Clinical Child Psychology and Psychiatry. 2003;8:503–12.

Higgins JP, Thompson SG. Quantifying heterogeneity in a meta-analysis. Statistics in Medicine. 2002;21:1539–58.

Higgins JPT, Green S. Cochrane Handbook for Systematic Reviews of Interventions. Version 5.1.0 [updated March 2011]: The Cochrane Collaboration. Available from www.cochrane-handbook.org; 2011.

Hill J. Biological, psychological and social processes in the conduct disorders. Journal of Child Psychology and Psychiatry. 2002;43:133–64.

Hilyer JC, Wilson DG, Dillon C, Caro L, Jenkins C, Spencer WA, et al. Physical fitness training and counseling as treatment for youthful offenders. Journal of Counseling Psychology. 1982;29:292–303.

HMSO. Mental Health Act 1983 (amended 1995 and 2007). London: The Stationery Office; 1983.

HMSO. Children Act 1989 (amended 2004). London: The Stationery Office; 1989.

HMSO. Mental Capacity Act 2005. London: The Stationery Office; 2005.

Hobson C, Scott S, Rubia K. Investigation of cool and hot executive function deficits in ODD/CD independently of ADHD. Journal of Child Psychology and Psychiatry. 2011;52:1035–43.

Howard GP. Effect of group counseling on at-risk African-American female students [dissertation]. Chicago, IL: Roosevelt University; 2008.

Hutchings J, Appleton P, Smith M, Lane E, Nash S. Evaluation of two treatments for children with severe behaviour problems: child behaviour and maternal mental health outcomes. Behavioural and Cognitive Psychotherapy. 2002;30:279–95.

Hutchings J, Gardner F, Bywater T, Daley D, Whitaker C, Jones K, et al. Parenting intervention in Sure Start services for children at risk of developing conduct disorder: pragmatic randomised controlled trial. BMJ. 2007;334:678–82.

Institute of Medicine. Crossing the Quality Chasm: A New Health System for the 21st Century. Washington, DC: National Academy Press; 2001.

Ireland JL, Sanders MR, Markie-Dodds C. The impact of parent training on marital functioning: a comparison of two group versions of the Triple P-Positive Parenting Program for parents of children with early-onset conduct problems. Behavioural and Cognitive Psychotherapy. 2003;31:127–42.

Irvine AB, Biglan A, Smolkowski K, Metzler CW, Ary DV. The effectiveness of a parenting skills program for parents of middle school students in small communities. Journal of Consulting and Clinical Psychology. 1999;67:811–25.

Ishikawa S, Raine A. Prefrontal deficits and antisocial behaviour: a causal model. In: Lahey B, Moffitt TE, Caspi A, eds. Causes of Conduct Disorder and Delinquency. New York, NY: Guilford Press; 2003. p. 277–304.

Ison MS. Training in social skills: an alternative technique for handling disruptive child behavior. Psychological Reports. 2001;88:903–11.

Izard CE, King K. Accelerating the development of emotion competence in Head Start children: effects on adaptive and maladaptive behavior. Development and Psychopathology. 2008;20:369–97.

Jadad AR, Moore RA, Carroll D, Jenkinson C, Reynolds DJM, Gavaghan DJ, et al. Assessing the quality of reports of randomised clinical trials: is blinding necessary? Controlled Clinical Trials. 1996;17:1–12.

Jaffee SR, Moffitt TE, Caspi A, Taylor A. Life with (or without) father: the benefits of living with two biological parents depend on the father's antisocial behavior. Child Development. 2003;74:109–26.

Johnson DL, Breckenridge JN. The Houston Parent–Child Development Center and the primary prevention of behavior problems in young children. American Journal of Community Psychology. 1982;10:305–16.

Jouriles EN, McDonald R, Spiller L, Norwood WD, Swank PR, Stephens N, et al. Reducing conduct problems among children of battered women. Journal of Consulting and Clinical Psychology. 2001;69:774–85.

Jouriles EN, McDonald R, Rosenfield D, Stephens N, Corbitt-Shindler D, Miller PC. Reducing conduct problems among children exposed to intimate partner violence: a randomized clinical trial examining effects of Project Support. Journal of Consulting and Clinical Psychology. 2009;77:705–17.

## References

Kable JA, Coles CD, Taddeo E. Socio-cognitive habilitation using the math interactive learning experience program for alcohol-affected children. Alcoholism: Clinical and Experimental Research. 2007;31:1425–34.

Kacir CD, Gordon DA. Parenting adolescents wisely: the effectiveness of an interactive videodisk parent training program in Appalachia. Child and Family Behavior Therapy. 1999;21:1–22.

Kannappan R, Bai RL. Efficacy of yoga: cognitive and human relationship training for correcting maladjustment behaviour in deviant school boys. Journal of the Indian Academy of Applied Psychology. 2008;34:60–65.

Kaplan S, Heiligenstein J, West S, Busner J, Harder D, Dittmann R, et al. Efficacy and safety of atomoxetine in childhood attention-deficit/hyperactivity disorder with comorbid oppositional defiant disorder. Journal of Attention Disorders. 2004;8:45–52.

Kazdin AE. Dropping out of child therapy: issues for research and implications for practice. Clinical Child Psychology and Psychiatry. 1996;1:133–56.

Kazdin AE, Esveldt-Dawson K, French N, Unis AS. Effects of parent management training and problem-solving skills training combined in the treatment of antisocial child behavior. Journal of the American Academy of Child and Adolescent Psychiatry. 1987;26:416–24.

Kazdin AE, Bass D, Siegel T, Thomas C. Cognitive-behavioral therapy and relationship therapy in the treatment of children referred for antisocial behavior. Journal of Consulting and Clinical Psychology. 1989;57:522–35.

Kazdin AE, Siegel TC, Bass D. Drawing upon clinical practice to inform research on child and adolescent psychotherapy: a survey of practitioners. Professional Psychology: Research and Practice. 1990;21:189–98.

Kazdin AE, Siegel TC, Bass D. Cognitive problem-solving skills training and parent management training in the treatment of antisocial behavior in children. Journal of Consulting and Clinical Psychology. 1992;60:733–47.

Keenan K, Shaw DS. Starting at the beginning: exploring the etiology of antisocial behaviour in the first years of life. In: Lahey B, Moffitt TE, Caspi A, eds. Causes of Conduct Disorder and Delinquency. New York, NY: Guilford Press; 2003. p. 153–81.

Kellam SG, Van Horn YV. Life course development, community epidemiology, and preventive trials: a scientific structure for prevention research. American Journal of Community Psychology. 1997;25:177–88.

Kelly PJ, Lesser J, Cheng A, Oscós-Sánchez M, Martinez E, Pineda D, et al. A prospective randomized controlled trial of an interpersonal violence prevention program with a Mexican American community. Family and Community Health. 2010;33:207–15.

Kendall PC, Reber M, McLeer S, Epps J, Ronan KR. Cognitive-behavioral treatment of conduct-disordered children. Cognitive Therapy and Research. 1990;14:279–97.

Kettlewell PW, Kausch DF. The generalization of the effects of a cognitive-behavioral treatment program for aggressive children. Journal of Abnormal Child Psychology. 1983;11:101–14.

Kim-Cohen J, Caspi A, Taylor A, Williams B, Newcombe R, Craig IW, et al. MAOA, maltreatment, and gene-environment interaction predicting children's mental health: new evidence and a meta-analysis. Molecular Psychiatry. 2006;11:903–13.

King CA, Kirschenbaum DS. An experimental evaluation of a school-based program for children at risk: Wisconsin early intervention. Journal of Community Psychology. 1990;18:167–77.

Kitzman H, Olds D, Henderson CJ, Hanks C, Cole R, Tatelbaum R, et al. Effect of prenatal and infancy home visitation by nurses on pregnancy outcomes, childhood injuries, and repeated childbearing. A randomized controlled trial. Journal of the American Medical Association. 1997;278:644–52.

Klein RG, Abikoff H, Klass E, Ganeles D, Seese LM, Pollack S. Clinical efficacy of methylphenidate in conduct disorder with and without attention deficit hyperactivity disorder. Archives of General Psychiatry. 1997;54:1073–80.

Klietz SJ, Borduin CM, Schaeffer CM. Cost-benefit analysis of multisystemic therapy with serious and violent juvenile offenders. Journal of Family Psychology. 2010;24:657–66.

Kliewer W, Lepore S, Farrell A, Allison K, Meyer A, Sullivan T, et al. A school-based expressive writing intervention for at-risk urban adolescents' aggressive behavior and emotional lability. Journal of Clinical Child and Adolescent Psychology. 2011;40:639–705.

Kling A, Forster M, Sundell K, Melin L. A randomized controlled effectiveness trial of parent management training with varying degrees of therapist support. Behavior Therapy. 2010;41:530–42.

Knapp M, Scott S, Davies J. The cost of antisocial behaviour in younger children. Clinical Child Psychology and Psychiatry. 1999;4:457–73.

Knapp M, McCrone P, Fombonne E, Beecham J, Wostear G. The Maudsley long-term follow-up of child and adolescent depression: 3. Impact of comorbid conduct disorder on service use and costs in adulthood. The British Journal of Psychiatry. 2002;180:19–23.

Knapp M, McDaid D, Parsonage M, (eds). Mental health promotion and mental illness prevention: the economic case. Personal Social Services Research Unit, London School of Economics and Political Science. London: Department of Health; 2011.

Knox L, Guerra N, Williams K, Toro R. Preventing children's aggression in immigrant Latino families: a mixed methods evaluation of the families and schools together program. American Journal of Community Psychology. 2011;48:65–76.

Kolko DJ, Dorn LD, Bukstein O, Burke JD. Clinically referred ODD children with or without CD and healthy controls: comparisons across contextual domains. Journal of Child and Family Studies. 2008;17:714–34.

Kolko DJ, Dorn L, Bukstein O, Pardini D, Holden E, Hart J. Community vs. clinic-based modular treatment of children with early-onset ODD or CD: a clinical trial with 3-year follow-up. Journal of Abnormal Child Psychology. 2009;37:591–609.

Kolko DJ, Campo J, Kelleher K, Cheng Y. Improving access to care and clinical outcome for pediatric behavioral problems: a randomized trial of a nurse-administered intervention in primary care. Journal of Developmental and Behavioral Pediatrics. 2010;31:393–404.

Koot HM. Longitudinal studies of general population and community samples. In: Verhulst FC, Koot HM, eds. The Epidemiology of Child and Adolescent Psychopathology. Oxford: Oxford University Press; 1995. p. 337–65.

Kratochwill TR, Elliott SN, Loitz PA, Sladeczek I, Carlson JS. Conjoint consultation using self-administered manual and videotape parent-teacher training: effects on children's behavioral difficulties. School Psychology Quarterly. 2003;18:269–302

Kratochwill TR, McDonald L, Levin JR, Young Bear-Tibbetts H, Demaray MK. Families and Schools Together: an experimental analysis of a parent-mediated multi-family group program for American Indian children. Journal of School Psychology. 2004;42:359–83.

Lahey BB, Loeber R, Hart EL, Frick PJ, Applegate B, Zhang Q, et al. Four-year longitudinal study of conduct disorder in boys: patterns and predictors of persistence. Journal of Abnormal Psychology. 1995;104:83–93.

Lahey BB, Schwab-Stone M, Goodman SH, Waldman ID, Canino G, Rathouz PJ, et al. Age and gender differences in oppositional behavior and conduct problems: a cross-sectional household study of middle childhood and adolescence. Journal of Abnormal Psychology. 2000;109:488–503.

Landsverk JA, Burns BJ, Stambaugh LF, Rolls Reutz JA. Psychosocial interventions for children and adolescents in foster care: review of research literature. Child Welfare. 2009;88:49–69.

Lane KL. Young students at risk for antisocial behavior: the utility of academic and social skills interventions. Journal of Emotional and Behavioral Disorders. 1999;7:211–23.

Lang JM, Waterman J, Baker BL. Computeen: a randomized trial of a preventive computer and psychosocial skills curriculum for at-risk adolescents. Journal of Primary Prevention. 2009;30:587–603.

Langberg JM. A pilot evaluation of small group Challenging Horizons Program (CHP): a randomized trial. Journal of Applied School Psychology. 2006;23:31–58.

Larkin R, Thyer BA. Evaluating cognitive-behavioral group counseling to improve elementary school students' self-esteem, self-control, and classroom behavior. Behavioral Interventions. 1999;14:147–61.

Larmar S, Dadds MR, Shochet IM. Successes and challenges in preventing conduct problems in Australian preschool-aged children through the Early Impact (EI) program. Behaviour Change. 2006;23:121–37.

Larsson B, Fossum S, Clifford G, Drugli M, Handegård B, Mørch W. Treatment of oppositional defiant and conduct problems in young Norwegian children: results of a randomized controlled trial. European Child and Adolescent Psychiatry. 2009;18:42–52.

Lau AS, Fung JJ, Ho LY, Liu LL, Gudiño OG. Parent training with high-risk immigrant chinese families: a pilot group randomized trial yielding practice-based evidence. Behavior Therapy. 2011;42:413–26.

Laub JH, Sampson RJ. Shared Beginnings, Divergent lives: Delinquent Boys to Age 70. Cambridge, MA: Harvard University Press; 2003.

Lavigne JV, Lebailly SA, Gouze KR, Cicchetti C, Jessup BW, Arend R, et al. Treating oppositional defiant disorder in primary care: a comparison of three models. Journal of Pediatric Psychology. 2008;33:449–61.

Leaf PJ, Alegria M, Cohen P, Goodman SH, Horwitz SM, Hoven CW, et al. Mental health service use in the community and schools: results from the four-community MECA Study. Methods for the Epidemiology of Child and Adolescent Mental Disorders Study. Journal of the American Academy of Child and Adolescent Psychiatry. 1996;35:889–97.

Leschied AW, Cunningham A. Seeking effective interventions for young offenders: interim results of a four-year randomized study of multisystemic therapy in Ontario, Canada. London, Ontario: Centre for Children; 2002.

Letourneau EJ, Henggeler SW, Borduin CM, Schewe PA, McCart MR, Chapman JE, et al. Multisystemic therapy for juvenile sexual offenders: 1-year results from a randomized effectiveness trial. Journal of Family Psychology. 2009;23:89–102.

Leung C, Sanders MR, Leung S, Mak R, Lau J. An outcome evaluation of the implementation of the Triple P-Positive Parenting Program in Hong Kong. Family Process. 2003;42:531–44.

Lewis RV. Scared straight–California style: evaluation of the San Quentin SQUIRES program. Criminal Justice and Behavior. 1983;10:209–26.

Li K-K, Washburn I, DuBois DL, Vuchinich S, Ji P, Brechling V, et al. Effects of the Positive Action programme on problem behaviours in elementary school students: a matched-pair randomised control trial in Chicago. Psychology and Health. 2011;26:187–204.

Liabø K, Richardson J. Conduct Disorder and Offending Behaviour in Young People: Findings from Research. London: Jessica Kingsley Publishers; 2007.

Linares LO, Montalto D, Li M, Oza VS. A promising parenting intervention in foster care. Journal of Consulting and Clinical Psychology. 2006;74:32–41.

Lipman EL, Boyle MH, Cunningham C, Kenny M, Sniderman C, Duku E, et al. Testing effectiveness of a community-based aggression management program for children 7 to 11 years old and their families. Journal of the American Academy of Child and Adolescent Psychiatry. 2006;45:1085–93.

Littell JH, Popa M, Forsythe B. Multisystemic therapy for social, emotional, and behavioral problems in youth aged 10–17. Cochrane Database of Systematic Reviews. 2005;19:Art. No.: CD004797. DOI: 10.1002/14651858.CD004797.pub4.

Lochman JE. Parent and family skills training in targeted prevention programs for at-risk youth. The Journal of Primary Prevention. 2000;21:253–65.

Lochman JE, Wells KC. The Coping Power program at the middle-school transition: universal and indicated prevention effects. Psychology of Addictive Behaviors. 2002;16:S40-S54.

Lochman JE, Wells KC. The Coping Power Program for preadolescent aggressive boys and their parents: outcome effects at the 1-year follow-up. Journal of Consulting and Clinical Psychology. 2004;72:571–78.

Lochman JE, Burch PR, Curry JF, Lampron LB. Treatment and generalization effects of cognitive-behavioral and goal-setting interventions with aggressive boys. Journal of Consulting and Clinical Psychology. 1984;52:915–16.

*References*

Loeber R, Burke JD, Lahey BB, Winters A, Zera M. Oppositional defiant and conduct disorder: a review of the past 10 years, part I. Journal of the American Academy of Child and Adolescent Psychiatry. 2000;39:1468–84.

Loomes G. Valuing reductions in the risks of being a victim of crime: the 'willingness to pay' approach to valuing the 'intangible' consequences of crime. International Review of Victimology. 2007;14:237–51.

Lopata C. Progressive muscle relaxation as aggression reduction for students classified as emotionally disturbed [dissertation]. Albany, NY: State University of New York; 2003.

Lösel F, Beelmann A. Effects of child skill training in preventing antisocial behavior: a systematic review of randomized evaluations. Annals of the American Academy of Political and Social Science. 2003;587:84–109.

Lowell DI, Carter AS, Godoy L, Paulicin B, Briggs-Gowan MJ, Lowell DI, et al. A randomized controlled trial of Child FIRST: a comprehensive home-based intervention translating research into early childhood practice. Child Development. 2011;82:193–208.

Loy JH, Merry SN, Hetrick SE, Stasiak K. Atypical antipsychotics for disruptive behaviour disorders in children and youths. Cochrane Database of Systematic Reviews. 2012; Issue 9:Art. No.: CD008559. DOI: 10.1002/14651858.CD008559.pub2.

Lynam DR, Henry W. The role of neuropsychological deficits in conduct disorders. In: Hill J, Maughan B, eds. Conduct Disorders in Childhood and Adolescence. Cambridge: Cambridge University Press; 2001.

Maayan L, Correll CU. Weight gain and metabolic risks associated with antipsychotic medications in children and adolescents. Journal of Child and Adolescent Psychopharmacology. 2011;21:517–35.

Macdonald G, Turner W. An experiment in helping foster-carers manage challenging behaviour. British Journal of Social Work. 2005;35:1265–82.

Maes HH, Silberg JL, Neale MC, Eaves LJ. Genetic and cultural transmission of antisocial behavior: an extended twin parent model. Twin Research and Human Genetics. 2007;10:136–50.

Magen RH. Parents in groups: problem solving versus behavioral skills training. Research on Social Work Practice. 1994;4:172–91.

Maguin E, Zucker RA, Fitzgerald HE. The path to alcohol problems through conduct problems: a family-based approach to early intervention with risk. Journal of Research on Adolescence. 1994;4:249–69.

Malone RP, Delaney MA, Luebbert JF, Carter J, Campbell M. A double-blind placebo-controlled study of lithium in hospitalized aggressive children and adolescents with conduct disorder. Archives of General Psychiatry. 2000;57:649–54.

Mann T. Clinical Guidelines: Using Clinical Guidelines to Improve Patient Care Within the NHS. London: NHS Executive; 1996.

Markie-Dadds C, Sanders MR. A controlled evaluation of an enhanced self-directed behavioural family intervention for parents of children with conduct problems in rural and remote areas. Behaviour Change. 2006a;23:55–72.

Markie-Dadds C, Sanders MR. Self-directed Triple P (Positive Parenting Program) for mothers with children at-risk of developing conduct problems. Behavioural and Cognitive Psychotherapy. 2006b;34:259–75.

Martin AJ, Sanders MR. Balancing work and family: a controlled evaluation of the Triple P-Positive Parenting Program as a work-site intervention. Child and Adolescent Mental Health. 2003;8:161–69.

Martinez CRJ, Eddy JM. Effects of culturally adapted parent management training on Latino youth behavioral health outcomes. Journal of Consulting and Clinical Psychology. 2005;73:841–51.

Martsch MD. A comparison of two cognitive-behavioral group treatments for adolescent aggression: high-process versus low-process [dissertation]. Springfield, IL: University of Illinois; 2000.

Mathai J, Anderson P, Bourne A. Comparing psychiatric diagnoses generated by the Strengths and Difficulties Questionnaire with diagnoses made by clinicians. Australian and New Zealand Journal of Psychiatry. 2004;38:639–43.

Maughan B, Rowe R, Messer J, Goodman R, Meltzer H. Conduct disorder and oppositional defiant disorder in a national sample: developmental epidemiology. Journal of Child Psychology and Psychiatry. 2004;45:609–21.

McArdle P, D. M, Quibell T, Johnson R, Allen A, Hammal D, et al. School-based indicated prevention: a randomised trial of group therapy. Journal of Child Psychology and Psychiatry. 2002;43:705–12.

McBurnett K, Raine A, Stouthamer LM, Loeber R, Kumar AM, Kumar M, et al. Mood and hormone responses to psychological challenge in adolescent males with conduct problems. Biological Psychiatry. 2005;57:1109–16.

McCabe C, Sutcliffe P, Kaltenthaler E. Parent-training programmes in the management of conduct disorder: a report from the NICE Decision Support Unit and the ScHARR Technology Assessment Group. Sheffield: NICE; 2005.

McCabe KM. The effects of yoga on symptoms associated with conduct disorder with callous unemotional traits as a moderator [dissertation]. Coral Gables, FL: University of Miami; 2009.

McCabe K, Yeh M. Parent-child interaction therapy for Mexican Americans: a randomized clinical trial. Journal of Clinical Child and Adolescent Psychology. 2009;38:753–59.

McCart MR. Reducing violence/victimization among assaulted urban youth [dissertation]. Milwaukee, WI: University of Wisconsin; 2006.

McCollister KE, French MT, Fang H. The cost of crime to society: new crime-specific estimates for policy and program evaluation. Drug and Alcohol Dependence. 2010;108:98–109.

McConaughy SH, Kay PJ, Fitzgerald M. The Achieving, Behaving, Caring Project for preventing ED: two-year outcomes. Journal of Emotional and Behavioral Disorders. 1999;7:224–39.

McCord J, Tremblay RE. Preventing Antisocial Behavior: Interventions from Birth through Adolescence. New York, NY: Guilford Press; 1992.

McDonald L, Moberg DP, Brown R, Rodriguez-Espiricueta I, Flores NI, Burke MP, et al. After-school multifamily groups: a randomized controlled trial involving low-income, urban, Latino children. Children and Schools. 2006;28:25–34.

McFarlane JM, Groff JY, O'Brien JA, Watson K. Behaviors of children following a randomized controlled treatment program for their abused mothers. Issues in Comprehensive Pediatric Nursing. 2005;28:195–211.

McGilloway S, Ni Mhaille G, Bywater T, Furlong M, Leckey Y, Kelly P, et al. A parenting intervention for childhood behavioral problems: a randomized controlled trial in disadvantaged community-based settings. Journal of Consulting and Clinical Psychology. 2012;80:116–27.

McMahon RJ, Estes AM. Conduct problems. In: Mash EJ, Terdal LG, eds. Assessment of Childhood Disorders. 3rd edn. New York, NY: Guilford Press; 1997. p. 130–93.

McMahon RJ, Forehand R, Griest DL. Effects of knowledge of social learning principles on enhancing treatment outcome and generalization in a parent training program. Journal of Consulting and Clinical Psychology. 1981;49:526–32.

McPherson SJ, McDonald LE, Ryer CW. Intensive counseling with families of juvenile offenders. Juvenile and Family Court Journal. 1983;34:27–32.

Melhuish E, Belsky J, Anning A, Ball M, Barnes J, Romaniuk H, et al. Variation in community intervention programmes and consequences for children and families: the example of Sure Start Local Programmes. Journal of Child Psychology and Psychiatry. 2007;48:543–51.

Meltzer H, Gatward R, Goodman R, Ford T. The mental health of children and adolescents in Great Britain: summary report. London: Office for National Statistics; 2000.

Metropolitan Area Child Study Research Group. A cognitive-ecological approach to preventing aggression in urban settings: initial outcomes for high-risk children. Journal of Consulting and Clinical Psychology. 2002;70:179–94.

Michelson L, Mannarino AP, Marchione KE, Stern M, Figueroa J, Beck S. A comparative outcome study of behavioral social-skills training, interpersonal-problem-solving and non-directive control treatments with child psychiatric outpatients. Behaviour Research and Therapy. 1983;21:545–56.

Millie A, Jacobson J, McDonals E, Hough M. Anti-social behaviour strategies: finding a balance [report]. Bristol: Joseph Rowntree Foundation; 2005.

Moffitt TE. Genetic and environmental influences on antisocial behaviors: evidence from behavioral-genetic research. Advances in Genetics. 2005;55:41–104.

Moffitt T. Life-course-persistent versus adolescence-limited antisocial behaviour: a 10-year research review and a research agenda. In: Cicchetti D, Cohen DJ, eds. Developmental Psychopathology, Vol 3: Risk, Disorder, and Adaptation. Hoboken, NJ: John Wiley; 2006. p. 570–98.

Moffitt TE, Caspi A, Rutter M, Silva P. Sex Differences in Antisocial Behvaviour: Conduct Disorder, Delinquency, and Violence in the Dunedin Longitudinal Study. Cambridge: Cambridge University Press; 2001.

Moffitt TE, Arseneault L, Jaffee SR, Kim-Cohen J, Koenen KC, Odgers CL, et al. Research review: DSM-V conduct disorder: research needs for an evidence base. Journal of Child Psychology and Psychiatry. 2008;49:3–33.

Montgomery P, Bjornstad GJ, Dennis JA. Media-based behavioural treatments for behavioural problems in children. Cochrane Database of Systematic Reviews. 2006; Issue 1:Art. No.: CD002206. DOI: 10.1002/14651858.CD002206.pub3.

Moore EAG, Gogerty PL. A twelve-year follow-up study of maltreated and at-risk children who received early therapeutic child care. Child Maltreatment. 1998;3:3–16.

Moran P, Rowe R, Flach C, Briskman J, Ford T, Maughan B, et al. Predictive value of callous-unemotional traits in a large community sample. Journal of the American Academy of Child and Adolescent Psychiatry. 2009;48:1079–84.

Morawska A, Haslam D, Milne D, Sanders MR. Evaluation of a brief parenting discussion group for parents of young children. Journal of Developmental and Behavioral Pediatrics. 2011;32:136–45.

Moss E, Dubois-Comtois K, Cyr C, Tarabulsy G. Efficacy of a home-visiting intervention aimed at improving maternal sensitivity, child attachment, and behavioral outcomes for maltreated children: a randomized control trial. Development and Psychopathology. 2011;23:195–210.

Mrazek P, Haggerty RJ, Committee on Prevention of Mental Disorders, Division of Biobehavioral Sciences and Mental Disorders, Institute of Medicine, eds. Reducing Risks for Mental Disorders: Frontiers for Preventive Intervention Research. Washington, DC: National Academy Press; 1994.

Muñoz RF, Mrazek PJ, Haggerty RJ. Institute of Medicine report on prevention of mental disorders. Summary and commentary. The American Psychologist. 1996;51:1116–22.

Muntz RH, Hutchings J, Edwards RT, Hounsome B, O'Céilleachair A. Economic evaluation of treatments for children with severe behavioural problems. Journal of Mental Health Policy and Economics. 2004;7:177–89.

Muris P, Maas A. Strengths and difficulties as correlates of attachment style in institutionalized and non-institutionalized children with below-average intellectual abilities. Child Psychiatry and Human Development. 2004;34:317–28.

Murray J, Farrington DP. Risk factors for conduct disorder and delinquency: key findings from longitudinal studies. Canadian Journal of Psychiatry. 2010;55:633–42.

Murray J, Irving B, Farrington DP, Colman I, Bloxsom CA. Very early predictors of conduct problems and crime: results from a national cohort study. Journal of Child Psychology and Psychiatry. 2010;51:1198–207.

National Audit Office. The cost of a cohort of young offenders to the criminal justice system. Technical paper. Ministry of Justice. London: The National Audit Office; 2011.

NCCMH. Antisocial Personality Disorder: Treatment, Management and Prevention. London & Leicester: The British Psychological Society & The Royal College of Psychiatrists; 2010.

NCCMH. Common Mental Health Disorders: Identification and Pathways to Care. London: The British Psychological Society & The Royal College of Psychiatrists; 2011.

NCCMH. Service User Experience in Adult Mental Health: NICE Guidance on Improving the Experience of Care for People Using Adult NHS Mental Health Services. Leicester & London: The British Psychological Society & The Royal College of Psychiatrists; 2012.

Nestler J, Goldbeck L. A pilot study of social competence group training for adolescents with borderline intellectual functioning and emotional and behavioural problems (SCT-ABI). Journal of Intellectual Disability Research. 2011;55:231–41.

Newcorn JH, Spencer TJ, Biederman MD, Milton DR, Michelson D. Atomoxetine treatment in children and adolescents with attention-deficit/ hyperactivity disorder and comorbid oppositional defiant disorder. Journal of the American Academy of Child and Adolescent Psychiatry. 2005;44:240–48.

NICE. Depression in Children and Young People: Identification and Management in Primary, Community and Secondary Care. NICE clinical guideline 28. Available from: www.nice.org.uk/guidance/CG28. 2005.

NICE. Parent-Training/Education Programmes in the Management of Children with Conduct Disorders. NICE technology appraisal guidance 102. Available from: http://publications.nice.org.uk/parent-trainingeducation-programmes-in-the-management-of-children-with-conduct-disorders-ta102. London: NICE/SCIE; 2006.

NICE. Antisocial Personality Disorder: Treatment, Management and Prevention. NICE clinical guideline 77. Available from: www.nice.org.uk/guidance/CG77. 2009a.

NICE. Attention Deficit Hyperactivity Disorder: Diagnosis and Management of ADHD in Children, Young People and Adults. NICE clinical guideline 72. Available from: http://guidance.nice.org.uk/uk/CG72/NICEguidance/pdf/English. 2009b.

NICE. The Guidelines Manual. Available from: www.nice.org.uk. London: NICE; 2009c.

NICE. National Costing Report: Antisocial Personality Disorder. London: NICE; 2009d.

NICE. Schizophrenia: Core Interventions in the Treatment and Management of Schizophrenia in Adults in Primary and Secondary Care (update). NICE clinical guideline 82. Available from: http://guidance.nice.org.uk/CG82/NICE guidance/pdf/English. 2009e.

NICE. Autism: Recognition, Referral and Diagnosis of Children and Young People on the Autism Spectrum. NICE clinical guideline 128. Available from: http://guidance.nice.org.uk/CG128/NICEGuidance/pdf/English. 2011a.

NICE. Common Mental Health Disorders: Identification and Pathways to Care. NICE clinical guideline 123. Available from: http://guidance.nice.org.uk/CG123NICE-Guidance/pdf/English. 2011b.

NICE. Service User Experience in Adult Mental Health: Improving the Experience of Care for People Using Adult NHS Mental Health Services. NICE clinical guidance 136. Available from http://guidance.nice.org.uk/CG136/NICEGuidance/pdf/English. 2011c.

NICE. Psychosis and Schizophrenia in Children and Young People: Recognition and Management. NICE clinical guideline 155. Available from: http://guidance.nice.org.uk/CG155/NICEGuidance/pdf/English. 2013.

Nicholson JM, Sanders MR. Randomized controlled trial of behavioral family intervention for the treatment of child behavior problems in stepfamilies. Journal of Divorce and Remarriage. 1999;30:1–23.

Nickel MK, Krawczyk J, Nickel C, Forthuber P, Kettler C, Leiberich P, et al. Anger, interpersonal relationships, and health-related quality of life in bullying boys who are treated with outpatient family therapy: a randomized, prospective, controlled trial with 1 year of follow-up. Pediatrics. 2005;116:e247–54.

Nickel M, Luley J, Krawczyk J, Nickel C, Widermann C, Lahmann C, et al. Bullying girls – changes after brief strategic family therapy: a randomized, prospective, controlled trial with one-year follow-up. Psychotherapy and Psychosomatics. 2006a;75:47–55.

Nickel MK, Muehlbacher M, Kaplan P, Krawczyk J, Buschmann W, Kettler C, et al. Influence of family therapy on bullying behaviour, cortisol secretion, anger, and quality of life in bullying male adolescents: a randomized, prospective, controlled study. Canadian Journal of Psychiatry. 2006b;51:355–62.

Ninness HC, Graben L, Miller B, Whaley D. The effect of contingency management strategies on the Bender Gestalt diagnostic indicators of emotionally disturbed children. Child Study Journal. 1985;15:13–28.

Nixon RD, Sweeney L, Erickson DB, Touyz SW. Parent-child interaction therapy: a comparison of standard and abbreviated treatments for oppositional defiant preschoolers. Journal of Consulting and Clinical Psychology. 2003;71:251–60.

Odgers CL, Milne BJ, Caspi A, Crump RP, Moffitt TE. Predicting prognosis for the conduct-problem boy: can family history help? Journal of the American Academy of Child and Adolescent Psychiatry. 2007;46:1240–49.

Office for National Statistics. Population Estimates for UK, England and Wales, Scotland and Northern Ireland, Population Estimates Time series 1971 to Current Year. Available from: www.ons.gov.uk/ons/rel/pop-estimate/population-estimates-for-uk–england-and-wales–scotland-and-northern-ireland/population-estimates-time-series-1971-to-current-year/index.html. Fareham: Office for National Statistics; 2011.

Offord D, Bennett KJ. Conduct disorder: long-term outcomes and intervention effectiveness. Journal of the American Academy of Child and Adolescent Psychiatry. 1994;33:1069–78.

Ogden T, Hagen KA. Treatment effectiveness of parent management training in Norway: a randomized controlled trial of children with conduct problems. Journal of Consulting and Clinical Psychology. 2008;76:607–21.

Ogden T, Halliday-Boykins C. Multisystemic treatment of antisocial adolescents in Norway: replication of clinical outcomes outside of the US. Child and Adolescent Mental Health. 2004;9:77–83.

Olds DL, Henderson CRJ, Tatelbaum R, Chamberlin R. Improving the delivery of prenatal care and outcomes of pregnancy: a randomized trial of nurse home visitation. Pediatrics. 1986;77:16–28.

Olds DL, Robinson J, O'Brien R, Luckey DW, Pettitt LM, Henderson CRJ, et al. Home visiting by paraprofessionals and by nurses: a randomized, controlled trial. Pediatrics. 2002;110:486–96.

Oliver S, Harden A, Rees R, Shepherd J, Brunton G, Oakley A. Young people and mental health: novel methods for systematic review of research on barriers and facilitators. Health Education Research. 2008;23:770–90.

Olsson TM. Intervening in youth problem behaviour in Sweden: a pragmatic cost analysis of MST from a randomized trial with conduct disordered youth. International Journal of Social Welfare. 2010a;19:194–205.

Olsson TM. MST with conduct disordered youth in Sweden: costs and benefits after 2 years. Research on Social Work Practice. 2010b;20:561–71.

*References*

Olweus D. Annotation: Bullying at school: basic facts and effects of a school based intervention program. Journal of Child Psychology and Psychiatry. 1994;35:1171–90.

Omizo MM, Hershberger JM, Omizo SA. Teaching children to cope with anger. Elementary School Guidance and Counseling. 1988;22:241–46.

Ortiz J, Raine A. Heart rate level and antisocial behavior in children and adolescents: a meta-analysis. Journal of the American Academy of Child and Adolescent Psychiatry. 2004;43:154–62.

Paediatric Formulary Committee. BNF for Children 2011–2012 (British National Formulary for Children). London: Pharmaceutical Press; 2011.

Pantin H, Prado G, Lopez B, Huang S, Tapia MI, Schwartz SJ, et al. A randomized controlled trial of Familias Unidas for Hispanic adolescents with behavior problems. Psychosomatic Medicine. 2009;71:987–95.

Patterson G. Coercive Family Process. Eugene, OR: Castalia; 1982.

Patterson J, Barlow J, Mockford C, Klimes I, Pyper C, Stewart-Brown S. Improving mental health through parenting programmes: block randomised controlled trial. Arcives of Disease in Childhood. 2002;87:472–77.

Pepler JP, King G, Craig W, Byrd B, Bream L. The development and evaluation of a multisystem social skills group training program for aggressive children. Child and Youth Care Forum. 1995;24:297–313.

Petit JA. The effects of an anger management program on aggressive adolescents: a cognitive-behavioral approach [dissertation]. New Orleans, LA: University of New Orleans; 1998.

Petra JR. The effects of a choice theory and reality therapy parenting program on children's behavior [dissertation]. Cincinatti, OH: The Union Institute; 2001.

Petrou S, Johnson S, Wolke D, Hollis C, Kochhar P, Marlow N. Economic costs and preference-based health-related quality of life outcomes associated with childhood psychiatric disorders. The British Journal of Psychiatry. 2010;197:395–404.

Pietrucha CA. A social-cognitive intervention program: toward the reduction of children's aggressive behavior through modification of social goals (peer acceptance) [dissertation]. Orono, ME: University of Maine; 1998.

Piquero A, Farrington D, Nagin D, Moffitt T. Trajectories of offending and their relation to life failure in late middle age: findings from the Cambridge Study in Delinquent Development. Journal of Research in Crime and Delinquency. 2010;47:151–73.

Pitts RP. The effectiveness and acceptability of the modified effective black parenting program with children exhibiting severe conduct problems [dissertation]. Bethlehem, PA: Lehigh University; 2001.

Prince's Trust. The cost of exclusion: counting the cost of youth disadvantage in the UK. Available from: www.princes-trust.org.uk/pdf/COE_full_report.pdf. London: The Prince's Trust; 2010.

Psychological Corporation. Wechsler Abbreviated Scale of Intelligence Manual. San Antonio, TX: Psychological Corporation; 1999.

Pullatz M, Bierman KL. Aggression, Antisocial Behaviour, and Violence Among Girls: A Developmental Perspective. New York, NY: Guilford Publications; 2004.

Querido JG, Eyberg SM. Psychometric properties of the Sutter-Eyberg Student Behavior Inventory-Revised with preschool children. Behavior Therapy. 2003;34:1–15.

Querido J, Eyberg S. Parent-child interaction therapy: maintaining treatment gains of pre-schoolers with disruptive behaviour disorders. In: Hibbs E, Jensen P, eds. Psychosocial Treatments for Child and Adolescent Disorders: Empirically Based Strategies for Clinical Practice. 2nd edn. Washington, DC: American Psychological Association; 2005.

Rao SA. The short-term impact of the family check-up: A brief motivational intervention for at-risk families [dissertation]. Eugene, OR: University of Oregon; 1998.

Rayfield A, Eyberg SM, Foote R. Revision of the Sutter-Eyberg Student Behavior Inventory: teacher rating of conduct problem behavior. Educational and Psychological Measurement. 1998;58:88–98.

Reid MJ, Webster-Stratton C, Hammond M. Enhancing a classroom social competence and problem-solving curriculum by offering parent training to families of moderate- to high-risk elementary school children. Journal of Clinical Child and Adolescent Psychology. 2007;36:605–20.

Reyes M, Buitelaar J, Toren P, Augustyns I, Eerdekens M. A randomized, double-blind, placebo-controlled study of risperidone maintenance treatment in children and adolescents with disruptive behavior disorders. American Journal of Psychiatry. 2006;163:402–10.

Rich BA, Eyberg SM. Accuracy of assessment: the discriminative and predictive power of the Eyberg Child Behavior Inventory. Ambulatory Child Health. 2001;7:249–57.

Rifkin A, Karajgi B, Dicker R, Perl E, Boppana V, Hasan N, et al. Lithium treatment of conduct disorders in adolescents. American Journal of Psychiatry. 1997;154:554–55.

Riggs PD, Mikulich-Gilbertson SK, Davies RD, Lochman M, Klein C, Stover SK. A randomized controlled trial of fluoxetine and cognitive behavioral therapy in adolescents with major depression, behavior problems, and substance use disorders. Archives of Pediatrics and Adolescent Medicine. 2007;161:1026–34.

Robertson AA, Grimes PW, Rogers KE. A short-run cost-benefit analysis of community-based interventions for juvenile offenders. Crime and Delinquency. 2001;47:265–84.

Robinson EA, Eyberg SM, Ross AW. Inventory of child problem behaviors: the standardization of an inventory of child conduct problem behaviors. Journal of Clinical Child Psychology. 1980;9:22–29.

Rohde P, Clarke GN, Mace DE, Jorgensen JS, Seeley JR. An efficacy/effectiveness study of cognitive-behavioral treatment for adolescents with comorbid major depression and conduct disorder. Journal of the American Academy of Child and Adolescent Psychiatry. 2004;43:660–68.

Romeo R, Knapp M, Scott S. Economic cost of severe antisocial behaviour in children–and who pays it. The British Journal of Psychiatry. 2006;188:547–53.

Rowe R, Maughan B, Pickles A, Costello EJ, Angold A. The relationship between DSM-IV oppositional defiant disorder and conduct disorder: findings from the Great Smoky Mountains Study. Journal of Child Psychology and Psychiatry. 2002;43:365–73.

Rowe R, Costello EJ, Angold A, Copeland WE, Maughan B. Developmental pathways in oppositional defiant disorder and conduct disorder. Journal of Abnormal Psychology. 2010;119:726–38.

Rowland MD, Halliday-Boykins CA, Henggeler SW, Cunningham PB, Lee TG, Kruesi MJP, et al. A randomized trial of multisystemic therapy with Hawaii's Felix Class youths. Journal of Emotional and Behavioral Disorders. 2005;13:13–23.

Sainsbury Centre for Mental Health. The chance of a lifetime: preventing early conduct problems and reducing crime. Available from: www.centreformentalhealth. org.uk/publications/chance_of_a_lifetime.aspx?ID=604. London: Sainsbury Centre for Mental Health; 2009.

Salmon K, Dadds MR, Allen J, Hawes DJ, Salmon K, Dadds MR, et al. Can emotional language skills be taught during parent training for conduct problem children? Child Psychiatry and Human Development. 2009;40:485–98.

Sanders MR, Christensen AP. A comparison of the effects of child management and planned activities training in five parenting environments. Journal of Abnormal Child Psychology. 1985;13:101–17.

Sanders MR, McFarland M. Treatment of depressed mothers with disruptive children: A controlled evaluation of cognitive behavioral family intervention. Behavior Therapy. 2000;31:89–112.

Sanders MR, Markie-Dadds C, Tully LA, Bor W. The Triple P-Positive Parenting Program: a comparison of enhanced, standard, and self-directed behavioral family intervention for parents of children with early onset conduct problems. Journal of Consulting and Clinical Psychology. 2000a;68:624–40.

Sanders MR, Montgomery DT, Brechman-Toussaint ML. The mass media and the prevention of child behavior problems: the evaluation of a television series to promote positive outcomes for parents and their children. Journal of Child Psychology and Psychiatry and Allied Disciplines. 2000b;41:939–48.

Sanders MR, Pidgeon AM, Gravestock F, Connors MD, Brown S, Young RW. Does parental attributional retraining and anger management enhance the effects of the Triple P-Positive Parenting Program with parents at risk of child maltreatment? Behavior Therapy. 2004;35:513–35.

Santisteban DA, Coatsworth JD, Perez-Vidal A, Kurtines WM, Schwartz SJ, LaPerriere A, et al. Efficacy of brief strategic family therapy in modifying Hispanic adolescent behavior problems and substance use. Journal of Family Psychology. 2003;17:121–33.

Sayger TV, Horne AM, Walker LM, Passmore JL. Social learning family therapy with aggressive children: treatment outcome and maintenance. Journal of Family Psychology. 1988;1:261–85.

Schaughency EA, Hurley LK, Yano KE, Seeley JR, Talarico B. Psychometric properties of the Sutter-Eyberg Student Behavior Inventory with clinic referred children. Annual meeting of the American Psychological Association, August 1989; New Orleans, LA.

Schuhmann EM, Durning PE, Eyberg SM, Boggs SR. Screening for conduct problem behavior in pediatric settings using the Eyberg Child Behavior Inventory. Ambulatory Child Health. 1996;2:35–41.

Schuhmann EM, Foote RC, Eyberg SM, Boggs SR, Algina J. Efficacy of parent-child interaction therapy: interim report of a randomized trial with short-term maintenance. Journal of Clinical Child Psychology. 1998;27:34–45.

Schumann BR. Effects of child-centered play therapy and curriculum-based small-group guidance on the behaviors of children referred for aggression in an elementary school setting (Texas) [dissertation]. Denton, TX: University of North Texas; 2004.

Schünemann HJ, Best D, Vist G, Oxman AD, GRADE Working Group. Letters, numbers, symbols and words: how to communicate grades of evidence and recommendations. Canadian Medical Association Journal. 2003;169:677–80. Correction in: 2004;30:1082.

Schünemann H, Broüek J, Oxman A. GRADE Handbook for Grading Quality of Evidence and Strength of Recommendation. Version 3.2 2 [updated March 2009]. Available from: www.cc-ims.net/gradepro: The GRADE Working Group; 2009.

Scott DD. Investigating the behavioral outcomes of an early literacy intervention for at-risk preschool children [dissertation]. Charlottesville, VA: University of Virginia; 2005.

Scott S. Conduct disorders in children. BMJ. 2007;334:646–47.

Scott S. Parent training programs. In: Rutter M, Bishop D, Pine D, Scott S, Stevenson J, Taylor E, et al., eds. Child and Adolescent Psychiatry Oxford: Blackwell; 2008.

Scott S. National dissemination of effective parenting programmes to improve child outcomes. The British Journal of Psychiatry. 2010;196:1–3.

Scott S, Dadds MR. Practitioner review: when parent training doesn't work: theory-driven clinical strategies. Journal of Child Psychology and Psychiatry. 2009;50:1441–50.

Scott S, Knapp M, Henderson J, Maughan B. Financial cost of social exclusion: follow up study of antisocial children into adulthood. BMJ. 2001;323:191.

Scott S, O'Connor TG, Futh A, Matias C, Price J, Doolan M. Impact of a parenting program in a high-risk, multi-ethnic community: the PALS trial. Journal of Child Psychology and Psychiatry. 2010a;51:1331–41.

Scott S, Sylva K, Doolan M, Price J, Jacobs B, Crook C, et al. Randomised controlled trial of parent groups for child antisocial behaviour targeting multiple risk factors: the SPOKES project. Journal of Child Psychology and Psychiatry. 2010b;51:48–57.

Scott S, Briskman J, Woolgar M, Humayun S, O'Connor TG. Attachment in adolescence: overlap with parenting and unique prediction of behavioural adjustment. Journal of Child Psychology and Psychiatry. 2011;52:1052–62.

Scotto Rosato N, Correll CU, Pappadopulos E, Chait A, Crystal S, Jensen PS, et al. Treatment of maladaptive aggression in youth: CERT guidelines II. Treatments and ongoing management. Pediatrics. 2012;129:e1577-e86.

Seda G, Jr. Stress inoculation versus social skills training for the treatment of aggression in emotionally disturbed children. La Mirada, CA: Biola University; 1992.

Semmens N. Towards an understanding of 'fear' as an intangible cost of crime. International Review of Victimology. 2007;14:219–35.

Sexton T, Turner CW. The effectiveness of functional family therapy for youth with behavioral problems in a community practice setting. Journal of Family Psychology. 2010;24:339–48.

*References*

Shapland J, Hall M. What do we know about the effects of crime on victims? International Review of Victimology. 2007;14:175–217.

Sharac J, McCrone P, Rushton A, Monck E. Enhancing adoptive parenting: a cost-effectiveness analysis. Child and Adolescent Mental Health. 2011;16:110–15.

Sharp C, Croudace TJ, Goodyer IM, Amtmann D. The Strength and Difficulties Questionnaire: predictive validity of parent and teacher ratings for help-seeking behaviour over one year. Educational and Child Psychology. 2005;22:28–44.

Shaw DS, Dishion TJ, Supplee L, Gardner F, Arnds K. Randomized trial of a family-centered approach to the prevention of early conduct problems: 2-year effects of the family check-up in early childhood. Journal of Consulting and Clinical Psychology. 2006;74:1–9.

Shechtman Z. An innovative intervention for treatment of child and adolescent aggression: an outcome study. Psychology in the Schools. 2000;37:157–67.

Shechtman Z. The contribution of bibliotherapy to the counseling of aggressive boys. Psychotherapy Research. 2006;16:645–51.

Shechtman Z, Birani-Nasaraladin D. Treating mothers of aggressive children: a research study. International Journal of Group Psychotherapy. 2006;56:93–112.

Shechtman Z, Ifargan M. School-based integrated and segregated interventions to reduce aggression. Aggressive Behavior. 2009;35:342–56.

Shepard SA, Dickstein S. Preventative intervention for early childhood behavioural problems: an ecological perspective. Child and Adolescent Psychiatry Clinics of North America. 2009;18:687–706.

Shin S-K. Effects of a solution-focused program on the reduction of aggressiveness and the improvement of social readjustment for Korean youth probationers. Journal of Social Service Research. 2009;35:274–84.

Shivram R, Bankart J, Meltzer H, Ford T, Vostanis P, Goodman R. Service utilization by children with conduct disorders: findings from the 2004 Great Britain child mental health survey. European Child and Adolescent Psychiatry. 2009;18:555–63.

Simonsen B, Myers D, Briere D. Comparing a behavioral check-in/check-out (CICO) intervention to standard practice in an urban middle school setting using an experimental group design. Journal of Positive Behavior Interventions. 2011;13:31–48.

Smith DK, Leve LD, Chamberlain P. Preventing internalizing and externalizing problems in girls in foster care as they enter middle school: impact of an intervention. Prevention Science. 2011;12:269–77.

Snyder KV, Kymissis P, Kessler K. Anger management for adolescents: Efficacy of brief group therapy. Journal of the American Academy of Child and Adolescent Psychiatry. 1999;38:1409–16.

Snyder R, Turgay A, Aman MB, C., Fisman S, Carroll A, Risperidone Conduct Study Group. Effects of risperidone on conduct and disruptive behavior disorders in children with subaverage IQs. Journal of the American Academy of Child and Adolescent Psychiatry. 2002;41:1026–36.

Soderlund J, Epstein MH, Quinn KP, Cumblad C, Petersen S. Parental perspectives on comprehensive services for children and youth with emotional and behavioral disorders. Behavioral Disorders. 1995;20:157–70.

Spencer TJ, Biederman J, Abikoff H, Pliszka SR, Boellner S, Lopez FA, et al. Safety and efficacy of mixed amphetamine salts extended release in children with oppositional defiant disorder (ODD). 157th Annual Meeting of the American Psychiatric Association, 1–6 May; New York, NY; 2004.

Stallman HM, Ralph A. Reducing risk factors for adolescent behavioural and emotional problems: a pilot randomised controlled trial of a self-administered parenting intervention. Australian e-Journal for the Advancement of Mental Health. 2007;6:125–37.

Stanger C, Ryan SR, Fu H, Budney AJ. Parent training plus contingency management for substance abusing families: a Complier Average Causal Effects (CACE) analysis. Drug and Alcohol Dependence. 2011;118:119–26.

StataCorp. Stata Statistical Software [Computer programme]. Version 12. College Station, TX: StataCorp; 2012.

Steiner H, Petersen ML, Saxena K, Ford S, Matthews Z. Divalproex sodium for the treatment of conduct disorder: a randomized controlled clinical trial. Journal of Clinical Psychiatry. 2003;64:1183–91.

Stolk MN, Mesman J, Zeijl J, Alink LRA, Bakermans-Kranenburg MJ, Ijzendoorn MH, et al. Early parenting intervention: family risk and first-time parenting related to intervention effectiveness. Journal of Child and Family Studies. 2008;17:55–83.

Strayhorn JM, Weidman CS. Reduction of attention deficit and internalizing symptoms in preschoolers through parent-child interaction training. Journal of the American Academy of Child and Adolescent Psychiatry. 1989;28:888–96.

Sukhodolsky DG, Solomon RM, Perine J. Cognitive-behavioral, anger-control intervention for elementary school children: a treatment outcome study. Journal of Child and Adolescent Group Therapy. 2000;10:159–70.

Sukhodolsky DG, Golub A, Stone EC, Orban L. Dismantling anger control training for children: A randomized pilot study of social problem-solving versus social skills training components. Behavior Therapy. 2005;36:15–23.

Sundell K, Hansson K, Löfholm CA, Olsson T, Gustle LH, Kadesjö C. The transportability of multisystemic therapy to Sweden: short-term results from a randomized trial of conduct-disordered youths. Journal of Family Psychology. 2008;22:550–60.

Swift MC, Roeger L, Walmsley C, Howard S, Furber G, Allison S. Rural children referred for conduct problems: evaluation of a collaborative program. Australian Journal of Primary Health. 2009;15:335–40.

Szapocznik J, Rio A, Murray E, Cohen R, Scopetta M, Rivas-Vazquez A, et al. Structural family versus psychodynamic child therapy for problematic Hispanic boys. Journal of Consulting and Clinical Psychology. 1989;57:571–78.

Taylor TK, Schmidt F, Pepler D, Hodgins H. A comparison of eclectic treatment with Webster-Stratton's Parents and Children Series in a children's mental health center: a randomized controlled trial. Behavior Therapy. 1998;29:221–40.

Tighe A, Pistrang N, Casdagli L, Baruch G, Butler S. Multisystemic therapy for young offenders: families' experiences of therapeutic processes and outcomes. Journal of Family Psychology. 2012;26:187–97.

Timmer SG, Zebell NM, Culver MA, Urquiza AJ. Efficacy of adjunct in-home coaching to improve outcomes in parent-child interaction therapy. Research on Social Work Practice. 2010;20:36–45.

Timmons-Mitchell J, Bender MB, Kishna MA, Mitchell CC. An independent effectiveness trial of multisystemic therapy with juvenile justice youth. Journal of Clinical Child and Adolescent Psychology. 2006;35:227–36.

Tolan P, Gorman-Smith D, Henry D. Supporting families in a high-risk setting: proximal effects of the SAFEChildren preventive intervention. Journal of Consulting and Clinical Psychology. 2004;72:855–69.

Trzesniewski K, Moffitt T, Caspi A, Taylor A, Maughan B. Revisiting the association between reading achievement and antisocial behavior: new evidence of an environmental explanation from a twin study. Child Development. 2006;77:72–88.

Turner KM, Sanders MR. Help when it's needed first: a controlled evaluation of brief, preventive behavioral family intervention in a primary care setting. Behavior Therapy. 2006;37:131–42.

Turner KM, Richards M, Sanders MR. Randomised clinical trial of a group parent education programme for Australian indigenous families. Journal of Paediactrics and Child Health. 2007;43:429–37.

Turgay A. Aggression and disruptive behavior disorders in children and adolescents. Expert Review of Neurotherapeutics. 2004;4:623–32.

Van De Wiel NM, Matthys W, Cohen-Kettenis PT, Maassen GH, Lochman JE, van Engeland H. The effectiveness of an experimental treatment when compared to care as usual depends on the type of care as usual. Behavior Modification. 2007;31:298–312.

Van Manen TG, Prins PJ, Emmelkamp PM. Reducing aggressive behavior in boys with a social cognitive group treatment: results of a randomized, controlled trial. Journal of the American Academy of Child and Adolescent Psychiatry. 2004;43:1478–87.

Verduyn CM, Lord W, Forrest GC. Social skills training in schools: an evaluation study. Journal of Adolescence. 1990;13:3–16.

Vostanis P, Meltzer H, Goodman R, Ford T. Service utilisation by children with conduct disorders: findings from the GB National Study. European Child and Adolescent Psychiatry. 2003;12:231–8.

Walker HM, Kavanagh K, Stiller B, Golly A, Severson HH, Feil EG. First step to success: an early intervention approach for preventing school antisocial behavior. Journal of Emotional and Behavioral Disorders. 1998;6:66–80.

Walton MA, Chermack ST, Shope JT, Bingham CR, Zimmerman MA, Blow FC, et al. Effects of a brief intervention for reducing violence and alcohol misuse among adolescents: a randomized controlled trial. Journal of the American Medical Association. 2010;304:527–35.

Wanders F, Serra M, de Jongh A. EMDR versus CBT for children with self-esteem and behavioral problems: a randomized controlled trial. Journal of EMDR Practice and Research. 2008;2:180–89.

Webster-Stratton C. Randomized trial of two parent-training programs for families with conduct-disordered children. Journal of Consulting and Clinical Psychology. 1984;52:666–78.

Webster-Stratton C. Enhancing the effectiveness of self-administered videotape parent training for families with conduct-problem children. Journal of Abnormal Child Psychology. 1990;18:479–92.

Webster-Stratton C. Individually administered videotape parent training: who benefits? Cognitive Therapy and Research. 1992;16:31–52.

Webster-Stratton C. Advancing videotape parent training: a comparison study. Journal of Consulting and Clinical Psychology. 1994;62:583–93.

Webster-Stratton C. Preventing conduct problems in head start children: Strengthening parenting competencies. Journal of Consulting and Clinical Psychology. 1998;66:715–30.

Webster-Stratton C, Hammond M. Treating children with early-onset conduct problems: a comparison of child and parent training interventions. Journal of Consulting and Clinical Psychology. 1997;65:93–109.

Webster-Stratton C, Kolpacoff M, Hollinsworth T. Self-administered videotape therapy for families with conduct-problem children: comparison with two cost-effective treatments and a control group. Journal of Consulting and Clinical Psychology. 1988;56:558–66.

Webster-Stratton C, Reid MJ, Hammond M. Preventing conduct problems, promoting social competence: a parent and teacher training partnership in head start. Journal of Clinical Child Psychology. 2001;30:283–302.

Webster-Stratton C, Reid MJ, Hammond M. Treating children with early-onset conduct problems: intervention outcomes for parent, child, and teacher training. Journal of Clinical Child and Adolescent Psychology. 2004;33:105–24.

Webster-Stratton C, Jamila Reid M, Stoolmiller M. Preventing conduct problems and improving school readiness: evaluation of the Incredible Years Teacher and Child Training Programs in high-risk schools. Journal of Child Psychology and Psychiatry. 2008;49:471–88.

Wechsler D. Wechsler Individual Achievement Test 2nd Edition (WIAT II). 2 edn. London: The Psychological Corp; 2005.

Weinblatt U, Omer H. Nonviolent resistance: a treatment for parents of children with acute behavior problems. Journal of Marital and Family Therapy. 2008;34:75–92.

Weis R, Lovejoy MC, Lundahl BW. Factor structure and discriminative validity of the Eyberg Child Behavior Inventory with young children. Journal of Psychopathology and Behavioral Assessment. 2005;27:269–78.

Welsh BC, Loeber R, Stevens BR, Stouthamer-Loeber M, Cohen MA, Farrington D. Costs of juvenile crime in urban areas: a longitudinal perspective. Youth Violence and Juvenile Justice. 2008;6:3–27.

Westermark PK, Hansson K, Olsson M. Multidimensional treatment foster care (MTFC): results from an independent replication. Journal of Family Therapy. 2011;33:20–41.

## References

Wiggins TL, Sofronoff K, Sanders MR. Pathways Triple P-Positive Parenting Program: effects on parent-child relationships and child behavior problems. Family Process. 2009;48:517–30.

Williams JH, Horvath VE, Wei H, Van Dorn RA, Jonson-Reid M. Teachers' perspectives of children's mental health service needs in urban elementary schools. Children and Schools. 2007;29:95–107.

Wilmshurst LA. Treatment programs for youth with emotional and behavioral disorders: an outcome study of two alternate approaches. Mental Health Services Research. 2002;4:85–96.

Wilson SJ, Lipsey MW, Derzon JH. The effects of school-based intervention programs on aggressive behavior: a meta-analysis. Journal of Consulting and Clinical Psychology. 2003;71:136–49.

Wolchik SA, West SG, Westover S, Sandler IN, Martin A, Lustig J, et al. The children of divorce parenting intervention: outcome evaluation of an empirically based program. American Journal of Community Psychology. 1993;21:293–31.

Wolchik SA, West SG, Sandler IN, Tein JY, Coatsworth D, Lengua L, et al. An experimental evaluation of theory-based mother and mother-child programs for children of divorce. Journal of Consulting and Clinical Psychology. 2000;68:843–56.

Woolfenden S, Williams KJ, Peat J. Family and parenting interventions in children and adolescents with conduct disorder and delinquency aged 10–17. Cochrane Database of Systematic Reviews. 1999; Issue 2:Art. No.: CD003015. DOI: 10.1002/14651858.CD003015.

World Health Organization. The ICD-10 Classification of Mental and Behavioural Disorders: Clinical Description and Diagnostic Guidelines. Geneva: WHO; 1992.

Youmans CW. Group counseling compared with individual counseling in the reduction of at-risk behaviors in black male students [dissertation]. Orangeburg, SC: South Carolina State University; 2001.

Zamora J, Abraira V, Muriel A, Khan KS, A. C. Meta-DiSc: a software for meta-analysis of test accuracy data. BMC Medical Research Methodology. 2006;6:31.

Zuddas A, Zanni R, Usala T. Second generation antipsychotics (SGAs) for non-psychotic disorders in children and adolescents: a review of the randomized controlled studies. European Neuropsychopharmacology. 2011;21:600–20.

# 12  ABBREVIATIONS

| | |
|---|---|
| β | regression coefficient |
| **ADHD** | attention deficit hyperactivity disorder |
| **AGREE** | Appraisal of Guidelines Research and Evaluation |
| **ASBO** | Anti-Social Behaviour Order |
| **AUC** | area under the curve |
| **BNF(C)** | *British National Formulary (for Children)* |
| **CAMHS** | child and adolescent mental health services |
| **CBCL** | Child Behavior Checklist |
| **CBT** | cognitive behavioural therapy |
| **CI** | confidence interval |
| **DSM-IV-TR** | *Diagnostic and Statistical Manual of Mental Disorders*, 4th Edition – Text Revision |
| **ECBI** | Eyberg Child Behavior Inventory |
| **EconLit** | American Economic Association's electronic bibliography |
| **Embase** | Excerpta Medica Database |
| **FN** | False negative |
| **FP** | False positive |
| **GAD** | generalised anxiety disorder |
| **GDG** | Guideline Development Group |
| **GP** | general practitioner |
| **GRADE** | Grading of Recommendations Assessment, Development, and Evaluation |
| **HbA1c** | glycosylated haemoglobin |
| **HTA** | Health Technology Assessment |
| **ICD-10** | *International Classification of Diseases*, 10th Revision |
| **ICER** | incremental cost-effectiveness ratio |
| **IQ** | intelligence quotient |
| **ITT** | intention to treat |
| **k** | number of trials |
| **MAOA** | monoamine oxidase type A |
| **MEDLINE** | Medical Literature Analysis and Retrieval System Online |
| **MTFC** | multidimensional treatment foster care |

*Abbreviations*

| | |
|---|---|
| **n/N** | number of participants |
| **NCCMH** | National Collaborating Centre for Mental Health |
| **NHS** | National Health Service |
| **NICE** | National Institute for Health and Care Excellence |
| **NNH** | number needed to harm |
| | |
| **OCD** | obsessive-compulsive disorder |
| **OIS** | optimal information size |
| | |
| **PICO** | population, intervention, comparison and outcome |
| **preMEDLINE** | in-process database for MEDLINE |
| **PSS** | personal social services |
| **PsycBOOKS** | full-text database of books and chapters in the American Psychological Association's electronic databases |
| **PsycEXTRA** | grey literature database, which is a companion to PsycINFO |
| **PsycINFO** | Psychological Information Database |
| **PTSD** | post-traumatic stress disorder |
| | |
| **QALY** | quality-adjusted life years |
| **QT interval** | the period from the start of the Q wave to the end of the T wave (duration of ventricular electrical activity) |
| | |
| **RCT** | randomised controlled trial |
| **ROC** | receiver operator characteristic |
| **RQ** | review question |
| **RR** | relative risk/risk ratio |
| | |
| **SCIE** | Social Care Institute for Excellence |
| **SD** | standard deviation |
| **SDQ** | Strengths and Difficulties Questionnaire |
| **SESBI-R** | Sutter–Eyberg Student Behavior Inventory-Revised |
| **SMD** | standardised mean difference |
| **SPC** | summary of product characteristics |
| | |
| **TN** | true negative |
| **TP** | true positive |
| | |
| **YOT** | youth offending team |